CLINICAL AND FIELDWORK PLACEMENT

IN THE HEALTH PROFESSIONS

Edited by Karen Stagnitti, Adrian Schoo & Dianne Welch

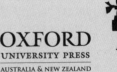

OXFORD
UNIVERSITY PRESS
AUSTRALIA & NEW ZEALAND

OXFORD
UNIVERSITY PRESS
AUSTRALIA & NEW ZEALAND

253 Normanby Road, South Melbourne, Victoria 3205, Australia

Oxford University Press is a department of the University of Oxford.
It furthers the University's objective of excellence in research,
scholarship, and education by publishing worldwide in

Oxford New York

Auckland Cape Town Dar es Salaam Hong Kong Karachi
Kuala Lumpur Madrid Melbourne Mexico City Nairobi
New Delhi Shanghai Taipei Toronto

With offices in

Argentina Austria Brazil Chile Czech Republic France Greece
Guatemala Hungary Italy Japan Poland Portugal Singapore
South Korea Switzerland Thailand Turkey Ukraine Vietnam

OXFORD is a trademark of Oxford University Press
in the UK and in certain other countries

National Library of Australia Cataloguing-in-Publication data

Stagnitti, Karen.

Clinical and fieldwork placement in the health professions/Karen Stagnitti, Adrian Schoo,
Dianne Welch.

9780195568462 (pbk.)

Includes index.
Bibliography.

Medical personnel—In-service training.
Clinical medicine—Study and teaching.
Fieldwork (Educational method)

Schoo, Adrian.
Welch, Dianne.

610.711

Edited by Bruce Gillespie
Text design by Peter Shaw
Typeset by diacriTech, Chennai, India
Proofread by Jamie Anderson
Indexed by Russell Brooks
Printed in China by Sheck Wah Tong Printing Press Ltd

CONTENTS

Lists of Figures, Tables and Case Studies   vi

Preface   ix

Acknowledgments   xi

Glossary   xii

Contributors   xxxi

PART 1: PREPARING FOR PLACEMENT   **1**

Chapter 1: Getting Ready for Placement   **3**
    Jane Maidment

Chapter 2: Working in Diverse Settings   **13**
    Sharleen O'Reilly

Chapter 3: Working with Mothers and Babies   **26**
    Joanne Gray

Chapter 4: Working with Children and Families   **37**
    Kelly Powell

Chapter 5: Working in Acute Settings   **50**
    Jo McDonall

Chapter 6: Working with Older People   **62**
    Jennifer Nitz

Chapter 7: Working in Mental Health   **76**
    Geneviève Pépin

Chapter 8: Working in Workplace Practice   **87**
    Michelle Conlan

Chapter 9: Working in Private Practice   **100**
    Tim Kauffman, Phoebe Maloney and Adrian Schoo

Chapter 10: Working in Rural and Remote Settings 108
Paul Tinley

Chapter 11: Working in Indigenous Health Settings 119
Deirdre Whitford, Angela Russell, Judy Taylor and Kym Thomas

Part 1 Checklist: Preparing for Placement 137

PART 2: MAKING THE MOST OF YOUR FIELDWORK PLACEMENT **143**

Chapter 12: Models of Supervision 145
Ronnie Egan and Doris Testa

Chapter 13: Making the Most of Your Fieldwork Learning Opportunity 159
Helen Larkin and Anita Hamilton

Chapter 14: Assessment of Clinical Learning 171
Megan Smith

Chapter 15: A Model for Alternative Fieldwork 186
Rachael Schmidt

Chapter 16: Interprofessional Learning: Working in Teams 199
Nick Stone

Chapter 17: Learning from Failure 218
Eva Nemeth and Lindy McAllister

Chapter 18: Using Online Technology 231
Anita Hamilton and Merrolee Penman

Part 2 Checklist: Making the Most of Your Fieldwork Placement 246

PART 3: ETHICS, LAW AND RESPONSIBILITIES **249**

Chapter 19: Fostering Partnerships with Action 251
Michelle Courtney and Jane Maidment

Chapter 20: Ethical and Supported Decision-making 263
Geneviève Pépin, Joanne Watson, Nick Hagiliassis and Helen Larkin

Chapter 21: The Three Rs: Roles, Rights and Responsibilities 281
Linda Wilson

Chapter 22: Legal Issues 299
Richard Ingleby

Part 3 Checklist: Ethics, Law and Responsibilities 309

PART 4: TRANSITION TO PRACTICE   **313**

Chapter 23: You Become the Supervisor   **315**
  Jennifer Pascoe, Uschi Bay and Michelle Courtney
Chapter 24: Starting Out in Supervision   **329**
  Liz Beddoe
Chapter 25: Health Workforce Recruitment   **345**
  Adrian Schoo and Karen Stagnitti
Part 4 Checklist: Transition to Practice   **355**

References   357
Useful Websites   367
Index   369

LISTS OF FIGURES, TABLES AND CASE STUDIES

FIGURES

2.1	The Australian hospital system	15
2.2	The iceberg concept of culture	22
3.1	Main functions of a health professional working with mothers and babies	28
4.1	The effective paediatric practitioner	41
4.2	Paediatric clinical reasoning process	47
4.3	The clinical reasoning process (thinking process) used by the health professional for Sarah	48
6.1	Scope of fieldwork settings when working with older people	63
8.1	Stakeholders in the occupational rehabilitation process	89
13.1	The fieldwork learning framework	160
16.1	IPL umbrella terms	203
16.2	Links between IPL and outcomes	207
17.1	Readiness to learn from failure in a fieldwork placement	225
18.1	Healthcare Blogger Code of Ethics symbol	233
18.2	HONcode symbol	233
18.3	RSS symbol	239
20.1	The doughnut principle	266
20.2	The person-centred risk assessment	267
20.3	The International Classification of Functioning, Disability and Health	270
20.4	The supported decision-making model	273
20.5	The decision-making pathway	275
21.1	Integration of stakeholders into a common direction	290
21.2	University mechanisms to address student concerns	296
24.1	The focus of supervision	330
24.2	The focus of the fieldwork placement supervision	331
24.3	Student and practitioner supervision: key differences	336

TABLES

1.1	Planning and organising for placement	6
1.2	First week: planning and organisation	7
2.1	Interdisciplinary team members	20
3.1	Learning another language	33
5.1	Preparation list before beginning an acute care placement	56
7.1	My proactive plan	80
7.2	Me as part of a team	83
10.1	Ratio of health professionals to population	111
12.1	Function and task checklist for you and your fieldwork educator	148
12.2	Five approaches to supervision	150
12.3	Strengths and limitations of the apprenticeship approach	151
12.4	Strengths and limitations of the growth therapeutic approach	151
12.5	Strengths and limitations of the role systems approach	152
12.6	Strengths and limitations of the competency-based approach	152
12.7	Critical incident technique	155
13.1	Personal attribute scenarios	162
13.2	Reframing generational attributes and behaviours	163
13.3	Alternative response types	165
13.4	Reflecting on practice window	166
14.1	Differences between clinical assessment and assessment in formal academic settings	173
14.2	Assessment criteria used during clinical placements and activities used to reveal achievement of these criteria	175
14.3	Developing self-assessment skills throughout a clinical placement	179
16.1	Terms associated with IPL	202
16.2	IPL myths and realities	204
16.3	Post-placement objectives and activities	216
17.1	Characteristics of students experiencing difficulties in fieldwork	219
18.1	Web 2.0 tools summary table	240
21.1	Examples of stakeholders' interests	283
21.2	Outline of stakeholder three Rs	284
24.1	The course of the supervision relationship	332
24.2	Supervisee levels of independence	337
24.3	Coping with uncertainty	340

CASE STUDIES

1.1	Grier's situation	10
2.1	Samuel the dietitian's first day on placement	19
3.1	Fragmented care	29

4.1	Sarah	38
5.1	What a day!	58
5.2	It's all in a day	60
6.1	Comparison of management for elective hip replacement surgery between a well and a frail elderly person	70
6.2	Comparison between two frail older persons who both have complex and chronic conditions	72
7.1	John Doe	83
8.1	A referral from the DVA	91
8.2	Workplace safety	92
8.3	The negotiation	94
9.1	Be quick in private practice	104
9.2	Pleasing the client	105
10.1	My first week	116
11.1	Nancy and Geoff	127
12.1	Working with Mr Omar	154
13.1	Jenna, Part 1	164
13.2	Jenna, Part 2	167
14.1	Nicole's midway assessment	171
15.1	The OWLS program	193
15.2	Eliot	195
16.1	Nice to meet you, too?	200
16.2	The Dean's savings scheme	201
16.3	An illustration of structured post-fieldwork IPL reflection	209
17.1	Chris's story of failing fieldwork	220
17.2	Rita's story of failing fieldwork	223
18.1	Meg the blogger	235
19.1	Forcefield analysis of the fieldwork enterprise	260
20.1	Lillian	271
20.2	Doug	274
20.3	Sarah	276
20.4	Sam	276
21.1	What information is missing in this situation?	290
21.2	Three scenarios	297
22.1	Julie	307
23.1	Jane's fieldwork experiences	318
23.2	Sri at work	322
23.3	Leah as a fieldwork educator	324
24.1	Let's do this together	335
24.2	Nita	338
24.3	Josie	341
25.1	John leaves home for the country	349

PREFACE

This book is aimed at students enrolled in a health profession. It is not a discipline-specific book. Clinical fieldwork placement or working in the field is experienced by all health students, and is an important part of education for those who are planning to start their career in a health-related area.

In all health professions, students are required to spend a certain number of hours in a healthcare setting working within their discipline-specific profession. This requirement is essential to becoming a competent health professional and practitioner. This experience is called various names, such as *authentic learning, work-situated learning* or *work-integrated learning*. While you may have thought that 'This is voluntary, so it is not that important to me, but since I have to pass it to pass the course, I'll have to go through with it!', the clinical fieldwork placement or clinical practicum is where you, as a student, start to understand how theory becomes applied when living people require your professional service.

Writing a book for all health professions has meant that we, the editors, have made some pragmatic decisions about terminology throughout the book. By using the same terminology throughout the book, we should be able to make it clear what is being referred to, and chapters can be compared using the same terminology.

The term *fieldwork placement*, which is used throughout this workbook, is the term that refers to the place where students are learning how to put in practice their knowledge and skills. *Fieldwork* was chosen, as it is a broader term than *clinical*: not all placements of all students are always in hospitals or clinical settings. Sometimes students are placed in a work setting or a school. Fieldwork placement has been used to represent the following: *fieldwork, clinical placement, clinical practicum, clinical education* and *fieldwork experience*.

Fieldwork educator is the term used for the person who supervises students in the placement setting. Depending on your profession, this person could also be called your *preceptor, clinical supervisor* or *clinical educator*. This is the supervisor in situ. Sometimes this person may also be an academic staff member from the university or educational institution that the student attends, but this is rare. The university staff involved in fieldwork organisation, collaboration or liaison are clearly identified in the text as university staff members.

Other terms used to refer to persons in this book are *health professional, patients and/or clients*, and *students*. *Health professional* refers to any person working in a health area and who has attained a minimum of a bachelor degree in their discipline area. *Patients* and *clients* are the people the student is assessing, treating, interviewing or working with. Both terms are used throughout the book, as some case studies refer to clinical situations (where *patient* is used) and other case studies refer to non-clinical situations (where *client* is used). The *student* is you. We use the term *entry-level degree*, as this encompasses both bachelor degrees and master's professional entry level degrees.

The term *work-integrated learning (WIL)* is used in this book. This is the buzz word (at the time of writing) for what we would call *fieldwork* or *practicum*. The Australian Learning and Teaching Council has just completed a large scoping study in 35 universities across Australia in relation to this topic, looking at it from the perspectives of universities and students. The term WIL has been defined by them as 'an umbrella term for a range of approaches and strategies that integrate theory with the practice of work within a purposefully designed curriculum' (Patrick et al. 2008: iv, cited in Smith et al. 2009: 23). In this sense WIL encompasses more than just fieldwork placements *per se*, and can be extended in meaning to how these are embedded and integrated within the whole student experience and how we endeavour within the curriculum to integrate the theory with the practice. We have referred to work integrated learning in some sections in some chapters when appropriate. The term is not always appropriate; hence we have used *fieldwork placement* to be more specific, and used *work-integrated learning* when references are to the student learning experience.

There are four parts to this book. Part 1 is called 'Preparing for Practice'. In this section, each chapter addresses a specific situated learning experience, and guides students through what to prepare for, what to expect and issues that it would be helpful to be aware of. Part 2, 'Making the Most of Your Fieldwork Placement', raises issues such as models of supervision, assessment, how to get the most out of your fieldwork experience, interprofessional learning, failure and online technology. Part 3 takes a broader view, placing fieldwork within the broader perspectives of the university, professional bodies and healthcare facilities. Legal issues that relate to fieldwork and the process of making ethical decisions are also covered. Part 4 covers the transition to practice, including aspects of becoming a fieldwork supervisor, and how to provide the basis for students returning to work in a particular area. At the end of each part is a checklist for easy reference.

We wish you all the best in your fieldwork placements.

Karen Stagnitti, Adrian Schoo and Dianne Welch

ACKNOWLEDGMENTS

We would like to acknowledge the invaluable help and assistance of Debra James from Oxford University Press in developing and preparing this book. Debra's advice has been much appreciated, and her enthusiasm for the project has made it a pleasurable experience. Without Debra, the book would not have become a reality.

We would also like to thank Bruce Gillespie whose editing and patience has made the process of the final stages of preparation of the manuscript an efficient and straightforward process. Thank you Bruce.

Finally, we would like to thank all the contributing authors, who have been enthusiastic about the concept of the book and whose depth of knowledge and passion for the field has made editing the book a delight.

Karen Stagnitti, Adrian Schoo and Dianne Welch

The authors and the publisher wish to thank the following copyright holders for reproduction of their material: Harvard Business School Publishing, for Figure 20.1 (page 266), 'The Doughnut Principle', from Handy, 1994, *The Age of Paradox*, Harvard Business School Press, reproduced by permission; Health on the Net Foundation, for Figure 18.2 (page 233), 'HONcode symbol', http://www.hon.ch/, reproduced by permission; Healthcare Blogger Code of Ethics, for Figure 18.1 (page 233), http://medbloggercode. com/, reproduced by permission; Paradigm, for Figure 20.2 (page 267), 'The person-centred risk assessment', from Kinsella, 2000, *Person Centred Risk Assessment*, Paradigm, Liverpool, reproduced by permission of the author; Shutterstock/VectorZilla, for Figure 18.3 (page 239), 'RSS symbol'; Taylor & Francis and Rightslink, for Figure 24.3 (page 336), 'Student and practitioner supervision: key differences', from Davys & Beddoe, 2000, 'Supervision of Students: A Map and a Model for the Decade to Come', *Social Work Education*, 19(5): 438–49, reproduced by permission; World Health Organization, for Figure 20.3 (page 272), 'The International Classification of Functioning, Disability and Health', from WHO, 2002, *Towards a Common Language for Functioning, Disability and Health: ICF The International Classification of Functioning, Disability and Health*, World Health Organization Press, Geneva, reproduced by permission.

Every effort has been made to trace the original source of copyright material contained in this book. The publisher will be pleased to hear from copyright holders to rectify any errors or omissions.

GLOSSARY

Aboriginal and Torres Strait Islander (ATSI) people
The people who occupied continental Australia, Tasmania and the Torres Strait Islands before the arrival of Europeans in 1788.

Aboriginal community-controlled health services
Primary health care services initiated and controlled by local Aboriginal communities to deliver holistic, comprehensive and locally appropriate health care (the term is understood to include both Aboriginal and Torres Strait Islander people).

Aboriginal health workers (AHWs)
Aboriginal and Torres Strait Islander healthcare workers, some with no clinical training, and others providing advanced clinical care to Aboriginal people in emerging areas of need, such as haemodialysis and midwifery.

Accommodation
A major problem faced by students investigating rural fieldwork placements; matters to be investigated before taking up a placement include cost (and possible subsidisation), cleanliness, service and food provision, air-conditioning, computer access, sharing and leisure.

Acute care
The treatment of patients for a relatively short period of time for an episode of illness that is brief but that can be severe, in a hospital's emergency department or ambulatory care clinic, or in another type of facility for the purpose of short stay.

Administrative function
The function of employees involved in organisational policies or protocols.

Adult learning principles
Principles that recognise (a) that the adult learner is an autonomous learner and able to direct her or his learning; (b) that the adult learner brings life experience to learning, which provides a valuable resource for new learning; and (c) new knowledge is directly applicable to real-life situations in the present rather than the future.

Alternative fieldwork
Fieldwork that offers the student a wide variety of learning experiences where service gaps have been identified by the agency that provides for the fieldwork placement.

Apprenticeship approach
The learning approach that gives primary emphasis to learning by doing, so that knowledge, skills, values and attitudes are transmitted by observing an experienced professional at work, and observing, emulating or modelling one's own behaviour on that of the experienced professional.

Articulated model of learning
The learning principle that competent practice relies on prior cognitive understanding; also known as the academic model.

Assessment
The measure of whether learning has taken place.

Assessment criteria
Since fieldwork cannot be assessed by exams or term papers, students need to show they are learning 'on the job', and that they are sufficiently flexible to take advantage of new situations. See Table 14.2 on page 175 for the full range of fieldwork assessment criteria.

Avatar
Within a virtual worlds computer program, a customisable graphical self-representation, which has its own name and can be adapted to have unique features.

Blog (weblog)
Websites that individuals known as bloggers create and maintain; usually a blog is about a single topic or theme, items are posted on a regular basis and opportunity is given to readers to reply directly to blog entries.

Bloggers
Computer users who post regularly on their own blogs, or reply to other users' blogs.

Capacity
An individual's ability to make a specific decision (rather than the contribution made by a healthcare professional or organisation).

Child and family nurse
A health professional working with mothers and children, whose scope of care extends from the antenatal period until the child is aged five years.

Chronic condition self-management program (CCSM)
A healthcare program that teaches participants how to better manage their chronic medical conditions, make informed decisions regarding their health and reduce their reliance on direct health care.

Clients and patients

The people the student is assessing, treating, interviewing or working with. Both terms are used throughout the book, as some case studies refer to clinical situations (where *patient* is used) and other case studies refer to nonclinical situations (where *client* is used).

Clinical placement, education or practicum

Fieldwork placement in a hospital or clinical setting; however, some health students are placed in a work setting, school or other type of organisation; hence *fieldwork placement* is the preferred term.

Clinical reasoning

The systematic application of a process of reasoning to the data collection of clients; an important element of clinical competence.

Collaborative writing tools

Computer programs that allow one or more persons to work on one project in real time or asynchronously; because each document is web based, and has its unique URL, groups of people can work on a document, spreadsheet or presentation, overcoming the need to keep track of different versions.

Communication

Usually of two types: (a) primary communication: between you and the patient or client; and (b) secondary communication: additional information gained by sharing information regarding the patient or client with other team members via medical files and by talking with the patient's or client's family or carer.

Community-based healthcare

Any healthcare service where students will be brought into contact with clients who 'come in off the street' rather than being hospital patients.

Community-building project

A project in which fieldwork students can contribute their skills to a wide range of skills and disciplines, while bringing into effect their own special abilities.

Competence

The range of abilities needed to become a successful professional, such as knowledge, skills, and attitudes (knows; knows how; shows how and does) (Miller 1990).

Competency-based approach

A learning model that defines learning objectives in specific, observable, behavioural terms, identified and expressed as behavioural skills.

Confidentiality

During fieldwork protects clients' rights to privacy and applies to all healthcare providers, whether they are professionals or students. It is an important issue, since private information is shared with other members of the care team to provide optimal care.

Consulting therapist
A therapist who visits schools, but who is often given very limited time to assess and establish recommendations for the child in school settings.

Constructive controversy
A planned approach to learning that enhances professional skills and knowledge after training and graduation. The encouragement of people to develop their skills to disagree respectfully, rather than assuming everyone needs to agree on everything all the time.

Continuing professional development
Opportunities for professional development available to students after graduation; one stimulating form of continuing professional development is to become a fieldwork educator to new students.

Continuity of care
The experience of care where various providers know what has happened before, agree on a management plan and guarantee care into the future.

Conventional fieldwork placements
Those placements where students have a fieldwork educator from the same profession, and placement occurs in a setting where that profession has had a presence for many years.

Core business
The core business of a profession is to define and assure standards of practice (including qualifying education) in the interests of the community, while concurrently advancing the standing of the profession within the community in the interests of the members of that profession.

Critical incident analysis
A learning method, based on *reflection* about a specific incident, using the following steps: (1) a description of the incident and those involved; (2) a description of the outcomes of the action for each involved in the incident; (3) a reflection on the process, naming the types of knowledge or experience that informed the actions, the skills used and the theories underpinning the actions; and (4) naming the learning from the incident, such as discipline-specific theory and knowledge; professional values and ethics; skills; personal beliefs and assumptions.

Critical reflection
The direction of health practice, based upon the questioning and challenging of knowledge generation, aimed at changing situations based upon a greater

appreciation of the political and potentially emancipatory aspects of those situations.

Cultural competence
The ability to relate effectively with individuals of different cultural backgrounds.

Critical reflection
The thinking process of analysing and reevaluating experiences and questioning outcomes.

Determinants of health
Factors associated with the health of individuals and communities, such as individuals' characteristics and behaviours, environment, genetics, income, level of education and social relations.

Disciplines
In this text: professional groups. In health care, client-focused teamwork ranges from multidisciplinary (working with separate disciplinary treatment plans) at the lower end of the scale to interdisciplinary (having a shared plan and monitoring progress together) or even transdisciplinary (with possibility of crossing professional boundaries) modes of service delivery at the higher end of the scale. The latter may involve two or more individuals, including family members, working together effectively and efficiently.

Discipline-specific knowledge or skills
Knowledge or skills that are specific to a particular profession.

Doughnut principle
A model for understanding the roles and responsibilities of those working in health and human services, especially when supporting someone with a disability through a decision-making process. The doughnut (see Chapter 20) has three concentric circles: (1) core responsibilities; (2) situations in which professionals have responsibility, but which require creativity and sound judgment; (3) aspects of a service user's life that are not the paid responsibility of health professionals, such as making moral decisions.

Duty of care
The obligation of a professional to adhere to an adequate standard of care while carrying out activities that could potentially be harmful.

Educative function
Learning skills based upon the discussion between students and fieldwork educators about the link between reading and practice within organisations.

Emotional intelligence (EI)
The ability, skill or capacity to identify, assess and manage emotions, whether they are personal, of others or of groups.

Entrepreneur
Health professional in private practice, running a small business, who is therefore dependent for his or her income on fees paid by clients.

Evidence-based approach
The systematic search for, and critical appraisal of, the most relevant evidence, combined with clinical expertise and client preferences and values, to answer a fieldwork question.

Experiential learning
A series of actions, such as observation and reflection, that assist in establishing meaning from direct experience.

Exclusion
The official removal of a student from a course for a set period of time; after which the student must reapply to complete the course. The return to the course is at the university's discretion.

Family-centred practice
Healthcare practice that involves parents in decision-making and fosters partnerships between parents and the professional(s).

Family services coordinator
The primary person responsible for the organisation of additional services, such as seeking funding and organising respite and family meetings.

Fieldwork
The placement of students in professional fields where they can gain hands-on experience before graduating; it (a) can occur at different levels of courses; for example, expectations for fieldwork placement at first year are very different from those required in a final year placement; (b) can occur in a variety of settings that have differing expectations; and (c) has specific requirements imposed by some professions.

Fieldwork education
A program of education of students undergoing fieldwork, which includes such aspects as students' roles; responsive and trend-setting practices; service enhancement, health promotion and program development; constructive peer evaluation and reflective practice.

Fieldwork education supervisor
The person who provides the same type of service to upcoming students as one's supervisor provided to oneself; including setting clear learning goals and expectations; providing feedback (formal and informal); facilitating self-directed learning opportunities; and undertaking an evaluation before the final evaluation to enable monitoring of progress.

Fieldwork educators
Professionals in the field who supervise students in their placement settings (in situ). They are also known as fieldwork education supervisors, field educators, fieldwork supervisors, clinical educators and clinical supervisors. This person can be an academic staff member from the student's university or educational institution. University staff involved in fieldwork organisation, collaboration or liaison are clearly identified in the text as university staff members.

Fieldwork learning framework
The personal and professional resources and attributes, developed during fieldwork, that contribute to developing skills, knowledge and behaviours for professional practice.

Fieldwork placement
The location where a student is sent to learn how to put in practice skills already studied in coursework; also known as clinical placement, clinical practicum, clinical education and fieldwork experience.

Fieldwork placement agency
Organisation that agrees to provide an industry learning experience for a student.

Final fieldwork placement
The final placement undertaken by a student before final assessment.

Forcefield analysis
An analytical tool for weighing up pros and cons in decision-making, by listing all of the components integral to an issue and giving each a weight in terms of its impact on potential outcomes.

Generic work skills
Abilities that are common across the professions.

Geriatric care (or geriatrics)
A branch of medicine or social science dealing with the health and care of old people (*Australian Oxford Dictionary*).

Goal-setting
Decisions made about where you want to be, and how you might get there (Chapter 13).

Governance
'A framework used by organisations to systematically develop accountability and continuous improvement of the quality of services' (Hafford-Letchfield 2006, p. 132).

Government
The organisation, whether federal or state, that provides the funding sources for higher education as well as for large areas of the Australian community's health and human services.

Growth therapeutic approach
A therapeutic approach that assumes, based on a high degree of self-awareness in the health worker, that therapy for both health worker and client is based on personal growth experience.

Healthcare Blogger Code of Ethics
Guidelines for ethical development of healthcare online tools that enable anyone to be the author within a website.

Health professional
Any person, working in a health area, who has attained a minimum of a bachelor degree in a discipline area.

Horizontal partnerships
Stakeholder partnerships where expertise is shared between partners, and the relationship is acknowledged as symbiotic.

Host centres
Community centres where identified gaps in services are addressed by student-directed projects to enhance and build on an existing service.

Impression management
The development of a professional online profile that is potentially visible to future employers, clients and colleagues.

Indigenous health settings
Healthcare services aimed at increasing the capacity of non-Indigenous students to improve Indigenous health outcomes, contribute to service delivery to Australian Aboriginal people and develop partnerships between Indigenous and non-Indigenous organisations and universities.

Individual professional
Individuals doing specialist work within health and human services, including occupational therapists, social workers, nurses, speech pathologists and physio-therapists.

Infection control

The measures that must be undertaken because patients are always at risk of acquiring infections in the healthcare environment because of lower resistance to infectious agents and an increased exposure to disease-causing microorganisms.

Injured workers

Individual workers who can be returned to the workforce following a work-related injury, through the efforts of rehabilitation consultants, as defined by the guidelines of the relevant Act.

In-placement review

Pre-set times during placements dedicated to evaluating progress, reflecting on student in-placement learning, and identifying any problems and ways to manage them; there should be one in-placement review during a typical fieldwork placement, preferably at least one a week.

Interdisciplinary team

The key unit within a person-centred care environment, which recognises the patient's or client's freedom to make his or her own decisions; with the patient or client at the centre of all care decisions.

Interprofessional education (IPE)

Program designed to help students from a variety of disciplines, who find themselves in the same team, to understand each other in order to avoid unnecessary misunderstandings that can cause team conflict and dysfunction.

Interprofessional learning (IPL)

A term used to describe interprofessional education (IPE) and interprofessional practice (IPP): 'Interprofessional education occurs when two or more professions learn with, from and about each other to improve collaboration and the quality of care' (Centre for the Advancement of Interprofessional Education 2002).

Job seeking

The assistance in finding jobs that can be provided by healthcare workers to disabled or work-injured workers, through such activities as clarifying suitable work areas; writing resumés; providing interview practice, education and/or counselling; answering questions in a way that avoids emotional distress during a job interview situation; identifying job vacancies; reviewing job application letters; and investigating and applying for employment incentives and specific employment-related programs if available.

Johari window

A reflective tool designed to develop and enhance self-awareness. It takes the form of a diagram (shown in Table 13.4 on page 166) that is divided into four panes or quadrants: open, blind, hidden and unknown.

Learning by doing
The learning approach that focuses on learning through observation and doing the work, rather than applying prior principles.

Learning in fieldwork
The interplay of a complex array of variables, which include students' knowledge, skills, attributes and dispositions; their capacity to manage time, tasks, themselves and others; reflective and clinical reasoning skills; a capacity to transform theoretical knowledge into practice; and the nature of fieldwork educator–student relationships.

Levels of supervision
The main levels of supervision exercised by fieldwork supervisors are (1) dependency; (2) fluctuation between dependency and greater independence; (3) proficiency and confident independence; and (4) professional autonomy.

Lifelong learning
The dynamic engagement of healthcare professionals with ideas, practices and people throughout their working lives.

Line management
A student's immediate supervisor or boss.

Medicare
A national insurance program that provides health insurance coverage in Australia.

Mental health
The successful performance of mental functions, in terms of thought, mood and behaviour, that results in productive activities, fulfilling relationships with others and the ability to adapt to change and cope with adversity.

Mentoring
The provision of a fully qualified healthcare professional to provide continuing advice and support for students, as much in general lifestyle directions as in specific practitioner skills.

Midway assessment
An assessment halfway through a placement that gives students an opportunity to learn from both successes and difficulties before facing final assessment.

Modernist perspective
The model that knowledge is understood in a linear, scientific and rational way, by which experts generate theory, and health professionals receive and apply this theory in practice.

Multiple language groups

The variety of group languages, histories, beliefs, practices and needs that may be found in any healthcare setting.

Narrative inquiry

The investigation of evidence provided by stakeholder narratives about personal experience, including stories told by students, fieldwork educators, clients and university educators.

Narrative record

The retelling of events about fieldwork placement from a personal perspective, in writing or conversation, or both.

Negligence

Failure to act with the caution a sensible person is expected to exercise in comparable circumstances.

Negotiation

Advice provided by healthcare consultants, often when forging agreements between injured workers seeking a suitable return-to-work plan and employers prescribing the limited options available.

Neonatal intensive care unit (NICU)

A specialised hospital unit that provides care for extremely premature babies, and babies who require surgical intervention.

Net Code of Conduct (HONCode)

A symbol accompanying a blog, podcast or wiki to indicate that it is reliable and trustworthy: that it is possible to identify who created the blog and what their credentials or experiences are.

Obligation

The legal obligation of the university for the actions of students on placement, even if the university is not implicated in or even aware of the act that might give rise to an action in negligence against the student.

Occupational rehabilitation

A program aimed at returning injured workers to work in a capacity that is in line with their functional and cognitive capacity.

Occupation Wellness Life Satisfaction (OWLS) program

A program designed to provide sufficient, relevant and valuable fieldwork opportunities for occupational therapy students within regional Victoria (see Chapter 15).

Online social networks

Online sites that support the maintenance of existing social networks, or help people connect with strangers who may share interests or activities, varying in the types of applications and communication tools they offer users, such as mobile connectivity, blogging and photo- or videosharing.

On placement
The measures and protocols that students should know before arriving at a new placement (see Chapter 5).

Open blog
A blog that is open to all viewers and participants, therefore should not carry confidential or identifying information.

Orientation
The supervisor's introduction of on placement students to facility settings and specific placement characteristics, such as caseload, in a way that may encourage students to return after graduation.

Pace of work
In the hospital setting, the combination of rapid patient movements and the variety of tasks that must be accomplished in a short time.

Paediatrics
The assessment and treatment of children who have a range of neurological, developmental, genetic and medical conditions that have an impact on their ability to participate in everyday situations.

Partnership
The relationship between stakeholders characterised by cooperation and mutual benefit.

Patients and clients
The people the student is assessing, treating, interviewing or working with. Both terms are used throughout the book, as some case studies refer to clinical situations (where *patient* is used) and other case studies refer to nonclinical situations (where *client* is used).

Peer skill performance evaluation
Evaluation of fieldwork students, in pairs or small groups, providing constructive student-driven feedback, aligned with specific learning goals of one's peers.

Personal attributes
The qualities that the student brings to the fieldwork placement, including traits such as age and gender, learning style, cultural and family background and the presence or not of a specific health condition or disability.

Personal authority
The personal quality that stems from an individual's demeanour and ability within professional relationships to exercise competence and enforce decisions. Too much

reliance on authority can lead to conflict in supervision, while too little exercise of legitimate authority can lead to collusion and the collapse of safe practice.

Person-centred care
A patient's or client's freedom to make his or her own decisions; it is a holistic view, with the patient or client at the centre of all care decisions.

Perspective transformation
The alteration of a student's or educator's viewpoint, such that the person experiences a changed and more accurate view of his or her performance.

Pharmaceutical Benefits Scheme (PBS)
The system that has been created by the Australian government to provide timely, reliable and affordable access to necessary and cost-effective medicines.

Placement contract
In fieldwork education, the document that addresses the specific expectations between the student, the supervisor and the education institution, including practical matters, the timeframe of the placement, agency conduct rules, arrangements for supervision and backup during the absence of the fieldwork educator.

Podcast
Named after Apple iPods, podcasts are downloadable audio or video files.

Police Record Check (PRC)
One of two certified documents (the other is the *Working With Children Check*) that students must complete and submit before the beginning of fieldwork placements each academic year. Without a PRC, students may not be granted permission to undertake fieldwork placement.

Post
Where a blog is about a single topic or theme, items are posted on a regular basis, with the most recent entries appearing at the top; each entry is called a post, with most bloggers allowing others to respond by posting comments.

Postmodernist perspective
The learning perspective that challenges the *modernist* understanding of knowledge: rather than understanding knowledge from only a theoretical perspective, postmodernists incorporate other types of knowledge generated by reflecting on personal experience and culture.

Post-placement
Students' and educators' review of the placement, preferably held immediately after each placement.

Practice-reflection–theory-reflection process
The process by which students can use a number of critical reflection tools, including critical incident analysis, journal keeping, think sheets and narrative records, leading to new insights or perspectives. *See also* Johari window.

Private practice
An autonomous, entrepreneurial and possibly lucrative health service provider business, which is established through the investment of capital and resources, and usually involves going into debt before an income can be derived.

Profession
The collective efforts of each specific work role undertaken by individual members of the health and human services workforce.

Professional standards and image
Those aspects of students' behaviour and appearance that allow fellow health professionals to evaluate performance and work successfully together within the placement (see Chapter 10).

Readiness to learn
Students' readiness to use the experience of success or failure in a fieldwork placement as a catalyst to alter perceptions of themselves or their worldview.

Reflection
A student's systematic consideration of fieldwork experience (positive and negative feelings) and the transition experience of moving into the workplace as a qualified health professional.

Rehabilitation provider
A health professional provided in most workplaces to meet with injured workers, the workers' supervisor and/or the return-to-work supervisor in order to assess the specific requirements of the injured worker, health practitioners, insurers and the employer.

Remote settings
Healthcare placements scattered widely throughout the hinterland of Australia, often forced to deal with workforce and facility shortages, but also providing intense social and healthcare experiences for students.

Return-to-work plan
A plan that is worked out, often with the healthcare workers as negotiators, to balance the interests of injured workers attempting to return to work, employers and other interested parties, such as insurers.

Risk assessment
As risk is the potential danger that might be posed to any person or organisation in the ordinary pursuit of daily activities, risk assessment looks not only at the risk

posed to individual persons, but also those supporting that person and on others within his or her community, including the impact of the activity on a person's reputation and any risk of lost opportunities for personal development if the person does not engage in an activity.

Role-emerging fieldwork
Activities of students that demonstrate and communicate the potential of their professional role within the fieldwork place and the community it serves.

Role systems approach
The learning approach that focuses on the interaction between the student and the fieldwork educator; it is the fieldwork educator's responsibility to ensure that the most appropriate type of learning and teaching occurs, a process that requires negotiation of the structure, process and content of fieldwork.

Royal Flying Doctor Service
A healthcare service, provided by pilots using small aircraft, that operates throughout remote areas of Australia.

RSS
Initials standing for Really Simple Syndication, Rich Site Summary or RDF Site Summary. RSS allows online users to subscribe to alerts from Internet news services, blogs or podcasts updates, journal table of contents alerts and even Pubmed searches. Subscribing to RSS feeds means that downloaders no longer need visit favourite websites or blogs for updates; rather, they are informed of updates.

Rurality (regional, rural and remote)
Any area in Australia that is not part of one of the state capitals, or other major cities, and is thus separated from many major services, industries and job opportunities.

Self-assessment
The development by students of the ability to assess their own performance and reduce their dependence upon external forms of assessment.

Self-awareness
Students' awareness of their own biases, assumptions and prejudices, and the ability to set appropriate professional boundaries, sustain self-respect and strike a balance between working independently and interdependently when required.

Self-regulation
The ability to demonstrate skills in time management, conflict management, impulse control and management of stressful situations and strong emotions without becoming overwhelmed.

Social software tools
Online tools used to support fieldwork learning, including weblogs (blogs), collaborative writing tools, online social networks, podcasts, syndication feeds (RSS), virtual worlds and wikis (see also Chapter 18).

Stakeholders
All those individuals and organisations who have something to contribute to or gain from any human activity. The health and human services profession includes such key stakeholders as universities, the government and individual professionals and students. Usually a partnership is formed that requires cooperation for a mutual benefit.

Stigma/stigmata
'A mark or sign of disgrace or discredit' (*Australian Oxford Dictionary*). Stigma labels a person as not being 'normal', not 'fitting in' the broader community.

Stress
As experienced by many health professionals, stress is mainly the result of high workload, poor job satisfaction, lack of skilled supporting staff and inadequate training and supervision.

Student
A person who is the consumer of higher education, including fieldwork placement. The term is used for entry-level degrees, as this encompasses both bachelor degrees and master's entry-level degrees.

Student supervision
The process occurring within a professional relationship in which the fieldwork educator assists students to prepare for, reflect upon and explore practice issues in order to develop competence in their professional practice.

Superclinic
A health centre that provides a raised level of healthcare services within one centre, often offering longer opening hours and additional healthcare providers, and services such as onsite pharmacies, pathology labs and radiography.

Supported decision-making
The principles that everyone is competent in making decisions, everyone communicates and we all seek support to make decisions from those we know and trust.

Supportive function
The fieldwork educator's assistance to the student to develop, maintain and enhance a professional sense of self; a process whereby the fieldwork educator acknowledges and responds to the student's emotional needs as these relate to the role of student.

Teamwork
The activities of a group of individuals who perform for a common purpose or goal and whose individual needs are of less importance than the needs of the group.

Think sheet
A structured, generalised writing exercise that encourages reflection on both behavioural and emotional responses to fieldwork placement experiences.

Three Rs
Roles, rights and responsibilities (see Chapter 21).

Transdisciplinary team
A group of health professionals from a variety of disciplines, carrying out treatment suggested by another health professional.

Transformative learning
A dynamic, individualised process of expanding consciousness, whereby an individual becomes critically aware of old and new self-views and chooses to integrate these views into a new self-definition (Wade 1998).

Transition
The transition experience usually implies a journey from one destination to another (from student to healthcare professional) and the arrival at an endpoint— but healthcare professionals are usually considered to be always in the process of 'becoming': continually learning, relearning and/or unlearning old assumptions to develop new ways of working with people.

Triple helix partnership model
The interconnected spiral relationship between major stakeholders in any enterprise, where spirals are rarely equal, with one party acting as the core around which the others rotate.

Tutorial programs
Programs for students, delivered face to face or online, designed to support students as well as challenging them in skill development, practice reflection and professional thinking.

Unit
A component of or subject within an entry level degree.

University
Facilities that deliver post-secondary education and advanced specialist knowledge through the integration of research and practice in health and human services.

University staff
Health professionals involved in fieldwork organisation, collaboration or liaison are clearly identified in the text as university staff members. The university fieldwork

liaison person is also known as university fieldwork education coordinator: a person who acts as the medium between the university and the education supervisor in the field.

Vertical partnerships
Partnerships between organisations, where one partner or group of partners acts as a consultant (commissioned expert) to others wishing to make changes in structure, functioning or methods of service delivery.

Vicarious liability
The responsibility employers have for the actions of their employees as they carry out their tasks.

Virtual worlds
Computer-based, simulated multimedia environments that are designed to enable users to interact with each other using digital objects; each user has a customisable graphical self-representation known as an *avatar*.

Vocational rehabilitation
The healthcare process that plans, in coordination with a clinical team, to enable people to return to work after an injury, including the provision of appropriate aids and accommodation, and assisting in accessing disability benefits as needed.

Vulnerable decision-makers
Adults with disabilities, such as developmental disabilities, psychiatric disorders and psychosocial difficulties, or neurological deficits, for whom the characteristics associated with their condition can affect decision-making.

Web 2.0
Online tools that have embraced the power of the Internet to harness collective intelligence. The Web 1.0 Internet changed from being a unidirectional repository into Web 2.0, with the ability to search and download information as a multidirectional virtual environment, where people can interact with each other, build networks, collaborate and share ideas, form questions, give information and create communities around topics of shared interest.

Wiki
('Hurry' in the Hawaiian language): a collection of linked webpages that can be contributed to, edited or updated by its users; the most famous example is Wikipedia.

Woman-centred care
Care that focuses on the woman's individual needs, aspirations and expectations, rather than the needs of the institution or professionals; and recognises the need for women to have choice, control and continuity from a known caregiver or caregivers.

Workforce recruitment

The graduate's application for a position, hoping to be recruited to the position. Workforce recruitment is important in both metropolitan and rural settings, and its success often depends on a student's positive placement experience.

Working With Children Check (WWC)

One of two forms (the other is the *Police Record Check (PRC)*) that students must complete satisfactorily, and provide certified copies of, before setting out on most fieldwork placements. The check is required once every five years.

Work-integrated learning (WIL)

A term synonymous with *fieldwork* or *practicum*, which has been defined by the Australian Learning and Teaching Council as 'an umbrella term for a range of approaches and strategies that integrate theory with the practice of work within a purposefully designed curriculum'. As such, WIL encompasses more than just fieldwork placement.

Workplace literacy

The sets of skills, attitudes and behaviours required to practise competently in any field or job.

Work practice

Workplace-based or work-related services provided to employers, insurers and other stakeholders, including services provided to an individual seeking employment or currently working.

CONTRIBUTORS

Uschi Bay, Lecturer, Social Work Department, Monash University, Victoria.

Liz Beddoe, Head of School of Counselling, Human Services and Social Work, Faculty of Education, University of Auckland, Auckland.

Michelle Conlan, Occupational Therapist, Bellarine Community Health Centre, Victoria.

Michelle Courtney, Senior Lecturer, Occupational Science and Therapy, School of Health and Social Development, Deakin University, Victoria.

Ronnie Egan, Social Work Unit, Victoria University, Melbourne, Victoria.

Joanne Gray, Senior Lecturer, Director of Midwifery Studies, Faculty of Nursing, Midwifery and Health, University of Technology, Sydney.

Nick Hagiliassis, Research Coordinator, Scope, Glenroy, Victoria.

Tim Kauffman, Kauffman Gamber Physical Therapy, Lancaster, Pennsylvania; and Adjunct Faculty, Columbia University, New York.

Lindy McAllister, Associate Professor and Deputy Head of School (Teaching and Learning), School of Medicine, University of Queensland.

Jo McDonall, Lecturer, School of Nursing, Deakin University, Victoria.

Anita Hamilton, Assistant Professor, Department of Occupational Therapy, University of Alberta, Edmonton.

Richard Ingleby, Barrister, Victoria; Visiting Professor, North China University of Technology, Beijing.

Helen Larkin, Lecturer, Occupational Science and Therapy, School of Health and Social Development, Deakin University, Victoria.

Jane Maidment, Senior Lecturer, School of Nursing and Human Services, Christchurch Polytechnic Institute of Technology, New Zealand.

Phoebe Maloney, Occupational Therapist, Heywood Rural Health, Victoria.

Eva Nemeth, Director of Clinical Education, Master of Speech and Language Program, Macquarie University, Sydney.

Jennifer Nitz, Geriatric Teaching and Research Team Leader, Division of Physiotherapy, School of Health and Rehabilitation Sciences, University of Queensland.

Sharleen O'Reilly, Lecturer, School of Exercise and Nutrition Sciences, Deakin University, Victoria.

Jennifer Pascoe, Occupational Therapist, Executive Assistant, World Federation of Occupational Therapists.

Merrolee Penman, Principal Lecturer, School of Occupational Therapy, Otago Polytechnic, Dunedin.

Geneviève Pépin, Senior Lecturer, Occupational Science and Therapy, School of Health and Social Development, Deakin University, Victoria.

Kelly Powell, Lecturer, Occupational Science and Therapy, School of Health and Social Development, Deakin University, Victoria.

Angela Russell, Student Coordinator and Special Projects, Spencer Gulf Rural Health School, in partnership with Pika Wiya Health Service, Port Augusta.

Rachael Schmidt, Lecturer, Occupational Science and Therapy, School of Health and Social Development, Deakin University, Victoria.

Adrian Schoo, Associate Professor of Physiotherapy, Faculty of Health Sciences, La Trobe University.

Megan Smith, Senior Lecturer, Course Leader, Physiotherapy, Sub Dean Professional Placements, Faculty of Science, Charles Sturt University, Albury.

Karen Stagnitti, Associate Professor, Occupational Science and Therapy Program, School of Health and Social Development, Deakin University, Victoria.

Nick Stone, Lecturer, Department of Management, University of Melbourne.

Judy Taylor, Senior Research Fellow, Spencer Gulf Rural Health School, Centre for Rural Health and Community Development, University of South Australia, Whyalla.

Kym Thomas, Coordinator: Aboriginal Health Unit, Spencer Gulf Rural Health School, University of South Australia.

Doris Testa, Social Work Unit, Field Education Coordinator, Victoria University, Victoria.

Paul Tinley, Associate Professor, Podiatry Course Coordinator, School of Community Health, Charles Sturt University, Albury.

Joanne Watson, Senior Speech Pathologist, and Research Fellow, Scope Victoria.

Dianne Welch, Associate, Head of School (Academic Programs), School of Nursing, Deakin University, Victoria.

Deirdre Whitford, Associate Professor, Head of Education, Spencer Gulf Rural Health School, South Australia.

Linda Wilson, Lecturer, School of Health and Social Development, Deakin University, Victoria.

PART 1
PREPARING FOR PLACEMENT

Chapter 1: Getting Ready for Placement   3

Chapter 2: Working in Diverse Settings   13

Chapter 3: Working with Mothers and Babies   26

Chapter 4: Working with Children and Families   37

Chapter 5: Working in Acute Settings   50

Chapter 6: Working with Older People   62

Chapter 7: Working in Mental Health   76

Chapter 8: Working in Workplace Practice   87

Chapter 9: Working in Private Practice   100

Chapter 10: Working in Rural and Remote Settings   108

Chapter 11: Working in Indigenous Health Settings   119

Most tertiary institutions endeavour to offer their students a broad fieldwork experience by giving the same student several placements throughout a course. This section provides information on a variety of fieldwork settings, and how to prepare for each. Chapter 1 gives information on getting ready for placement and provides a general introduction for any placement that you may undertake. The next ten chapters provide information on specific contexts of practice, from geographical locations (such as rural or remote placements) to specific client-based settings (such as mothers and babies). In each of these chapters you will be introduced to what you need to prepare for each setting, what you might expect, and the type of knowledge you are likely to develop over your fieldwork placement in that setting. Fieldwork placements introduce you to the complexity of practice in your health field. We hope you enjoy your experience, and can integrate academic learning successfully with practical experience.

CHAPTER 1
GETTING READY FOR PLACEMENT

Jane Maidment

LEARNING OUTCOMES

After reading this chapter, you should be able to:
- understand the purpose and scope of work-integrated learning
- be aware of the practical steps to take in preparing for the fieldwork placement
- analyse aspects of workplace literacy with reference to oneself and the team
- raise self-awareness about being a student on placement.

KEY TERMS

Emotional intelligence (EI)
Experiential learning
Fieldwork educator
Fieldwork placement
Self-awareness
Self-regulation
Work-integrated learning
Workplace literacy

INTRODUCTION

This chapter outlines a range of factors to consider before embarking on a fieldwork placement. These considerations focus mainly on practical matters, and will be relevant to you, regardless of your health-related discipline. Work-integrated learning has a long and strong tradition in most health-related disciplines. Many seasoned health professionals consider their past student fieldwork placement as the most significant and memorable learning experience in their early careers, shaping and radically influencing their style of working, future career choices and identification with their chosen discipline. Engaging with real clients in the context of a bona fide workplace brings a critical edge to learning that cannot be captured in the classroom. Together, these factors create an exciting, dynamic and challenging milieu. In order to make the most of the learning opportunities offered in the field it is important to build a sound foundation from which to begin your fieldwork placement. Understanding the scope and purpose of the fieldwork placement is the logical place to start.

SCOPE AND PURPOSE OF WORK-INTEGRATED LEARNING

The scope of the profession

It may seem self-evident that the purpose of 'going out on placement' is to learn how to practise one's discipline. Learning to practise, however, involves more than demonstrating the technical skills associated with your discipline, such as conducting an intake assessment, constructing a splint or charting a patient's medication. It entails:

- discovering and articulating the connections between the theory you have learned in the classroom and the client situations you encounter on fieldwork placement
- developing greater awareness and analysis of your own professional values in situ, where challenging ethical dilemmas can arise
- learning how interdisciplinary teamwork operates, and about ways you and people from your discipline might contribute to the team in order to better serve the client population.

The scope of work-integrated learning is broad, influenced by the cultural norms of the workplace, and complex in terms of incorporating a range of stakeholders.

Much has been written about this type of experiential learning, leading to a plethora of terminology to describe the activities associated with work-integrated learning. Stints of structured learning in the field have been variously described as clinical rounds, placement, field education and the practicum. Similarly, the roles of those people primarily responsible for facilitating the learning of students in the field are referred to as 'preceptors' in nursing, 'field educators' in social work, 'fieldwork supervisors' in occupational therapy and 'clinical supervisors' in other disciplines. While the names for the fieldwork placement and the names given to your principal supervisor differ from discipline to discipline, the functions of the fieldwork placement and the key people in the process remain the same: to provide a milieu in which you can engage in authentic work-integrated learning, with structured professional guidance and supervision. In this context, the term *fieldwork placement* is used for placement or practicum, and *fieldwork educator* is used for the person who directly supervises you when you are at the placement.

There are a diverse range of agency settings in which you may be placed, including large hospital settings, community health and non-government organisations. The client group you work with will be determined by the setting of your fieldwork placement, and might include but will not be limited to, older persons, mothers with babies, people with mental health issues or those attending rehabilitation. Throughout your degree program you will have opportunities to learn about and experience work in a variety of settings.

The duration of a fieldwork placement can vary, and may include individual days in an agency, blocks of several weeks in full-time or part-time work, or year-long internships. Student fieldwork placement opportunities usually increase in length and intensity over the course of a degree program, with many prescribing regulations for the numbers of days and hours that must be completed. These guidelines are set down by professional accreditation bodies such as the Australian Association of Social Work, the Australian Nursing and Midwifery Council, the World Federation of Occupational Therapy and the World Confederation of Physical Therapists. In Chapter 19 you will be able to read more about the significant role of professional associations in providing governance and regulation influencing health education and practice.

THINK AND LINK 1.1

You are gaining the knowledge and learning the skills to become a member of your profession. Chapter 19 discusses how professional associations, universities and government work together to enable you to take part in fieldwork education.

While you may have entered the program with the goal of working in a specific field such as disability or mental health, it is important to be open to the professional opportunities that can be generated in all settings. Frequently students, after having been on placement, become passionate about working in fields they had not previously thought about. It is important not to hold tight to preconceived ideas about a specific place or client group you want to work with until you have finished your degree. If you are placed in an agency that differs from your preferred choice (which happens frequently), demonstrating annoyance or lack of interest will have a negative impact upon your engagement with the staff and clients in that agency. This standpoint can also lead to you becoming less open to exciting alternative learning and career possibilities.

Wherever you go on placement, paying attention to planning and organising is a key to successful completion. Research on problems experienced by students on fieldwork placement identifies common stressors that can be addressed with some forward planning. These include issues such as financial constraints, managing child care, travel arrangements and attending to personal safety (Maidment 2003).

GETTING READY

Planning for the placement begins well before your actual start date. Table 1.1 lists a series of factors to consider, and strategies that past students have utilised.

Table 1.1: Planning and organising for placement

Preplacement Planning and Organisation	
Finances	Being out on placement incurs additional costs. Start budgeting early for travel to and from your placement, purchase of work-appropriate clothing, any required equipment or books, additional child care expenses, accommodation and depleted wages if you need to cut back on paid work hours. Some students have applied for bank loans to cover extra costs during this time.
Program administration	All programs organising fieldwork placements require you to complete a set of paperwork beforehand. Ensure that you submit this material to the field coordinator by the dates required and that you attend any information sessions offered by the institution.
Police checks	Most institutions require students to produce a *police check* at the time of interview or on the start date. These can take several weeks to process. Make an application for a police check well in advance of beginning placement. A police check must be completed for each current year of your course.
Working with children check	Most states now also require students to provide a *working with children check* before placement with minors. These checks also take some time to process, so begin the process at least two months before placement begins.
Child care	Students with children frequently need to find additional child care while on placement. Discuss this need well in advance with your family members, local child care centre and other potential minders. You may need to use after-school care or employ a caregiver in your home.
Travel	Think about how you will get to your placement, whether by car, car pooling, public transport or bike. Plan your route from home to the placement agency if you are travelling to an unfamiliar location, allowing for extra time on the first day.
Dress code	Find out if there is a prescribed agency dress code or uniform you are expected to wear on placement. Standard of dress in an agency setting is likely to be more formal than the casual clothes you would wear to university.
Placement interviews	Some fieldwork placement programs require students to attend an interview before beginning. Prepare a curriculum vitae to take with you. Ensure you also take your driver's licence, police check and working with children check. Before attending an interview make sure you know the location of the agency, and familiarise yourself about the work of the agency from the web or by requesting information to be sent by post. Have some ideas about what you are wanting to learn during the placement, and prepare some questions to ask at the interview.
	If you do not need to have an interview, but are simply given a start date, make contact with your fieldwork educator over the telephone to introduce yourself before you begin. Be informed about the purpose of the agency and the scope of the work before you start.

Table 1.2 outlines matters you need to familiarise yourself with during your first week on placement.

Table 1.2: First week: planning and organisation

Agency administration	During the first week on placement students frequently need to complete agency confidentiality contracts, provide personal ID to collect and sign for keys or building security cards, be supplied with a computer password or security code, learn the systems for car and room bookings, and become informed on office procedure for recording your whereabouts during the day.
Safety	Most agencies have policies and procedures to address personal and occupational safety in the workplace. Ask to read these and discuss key safety processes associated with office appointments and home visits with your fieldwork educator during the first week.
Orientation	It is usual to have an orientation phase to the physical surroundings and the work of the agency, and to meet your new colleagues. By the end of the first few days in the agency you should know where you can leave your personal belongings, use desk space and who to approach when you have questions or issues to address. Ask what people normally do at lunchtime and how long you have for this break. As the placement progresses you will continue with your orientation to the field of practice and organisational policy, and learn agency information recording and storage procedures.
First client contact	It is usual at the beginning of a placement to spend some time observing your supervisor or other practitioners working with clients. In order to prepare for this observation it is helpful to have read the client file and spoken with the fieldwork educator about particular points to look out for during your observation. Debriefing with the fieldwork educator after these client sessions is the time to ask questions, and discuss ideas. Having observed a number of sessions, you may then often work with an experienced practitioner. Students in their final years of training can be expected to work relatively independently with clients, while continuing to receive professional supervision.

Once you arrive at the agency to begin your fieldwork placement, it is important from the outset to demonstrate your workplace literacy.

WORKPLACE LITERACY

Traditionally the term *workplace literacy* has been adopted to describe 'the written and spoken language, math [maths] and thinking skills that workers and trainees use to perform job tasks or training' (Askov et al. 1989 cited in O'Conner 1993: 196). In this discussion the notion of workplace literacy is broadened, and defined as

REFLECTION 1.1

Discussing emotional intelligence

Complete this exercise before you go out on placement. Listed below are sets of attributes associated with self-awareness, self-regulation, self-motivation, social awareness and social skills. Identify the specific attributes that you are confident you can demonstrate while you are on placement, and those that you feel you need to develop. Discuss your self-assessment with a partner or group members. When doing this exercise, be mindful of the feedback you have already received from your peers, friends, family and lecturers about the way you communicate, behave and work with others.

During the early meetings you have with your fieldwork educator, it may be helpful to share the list of attributes below, and discuss your strengths and weaknesses in these areas.

Attributes of emotional intelligence

Self-awareness
- Being aware of own bias, assumptions, and prejudices
- Setting appropriate professional boundaries
- Having self-respect
- Striking the balance between working independently and interdependently when required.

Self-regulation
- Demonstrating skills in time management
- Applying conflict management strategies when needed
- Exercising impulse control
- Managing stressful situations and strong emotions without becoming overwhelmed
- Being free from emotional dependence.

Self-motivation
- Initiating your own learning and practice responses in the workplace
- Being positively responsive to feedback
- Being proactive in addressing injustice at micro, meso and macro levels.

Social awareness
- Recognising the social norms of the workplace setting and responding appropriately to them
- Demonstrating personal temperament conducive to working in an agency and teamwork setting
- Applying moral courage and demonstrating social responsibility.

Social skills
- Showing respect, and responding with empathy
- Demonstrating a genuine interest in the lives of others
- Understanding and using a range of nonverbal behaviours to put clients and colleagues at ease.

Source: Beddoe & Maidment 2009: 27–8. Reprinted by permission, Cengage Learning Australia

CLINICAL REASONING 1.1

Clinical reasoning includes using all the skills and knowledge you have to help you interpret a client's situation and the course of action (or not) you should take. Self-awareness, social skills and social awareness are some of the skills involved in clinical reasoning.

being the sets of *skills, attitudes and behaviours* required to practise competently in the field. This definition incorporates the spectrum of attributes that have been written about extensively under the umbrella term of *emotional intelligence (EI)*, including demonstrating self-awareness, self-regulation, self-motivation, social awareness and social skills (Cherniss 2000: 434). It is now recognised that bringing these particular attributes to practice when working within teams and with clients can enhance service delivery outcomes in healthcare settings (Meyer et al. 2004).

Emotional intelligence

Clearly, factors associated with EI include aspects of behaviour that are quite personal and sometimes difficult to discuss, but have significant bearing on how student performance is assessed. Simple things like being on time for work and meetings, being open to constructive feedback, attending to personal hygiene, having sound communication skills and respecting established lines of authority are all part of demonstrating workplace literacy. Familiarising yourself with the guidelines and attendant expectations set out by your educational institution and placement agency will enable you to 'know the rules' and requirements for successful completion of your placement. However, in most workplaces there are some unwritten rules. As a student your role during the early days on placement is to become aware of these unwritten rules. Use your supervision time to discuss your observations in private before commenting in a team meeting or the tearoom about what you see. In this way you respect the established workplace culture and give yourself the time and opportunity to become informed. At first, however, remain silently curious.

It can be challenging negotiating your student role at the beginning of fieldwork placement in an unfamiliar context, while also feeling the pressure of being assessed and needing to demonstrate competence. These conditions frequently result in students feeling stressed during the first placement (Zupiria Gorostidi et al. 2007)

MANAGING THOUGHTS AND FEELINGS

Going out on placement can be exciting, scary and challenging, all at once. Often you are juggling multiple responsibilities with working in paid employment, continuing sporting commitments, providing child care as well as being on placement. It is important therefore to give some thought and preparation to how you might manage the levels of stress that students commonly associate with this experience. Past studies in this field (Murray-Harvey et al. 2000; Maidment 2003; Zupiria Gorostidi et al. 2007) cite students using the following techniques to manage stress:

- taking care of the practical arrangements such as organising travel, child care and other work commitments before fieldwork placement
- framing the placement as a *time to learn* rather than viewing the experience as primarily a time to demonstrate proficiency and competence
- being prepared and organised to meet workplace commitments and deadlines (using a diary to record meetings and assignment commitments)
- focusing on developing supportive collegial relationships with other team members in the agency
- using problem-solving techniques such as consultation, sourcing new information, prioritising and asking for help
- giving time to maintaining personal interests (such as sport and hobbies) and friendships outside of the placement
- learning relaxation techniques, including breathing and meditation exercises.

Case Study 1.1   **Grier's situation**

Read the following case study and identify strategies you might use if you found yourself in Grier's situation.

Grier, 21 years old, has just started out in her first fieldwork placement in a community health centre. She has been looking forward to having some hands-on experience with real clients, but is also feeling nervous. She has read all of the materials about what she is supposed to do on placement, and has been told that the agency is a very busy place. However, she had not quite realised how busy everyone would be, and now feels she is in the way. At the team meetings where client situations are discussed, each team member gives a brief summary of who she or he has seen and provides a progress report. These contributions are snappy and to the point. Everyone seems very organised and efficient, confident and outspoken. The staff talk about how 'stretched' they are and how they do not have enough time or resources to do everything required. Grier is feeling nervous about taking up people's time, not making a useful contribution, being in the way and worried about eventually needing to speak up in the team meeting.

Questions

1 What other words could you use to describe Grier's emotional state?

2 Refer back to the emotional intelligence list. What emotional intelligence attributes do you think Grier should call upon?

3 What action should Grier take to feel more at ease in the setting?

SUMMARY

This chapter outlines the factors to consider when getting ready for your fieldwork placement, while identifying key features for working with others and managing well during the fieldwork placement. Planning, organisation and time management are key skills that will contribute to success in the field, along with having effective interpersonal skills such as those identified under workplace literacy. Being on placement is frequently a time of considerable personal and professional challenge and change.

In closing I am reminded of an observation made by a professor of engineering some years ago, when he observed that students returned from field placement 'six months older but two years wiser'.

DISCUSSION QUESTIONS

1 Note how you feel about going out on your first placement. Identify what you think might be your major challenges. Think about ways you might address these challenges.

2 What would you put on a list of considerations to work through to ensure you are prepared? (Hint: there is a checklist at the end of this section which may assist you here.)

3 On placement you are likely to encounter clients from diverse backgrounds. What strategies do you think you would use to communicate effectively with people who are quite different from yourself?

4 When you first start working in the field it is sometimes hard to stop thinking about client situations when you go home. How do you think you might manage this issue?

References

Beddoe, E. & Maidment, J. (2009). *Mapping Knowledge for Social Work Practice: Critical Interactions*. Cengage Learning, Melbourne.

Chermiss, C. (2000). 'Social and Emotional Competence in the Workplace'. In R. Bar-On and J. D. A. Parker (eds), *The Handbook of Emotional Intelligence: Theory, Development,*

Assessment, and Application in the Home, School and in the Workplace. Jossey-Bass, San Francisco: 433–58.

Maidment, J. (2003). 'Problems Experienced by Students on Field Placement: Using Research Findings to Inform Curriculum Design and Content'. *Australian Social Work*, 56(1), 50–60.

Meyer, B., Fletcher, T. & Parker, S. (2004). 'Enhancing Emotional Intelligence in the Health Care Environment'. *Health Care Manager*, 23(3), 225–34.

Murray-Harvey, R., Slee, P., Lawson, M., Silins, H., Banfield, G. & Russell, A. (2000). 'Under Stress: The Concerns and Coping Strategies of Teacher Education Students'. *European Journal of Teacher Education*, 23(1), 19–35.

O'Connor, P. (1992). 'Workplace Literacy in Australia: Competing Agenda'. In A. Welch and P. Freebody, *Knowledge, Culture and Power: International Perspectives on Literacy as Policy and Practice*. Routledge, London.

Zupiria Gorostidi, X., Huitzi Egilegor, M., Jose Alberdi Erice, M., Jose Uranga Iturriotz, I., Eizmendi Garate, M. et al. (2007). 'Stress Sources in Nursing Practice. Evolution During Nursing Training'. *Nurse Education Today*, 27(7), 777.

CHAPTER 2
WORKING IN DIVERSE SETTINGS

Sharleen O'Reilly

LEARNING OUTCOMES

After reading this chapter, you should be able to:
- adapt to diverse work settings
- understand the structure of the healthcare setting in Australia
- define some key elements involved in successful orientation on placement
- understand the meanings of cultural awareness and cultural competence
- work with interpreters.

KEY TERMS

Confidentiality
Cultural competence
Interdisciplinary team
Medicare
Person-centred care
Pharmaceutical Benefits Scheme
Superclinic

INTRODUCTION

Starting any work-integrated learning can be a time of change and transition for you. It may be the first time that you will enter your future work environment, your first exposure to working with clients or even be your first time entering a healthcare setting in Australia. The result can be high levels of anxiety, stress and uncertainty. The aim of this chapter is to help you adapt to diverse workplace settings through addressing common issues faced by students within these environments.

AUSTRALIAN HEALTHCARE SYSTEM

Overall structure

Australia has two levels of government (state/territory and federal). This division affects the healthcare system and the way that it is run. The federal government, usually referred to as the Commonwealth government, has responsibility for policy setting and budget allocation for the whole of Australia. The states and territories are largely responsible for the funding, delivery and management of the healthcare services. In 2009 this division is under review, with the Commonwealth government putting forward arguments that healthcare should be managed federally. At the time of writing this debate is just beginning.

Healthcare services include acute and psychiatric hospital services and other public health services, such as dental health, school health, environmental health, maternal and child health programs. The federal government funds most health research and medical services outside the hospital setting, while both state and federal governments fund public hospitals and community care for aged and disabled persons. The care of older persons is divided into two main areas: residential (such as accommodation provided by nursing homes or hostels) and community care (such as services provided in the form of delivered meals, home help or transport). The funding of older persons care is divided amongst a variety of sources. They include all levels of government, and non-government bodies such as charitable, religious and commercial providers. Residential aged care is funded and regulated by the federal government. Both public and non-government (mostly religious and charitable) organisations provide community care services, under the Home and Community Care (HACC) Program, which aims to keep individuals independent of residential care and out of hospitals through increased provision of services to at-risk persons.

The Australian Red Cross is funded by the federal and state governments to operate the Blood Bank and organ donation system. Because of the vast size of Australia, several specialised services, such as the Royal Flying Doctor Service (delivering care to remote areas by aircraft), Aboriginal and Torres Strait Islander peoples community-controlled health services (providing for indigenous specific health needs) and Regional Health Services (providing for community-identified priorities in health and ageing services), funded by state and federal governments, reach out to regional and remote communities.

Public hospitals

The public health system in Australia is called Medicare. It allows for public hospital services to be provided at no cost, substantial reductions to the cost of prescription medicines (with a safety net providing free medicines for the chronically ill) and free or subsidised treatment by doctors, and some optometrist and dentist services. Medicare covers all people residing in Australia who are Australian citizens, New Zealand citizens or holders of permanent visas (see Figure 2.1). Australia does have a number of reciprocal agreements with other countries, allowing people from those countries various levels of access to the Medicare system.

Most public hospitals provide acute-care beds and emergency outpatient clinics with those in urban areas generally providing a more complex level of care, such as organ transplant, burns management, paediatrics, intensive care and specialist services. Private hospitals are generally involved in the delivery of less complex

Figure 2.1: The Australian hospital system

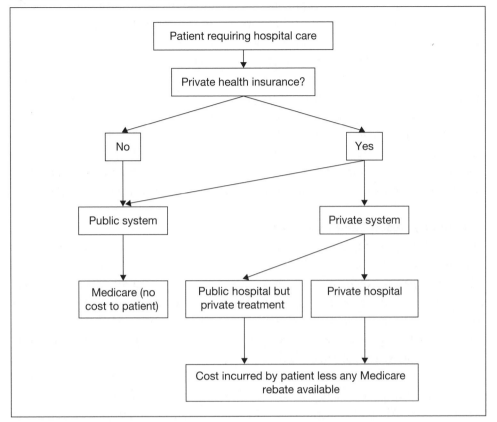

Source: O'Reilly, S. 2009

non-emergency care, although there are some that specialise in delivery of complex and high technology care. Independent centres for the provision of same-day outpatient surgery and other procedures, such as endoscopy, are mostly run privately, although public hospitals may also provide these services. Unlike other countries, Australia has no system of unique patient identifiers. Each hospital allocates a unique record number (URN) to each patient, and this number varies from hospital to hospital, making tracking of patient records difficult between sites. Pathology and diagnostic imaging is also predominantly privately run. Mental health has historically been operated separately from other healthcare services, but there is a current federal investigation aimed at integrating mental health back into the mainstream healthcare system.

The private system
Australia also has a strong private health sector that consumers access through having private health insurance. The federal government encourages people, especially those over 30 years of age, to hold private health insurance through a

30 per cent subsidy to the cost, and reduced Medicare levy in the individual taxation system for those who hold private health insurance. Holding private health insurance allows individuals to choose how they access the healthcare system. They can either remain within the public system or elect to be treated privately. Public hospitals will charge patients private fees and a portion of the medical inpatient fees if they want to access a treatment through a doctor of their choice or have a specific accommodation arrangement, for example their own room. Private hospital access is the other option available to those with private health insurance. These hospitals can be run by commercial or not-for-profit organisations, such as religious bodies, or private health insurance funds. Private health insurance can also be used to cover allied health services and some medical appliances such as hearing aids and glasses.

Community-based health services

Outside of hospital care, patients may need to access general practitioners, private specialists, or other allied health practitioners or services. The Medicare system allows for the cost to be either fully reimbursed or substantially covered (patient pays the 'gap' between the full cost and the Medicare rebate). Patients can choose to pay for the service upfront and apply for a rebate through Medicare offices, or where 'bulk billing' is offered: the service bills Medicare directly, so there is no out-of-pocket expense for patients when they receive the service.

Prescription medicines dispensed in the community receive a direct subsidy from the federal government through a scheme called the Pharmaceutical Benefits Scheme (PBS). All public hospitals provide medicines free of charge and do not use the PBS. Non-prescription medicines are made available mainly through pharmacies, although some are available through other suppliers, such as supermarkets. There are two categories within the PBS: concessional (war veterans, pensioners, certain disadvantaged groups) and general; the difference is that a smaller 'gap' amount is paid by the concessional group for each medicine received.

Community-level healthcare is delivered mainly through health centres, which provide a variety of services, depending on the focus of that centre, although generally they offer services from general practitioners, allied health professionals (such as social workers, dietitians, podiatrists, physiotherapists, occupational therapists and speech pathologists) and nurses. People who access community-level care are commonly referred to as 'clients', reflecting the fact that individuals are actively involved in their own care.

Community-level healthcare also has a health promotion focus, and may be part of a Primary Care Partnership (PCP) within a region. PCPs were formed to make health promotion work more effective within the region where healthcare centres are located, and to offer a coordinated approach to meeting the health needs of the communities they serve. The PCP receives all the funding to coordinate and run health-promotion activities within their communities from a central location.

Superclinics are part of a new initiative in Australia, providing a raised level of healthcare services within one centre, and often offering longer opening hours and additional healthcare providers, and services such as onsite pharmacies, pathology labs and radiography (Commonwealth Department of Health and Ageing 2000).

REFLECTION 2.1

Australian healthcare system
1 Do you have any experience with the Australian healthcare system, either as a health professional or from the perspective of a patient or client?
2 Do you have any experience of healthcare systems in other countries?
3 What do you think are the major benefits and drawbacks of the Australian system from the perspective of a health professional and a patient or client?

ORIENTATION TO NEW SETTINGS

Entering a new environment is always a time for increased anxiety and uncertainty. The most important point to remember is that you are going on fieldwork placement as a student and you are not expected to know everything in your first week! Your fieldwork placement will give you the time to develop your skills and knowledge in a practical environment, and your fieldwork educator will be there throughout your placement to provide you with support and guidance.

Important points to remember are:

1 **Ask for help**

Ask for help in getting directions, advice or finding out someone's name. Aim to use any resources that you have to hand, for example, a student orientation manual. Ask a fellow student, or if that fails, ask staff members, as they will usually respond positively and can remember what it was like to be unfamiliar with their workplace. Staff may be less inclined to help in situations where the same questions are asked repeatedly, when questions are posed at inappropriate times or where the answer is easily available.

2 **Observe, observe, observe!**

While on fieldwork placement, take time to observe and remember names, faces and positions, as well as department names, services and the roles held within them. This can help orientate you to your new setting and the people you will be working with.

3 **Record**

Keep a diary or notebook with you. It can be used to write down any learning issues you encounter, jot down any questions you have for your supervisor or keep lists of important information within reach. Write your daily to-do list, or simply use it as a reflective tool to help process your experiences on placement.

4 Read

Most orientation processes involve a fair amount of reading, as you will need to become familiar with the placement site procedures and policies. Although this can be overwhelming and boring to do, it will pay dividends when you actually start interacting with patients or clients and the interdisciplinary team, and as you gain more confidence about how the placement site works and care is administered. Each placement site operates differently, including such aspects as medical record-keeping and storage, admission and discharge procedures and mealtime and workplace norms, such as start and finish times, meal break allocation and reporting illness procedures.

5 Communicate

A key to a successful placement is maintaining open communication channels. Both you and your supervisors need to be aware of your learning goals and how you are progressing with them. Supervisors are not mind readers! You will need to express your fears, concerns or needs as 'I' statements, then express preferences as possibilities, not as if they are the only option. Negotiate together the possible options to arrive at the best possible outcome, and act in a responsible manner while working through them, rather than blaming others for any issues that arise. Regular meetings and clear learning goals are core aspects to a successful placement and open communication (Cleak & Wilson 2007: 26–7).

6 First impressions

As you enter a workplace, remember that first impressions do last. Your appearance will reflect on your profession, even though you are still a student. Most fieldwork placement sites will have a dress code that will include either a uniform or required standard of appearance in conjunction with appropriate identification of who you are. *Smart casual* is the term commonly used: don't wear jeans or revealing clothing. Look at how your supervisor and peers dress for guidance. Is the way you are dressed a good reflection on how you would like to see a health professional dress if you were a patient or client? Comfortable, enclosed shoes and clean, ironed clothes, in conjunction with a neat appearance (tidy hair, makeup and jewellery) can help make your first impression with patients and co-workers a positive one.

7 Confidentiality

While you are on placement you will have access to sensitive, personal and privileged information. It is your obligation as a healthcare professional to respect that the information was provided in confidence, and should not be shared unless consent is given by the patient or client. Patient information or experiences should not be used as conversation pieces, and any notes taken for learning purposes should not contain identifying information. They should be kept for your use alone, and disposed of correctly.

THINK AND LINK 2.1

Confidentiality

Confidentiality is an important concept to understand throughout your fieldwork experiences and in professional practice. Chapter 22 places confidentiality into a legal context and emphasises the importance of not using patient information as conversation pieces. Consider Samuel's actions on his first day of placement: see Case Study 2.1.

Case Study 2.1	Samuel the dietitian's first day on placement

Samuel is a student dietitian on his first placement in a large teaching hospital. He has arrived on his first day a bit late and tired from working the previous evening in his part-time job. His fieldwork educator is in charge of a busy gastrointestinal ward, and has already left for the early morning ward round. She has given a list of possible procedures for a colleague to hand to Samuel. He should observe these procedures either that morning or afternoon. He also needs to read a folder on the policies and procedures of the dietetic department. Samuel is keen to experience what the workplace has to offer. Later that morning he volunteers to observe a nasogastric feeding tube being placed. Reading the policies and procedures are the task he has elected to do that afternoon, provided he has time.

The placement of the tube was a success and the patient was able to start feeding. Samuel found that the whole experience helped him see the relationship between the process of placing a tube and the dietitian's role of providing adequate nutrition to the patient. He is keen to share this experience with his peers. When he meets one of them in the elevator, he describes the event in detail, including the ward and patient's name.

Questions

1　What are the areas of concern about Samuel's first day?
2　What could Samuel have done differently to improve it?
3　What could his supervisor have done differently to improve it?

INTERDISCIPLINARY TEAM

In Australian healthcare settings, the interdisciplinary team is seen as the key unit within a 'person-centred' care environment. *Person-centred care* involves recognising the person's freedom to make his or her own decisions; it is a holistic view, with the patient or client at the centre of all care decisions. The interdisciplinary team approach acknowledges the diverse skill base and understandings that each profession offers when caring for patients or clients. It seeks to use these in the most effective manner possible to achieve the best possible health outcomes for the patient or client. A variety of members may make up a team. Table 2.1 outlines some of the team members you may encounter on placement, as well as their levels and roles.

Table 2.1: Interdisciplinary team members

Title	Levels	Role
Nursing staff	• Student • Enrolled nurse • Registered nurse (RN) • Midwife • Nurse practitioner • Nurse manager	Primary care delivery to patients or clients. Students and enrolled nurses are not registered to practise independently. Midwives are trained in the care of pregnancy and birth. Nurse practitioners have advanced training in specialised areas. Nurse managers are generally responsible for the running of a ward or unit and the nursing staff within it
Medical staff[1]	• Intern or student • Resident • Registrar • Senior registrar • Consultant	Responsible for primary care of patients or clients. Interns or students are not registered to practise independently, and are supervised. Residents are registered to practise independently. Registrars are registered medical staff training in a specialty area. Consultants are fully registered specialists with the ultimate responsibility for primary care of patients or clients within their specialty area, and manage the medical staff under them
Care Assistant		Supporting the care of patients or clients in roles possibly delegated by nursing staff or other healthcare professions, for example, attending personal needs of patients, moving patients or equipment, or collection and distribution of food orders
Technician		Involved in the provision and running of specialist equipment or services, for example, sterile supply, anaesthetic assistance, cardiac monitoring

Healthcare worker		May function independently or as part of interdisciplinary team. Various roles can be undertaken; for example, that of an Aboriginal healthcare worker
Social worker[2]		Responsible for linking of patients or clients with social supports available such as housing or Centrelink (government support services)
Dietitian[2]		Responsible for the provision of adequate nutrition and nutrition education to patients or clients
Physiotherapist[2]		Responsible for patient or client care and education in the areas of mobility, rehabilitation and ventilation
Occupational therapist[2]		Responsible for therapy involved in recuperation from injury or disease and performance of activities of daily living such as washing, dressing, eating and hobbies
Podiatrist[2]		Responsible for assessment and treatment of feet and associated conditions
Speech pathologist or therapist[2]		Responsible for study and treatment of speech, communication, language and swallowing problems
Psychologist[2]		Responsible for assessment and treatment of mind and behaviour problems
Counsellor		Responsible for supporting patients or clients in dealing with personal and non-psychological problems

Source: O'Reilly 2009, content adapted from Levett-Jones & Bourgeois 2007: 36–8

1 *The level of medical staff present in different healthcare settings will vary. For example, some private settings will only employ consultants and senior registrars, whereas other settings can be training hospitals, which will have interns through to consultants.*
2 *Students require supervision and are not qualified to practise independently.*

REFLECTION 2.2

Working in teams
When learning about interdisciplinary teams, some activities that will help facilitate your learning are:
- attending team meetings where possible, as they give you real insight into how the team works
- becoming familiar with how different staff roles interact within different teams
- developing an understanding of how the team communicates and works together to provide patient-centred care.

DIVERSITY AND CULTURAL COMPETENCE

Australia is a diverse country, especially in terms of culture. This presents its own challenges to the student. Culture is a loose term for the patterns of human behaviour exhibited by social or ethnic groups, allowing them to identify as a unique group. The iceberg concept of culture is shown in Figure 2.2. It illustrates that the visible portion of a person's culture is only a small part of what is actually below that surface.

Cultural competence is defined as 'the demonstration of knowledge, attitudes and behaviours based on diverse, relevant, cultural experiences' (Schim et al. 2005: 355). To work in a culturally competent manner, it is important that you become culturally aware. The first step in this process is to look at your own cultural background, so that you can have insight into how this affects your view of the world around you. Then look at your peers, notice how diverse their cultural backgrounds are, and learn from them about their cultures (Baird 2008, 105–8).

Figure 2.2: The iceberg concept of culture

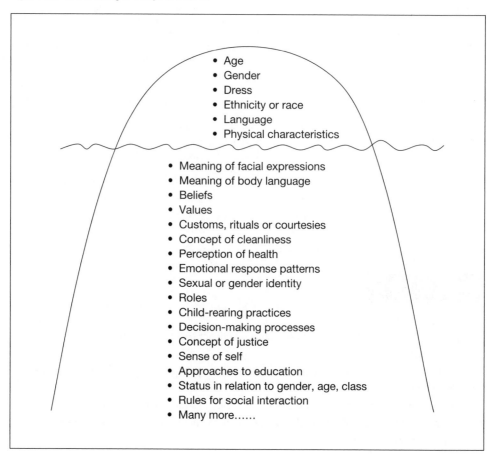

Source: Adapted from the National Center for Cultural Competence 2005

REFLECTION 2.3

Cultural competence

In order to achieve cultural competence it is important to consider:

- taking a firm grasp of what culture is and what it is not
- gaining insight into intracultural variation; do not assume each person from a certain culture will identify with what you understand that culture to be
- understanding how people acquire their culture, and culture's important role in personal identities, ways of life and mental and physical health of individuals and their communities
- being conscious of your own culturally shaped values, beliefs, perceptions and biases
- observing your reactions to people whose cultures differ from your own, and reflecting upon these responses
- seeking and participating in meaningful interactions with people of a variety of cultural backgrounds
- becoming aware of the cultural implications of personal space, body language, silence, eye contact and touch in your interactions with patients or clients
- examining policies and implementing practices in your care to tailor your interactions to meet patients' social, cultural, religious and linguistic needs.

WORKING WITH INTERPRETERS

Most students will require the services of an interpreter over the course of their placement or professional career. Interpreters are a service that is provided free of charge by healthcare institutions, and all interpreters will be fully qualified to work in the languages or dialects they specialise in. It is preferable to use the services of an interpreter rather than family members, as the information being translated may be subject to censoring or inaccurate translation when not undertaken by a trained translator. It is also important to consider the setting where the translation is occurring especially if sensitive information will be discussed.

Points to remember when working with an interpreter:

- Working with an interpreter requires planning, as he or she needs to be booked in advance
- Think about where you are going to hold the session, and any other events that may affect the session, for example, other tests or appointments
- A session with an interpreter takes double the length of time compared to normal session time, and is tiring for all involved. You will normally only cover half the aimed for content
- There is no need to shout or use 'pidgin' (oversimplified) English
- Talk to the patient or client, not the translator

- Maintain eye contact and positive body language with the patient or client, who is the person you are working with. The interpreter is simply there to help your communication
- Use short sentences and questions
- There is no need to speak English with an accent. It will not help the person to understand you better.

SUMMARY

All new environments require personal adjustment, especially the Australian healthcare system. Allow adequate time and space to orientate yourself to the workplace where you are going to be undertaking your fieldwork placement. Key points for consideration are: learn how the workplace interacts with clients, how the workplace links with other services or healthcare settings, what makes members of the interdisciplinary team work together in that workplace, and what is expected of the student within that interdisciplinary team and the placement. Australia, along with many other countries, has a culturally diverse population. This means that you need to become culturally aware and competent in working with people from diverse backgrounds. This involves examining your own cultural background, opening yourself to the influence that culture has on a person's environment, and using this knowledge to improve the level of communication between clients, you and healthcare professionals. Develop the skill of using an interpreter.

DISCUSSION QUESTIONS

1   Think about the fieldwork placement you will be entering. How does it fit into the larger picture of the Australian healthcare sector? What services and healthcare professionals are linked to your placement setting? How do patients or clients access your placement setting? Is it a private or public service?

2   With the help of one of your peers, chat about their feelings about going on placement and what they have done to prepare themselves for this new experience. Was their preparation similar to yours? What was different, and how do you think their experiences could help you?

3   Identify five characteristics that are visible aspects of your cultural identity. Do these aspects accurately define what you would classify as who you are and where you come from? Which aspects are not easily apparent, and are these important to you? Ask your peer the same questions, and examine the cultural differences that may exist. If so, how could you best work with them in a healthcare setting, with one of you as a health professional and the other as a client or patient?

References

Baird, B. N. (2008). *The Internship, Practicum and Field Placement Handbook: A Guide for The Helping Professions* (5th edn). Pearson Prentice Hall, NJ.

Cleak, H. & Wilson, J. (2007). *Making the Most of Field Placement* (2nd edn). Thomson, Melbourne.

Commonwealth Department of Health and Ageing (2000). *The Australian Healthcare System: An outline.* <http://www.health.gov.au/internet/main/publishing.nsf/Content/EBA6536E92A7D2D2CA256F9D007D8066/$File/ozhealth.pdf>. Accessed 12 January 2009.

Levett-Jones, T. & Bourgeois, S. (2007). *The Clinical Placement: An Essential Guide for Nursing Students.* Churchill Livingstone, Sydney.

National Centre for Cultural Competence (2005). *Cultural Awareness: Teaching Tools, Strategies and Resources* <http://www.nccccurricula.info/awareness/D16.html>. Accessed 12 January 2009.

Schim, S., Doorenbos, A. & Borse, N. (2005). 'Cultural Competence among Ontario and Michigan Healthcare Providers'. *Journal of Nursing Scholarship.* 37(4), 354–60.

Useful Websites

Self directed learning modules on cultural awareness and cultural competency for health professionals <www.nccccurricula.info/modules.html>.

Australian Department of Health and Ageing <www.health.gov.au>

CHAPTER 3
WORKING WITH MOTHERS AND BABIES

Joanne Gray

LEARNING OUTCOMES

After reading this chapter, you should be able to:
- describe the key constructs of working with mothers and babies
- reflect on the nature of woman-centred care
- appreciate the importance of continuity of care for women
- commence your fieldwork placement with an understanding of the primacy of the woman and the family unit in working with mothers and babies
- identify the importance of the family unit as the foundation of support for mothers and babies
- recognise that pregnancy and childbirth are normal physiological processes
- understand the structures of a maternity unit

KEY TERMS

Child and family health
Child and family nurse
Confidentiality
Continuity of care
Family-centred practice
Midwifery
Neonatal intensive care unit (NICU)
Woman-centred care

INTRODUCTION

On hearing that you will be working in a fieldwork placement with mothers and babies, many will tell you how wonderful this experience will be and how much you will enjoy it. This is very true, and being prepared for this placement by understanding the philosophy that guides the practice in these areas will ensure that you do indeed enjoy your experience.

This chapter will introduce key philosophical underpinnings in these areas of health practice. You will find that these differ from other areas you may work in. Working with mothers and babies requires a set of skills that are different from working with other client groups.

This chapter is divided into the different areas of practice that you may encounter when working with mothers and babies. Care of pregnant women can take place in a range of settings. Your placement will, most probably, be with pregnant women in the hospital or community setting. Following the birth of the baby, you may be required to work with mothers during this early postnatal period. Again this may occur in the hospital or community setting, or perhaps in the woman's home. If you are working with babies who are unwell, your placement will occur in the special care baby unit, or neonatal intensive care unit in a hospital. Once mothers and babies are at home together, your placement is likely to be in a community setting.

There is something quite special about being given the opportunity to work with mothers and babies in your fieldwork placement. These experiences will enable you to put the theory that you have learnt into practice and to understand the realities of the profession you have chosen. Your fieldwork placement is a unique opportunity to communicate with women, learn about their experiences as a mother and gain an insight into parenting.

Good communication is a key skill in this placement. You will also discover what it is that you do not know, or are not sure about during this placement. Pursue this knowledge, then take this new understanding with you to your next placement, ensuring that your practice is informed by theory, and that theory informs your practice.

REFLECTION 3.1

Reflect on the following, then identify:
- What are the main considerations when you are working with mothers and babies?
- What do you think the role of the mother involves? List some key activities that you believe are part of the mothering role.
- Think about what a family means to you. Families come in a variety of forms, so it is interesting to reflect on what you believe a family to be. Jot down the different family structures that you know of.

AUSTRALIA'S MOTHERS AND BABIES

The National Perinatal Statistics Unit of the Australian Institute of Health and Welfare publishes data related to mothers and babies. Its most recent report (Laws et al. 2007) indicates that in 2005, 267,793 women gave birth in Australia to 272,419 babies. This was an increase of 5.9 per cent from the previous year. The mean age of these women was 29.8 years, with Aboriginal or Torres Strait Islander women accounting for 3.7 per cent of all mothers. Spontaneous vaginal birth occurred in 58.5 per cent of births, with 30.3 per cent of women having a caesarean section. The caesarean section rate is compared to that of 1996, when it was 19.5 per cent.

These statistics on women and babies tell us quite a lot about the maternity health setting. You will be working with young, well women, who mostly experience a normal life event of giving birth. You will also find that there is an increasing incidence of caesarean birth, which has an impact on the care required for women and babies. If you work with Aboriginal and Torres Strait Islander women, you will find that the maternal and infant mortality rate is much higher than that for non-Indigenous Australian women, and these women will often have other health problems that lead to complications in pregnancy.

Australia has a strong reputation for providing safe care to mothers and babies. Australian women experience low mortality and morbidity for maternity care, though this is not shared by women in rural communities, or by Indigenous women. It would be valuable to obtain a copy of the review of maternity services in Australia discussion paper (Department of Health and Ageing 2009), as this provides a comprehensive overview of the Australian maternity system and its current challenges.

Key skills of the health professional working with mothers and babies

The following diagram depicts key skills that are essential when working with mothers and babies.

Figure 3.1: Main functions of a health professional working with mothers and babies

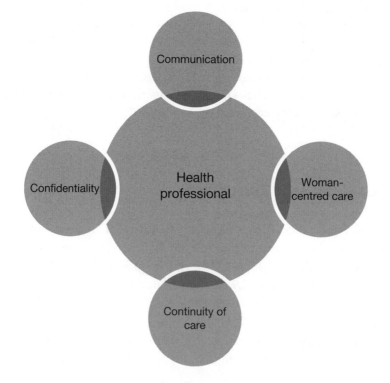

WOMAN-CENTRED CARE

Woman-centred care is a key philosophical approach underpinning working with mothers and babies. This approach recognises the primacy of the woman and the woman as the centre of care provision. It has been defined as follows:

Woman-centred care is a concept. It implies that midwifery:
- Focuses on the woman's individual needs, aspirations and expectations, rather than the needs of the institution or professionals;
- Recognises the need for women to have choice, control and continuity from a known caregiver or caregivers;
- Encompasses the needs of the baby, the woman's family and other people important to the woman, as defined and negotiated by the woman herself;
- Follows the woman across the interface of community and acute settings;
- Addresses social, emotional, physical, psychological, spiritual and cultural needs and expectations;
- Recognizes the woman's expertise in decision making

(Leap 2009: 12)

Recognising woman-centred care as a key construct in working with mothers and babies will enable you to understand the differences inherent in this fieldwork placement. The identification of the woman, and those who are important to her as her family unit, is fundamental to providing care. Women are mostly self-determining in the care of themselves and their baby, and their choices should be respected.

CONTINUITY OF CARE

Case Study 3.1 | **Fragmented care**

Donna is a 36-year-old woman and she is expecting her first child. Donna visits her local GP (1) to have her pregnancy diagnosed. Donna is then sent to the local pathology service (2) for her routine pregnancy blood tests. Donna, accompanied by her partner Michael, also has an ultrasound scan (3) to determine her estimated date of birth. Donna and Michael have decided to access the local maternity unit in a public hospital. Donna organises an appointment for the booking-in visit (4). At this visit, Donna provides a comprehensive personal history, and she is given a number of resources for reading during her pregnancy. Donna makes her first appointment at the antenatal clinic, and she is seen by a midwife (5). As Donna has some concerns about her age and the possible effects on her baby, she is seen by the obstetric registrar (6). Donna decides to have further antenatal screening (7). Donna and Michael are relieved to learn that the screening test indicates that all is well and Donna's pregnancy continues without complication. She has a further eight visits at the antenatal clinic, and sees a different midwife every time (15). Donna commences labour at home just after her due date and presents to the birthing unit (16) to find she is established in labour. She labours well, and her period of time in the birthing unit goes over a change of shift so she is cared for by another two midwives (18). After birth Donna requires some intravenous fluids and the cannula for venous access is inserted by the resident (19). Donna is reviewed by the obstetric registrar (20), and she is then transferred to the postnatal unit.

As you can see from this case study, Donna, who is a well woman, experiencing a healthy, uncomplicated pregnancy, was seen by at least 20 health professionals. This case study did not calculate the students she is likely to have met, or the care that she received in the postnatal unit.

Questions
1   What do you see as the concerns related to this fragmentation of care?
2   Reflect on how Donna may feel about having to share her story, and the personal journey of her pregnancy, with so many different health professionals.

As the case study above has shown, women may experience a very fragmented approach to their care during pregnancy and birth. *Continuity of care*, which is known to confer benefits when working with mothers and babies, is broadly defined as: 'For continuity to exist, care must be experienced as connected and coherent. For patients and their families, the experience of continuity is the perception that providers know what has happened before, that different providers agree on a management plan, and that a provider who knows them will care for them in the future' (Haggerty et al. 2003: 1221). In maternity care, evidence tells us that women have better outcomes when they experience continuity of care with a midwife (Hatem et al. 2008).

What does this mean for you working with mothers and babies? Having an appreciation of the value of continuity of care will assist you when you establish a relationship with women. Simply by acknowledging to the woman that 'you have probably already told someone your history before' indicates to the woman that you are aware of what she may have experienced. You can also try to have continuity for yourself by, wherever possible, trying to provide care to the same women and babies you have previously met.

REFLECTION 3.2

Communication: the language of maternity care
The words we use when communicating with women are important. For example, what message do you think the following words and phrases send to women?
- failure to progress
- incompetent cervix
- delivery (as opposed to birth).

It is important to be careful with our language when communicating with women. Convey positive messages to show that we are not condescending or dismissive. Calling every woman 'dear' or referring to them as 'ladies' can sound condescending and inappropriate, and not woman-centred.

When you enter your fieldwork placement, think about the language that you use, and the language you hear around you.

1   What messages are conveyed about women in the handover reports?

2   Do health professionals make judgments about women simply by the language they use?

CONFIDENTIALITY

The concept of *confidentiality*, which includes elements of privacy, is an ethical responsibility for health professionals. Patients will often share very personal details with their health care professional, so it is essential that we respect their right to confidentiality.

Having a baby is a very exciting, but also a very private time in a woman's life. The family often wish to be the ones who share the news of the arrival of a new baby. As health professionals, we need to respect this, and ensure we do not accidentally inform family members or friends. Family dynamics can be complex: the choices that women make around who is told about the birth of their baby, and when, can be difficult decisions.

When you work in smaller communities, for example in a rural area, members of the community are often well known to each other. Therefore it is important that you are very careful about the information you share with others and what you discuss in public areas. It might be that, when you are sharing a story from your workday with a colleague, you mention that you were working with a woman who had twins that day. Although you have not mentioned the woman, or the hospital, or anyone by name, it is likely that only one woman in that community had twins that day, so that woman and her family are automatically identified.

Women also share very confidential information with their midwife or obstetrician, and this may be recorded on her health record. A woman, for example, may identify her previous pregnancy history, including any terminations of pregnancy. Some women choose not to share this information with their partner. It is important, therefore, that you respect the woman's wishes to keep this information confidential. In other circumstances pregnancy screening may have identified the gender of the baby. Some parents choose not to be told this. Again, it is essential that you respect this and do not accidentally disclose confidential information.

THINK AND LINK 3.1

Chapter 20 discusses ethical issues in more depth and Chapter 22 discusses confidentiality within a legal framework. These chapters link to the concept of confidentiality, including privacy and ethical responsibility when working with mothers and babies.

WHO'S WHO: THE MATERNITY CARE WORKFORCE

Every fieldwork placement that you attend will have different staff. It is helpful for you to understand who they are and what they are responsible for. Within a hospital maternity unit there will be unit managers (titled either midwife or, sometimes, nurse). The managers of each unit, or area, hold the overall responsibility for the day-to-day operation of the unit. Midwives are the most prevalent health workers in maternity services.

In Australia it was traditional that midwives were prepared for practice after first gaining a nursing qualification. However, in 2002 South Australia and Victoria commenced Bachelor of Midwifery programs, and most other states and territories have now followed. These programs (sometimes referred to as *direct-entry*) are becoming the preferred route to midwifery registration in Australia. You will be working alongside midwives then, who are not nurses. Midwives have a defined scope of practice, and are registered on a separate register to nurses. As a distinct discipline, they are able to provide care, independently, to women during their pregnancy, labour and birth, and into the early parenting period. While working in a maternity unit you will also work alongside other students, such as midwives, doctors and nurses. Occasionally registered nurses also work in the maternity setting, but their practice is restricted to the antenatal and postnatal periods.

You will also work with medical residents, registrars who are in obstetrics training programs, and obstetricians. The maternity setting is multidisciplinary, depending on the needs of each woman, so you will also encounter anaesthetists, members of the endocrinology team or other medical specialists.

REFLECTION 3.3

Learning another language

You may not be familiar with many words that are associated with maternity care. It would be helpful to find the meaning of some of the common words or phrases that you will find used every day in relation to mothers and babies.

Table 3.1: Learning another language

Word	Definition
Antenatal period	
Postnatal period	
Parity	
Gravid	
Primipara	
Multipara	
First stage of labour	
Second stage of labour	
Third stage of labour	
Postpartum haemorrhage	
Forceps birth	
Vacuum birth	
Caesarean section	
Gestation	
Term	
Postdates	
Preterm	
Fundus	
Involution	
Puerperium	

Source: Gray et al. 2009

The maternity unit

Most of the work that you do with women and babies will occur in the hospital maternity unit. These units differ from the typical hospital ward unit. Most women are well and are able to move freely around the unit without the need of assistance. Indeed, the maternity unit should be designed to enable women to provide their own care and also to provide care to their babies.

The maternity unit is a busy place. Over recent years, with the increasing rate of caesarean sections in Australia, the care required by women in the immediate postnatal period has changed. Women who are well following birth can often be cared for at home with the support of a community midwife and their family. These women may be discharged from hospital care within 48 hours following birth. Women who have had a caesarean section usually remain in hospital for a period of three to four days. This short length of stay in hospital means that mothers are often overwhelmed with the information that they are given in relation to their new role as mothers. This information can often be confusing, and sometimes even conflicting. A considered approach to the care of women at this time is vital so that women gain the skills and confidence required to adjust to their role as a parent.

The unwell baby

Sick babies are cared for in the hospital in the *neonatal intensive care unit (NICU)*. The type of care provided to the unwell baby depends on the specifications of the NICU, with specialised units being able to care for extremely premature babies, and babies who require surgical intervention. All maternity units are able to provide care for well babies, and some can also then care for babies once they no longer require the specialised skills of a NICU.

Having a baby in the neonatal intensive care unit is a most distressing time for new parents. Some parents may have had some forewarning of the need for their baby to be admitted to a NICU. For other parents, the birth of an unwell baby is completely unanticipated. If women are aware that they will give birth to a baby who requires admission to a NICU, they will have probably been given a tour of the unit and have met the staff who work there. Staff in the NICU are very aware of the need to keep the family unit together during this difficult period. Cooper and colleagues (2007) suggest that family-centred care is about 'viewing the family as the child's primary source of strength and support'. They further suggest that 'this philosophy incorporates respect, information, choice, flexibility, empowerment, collaboration and support into all levels of service delivery' (Cooper et al. 2007: S32).

CHALLENGES WHEN WORKING WITH MOTHERS AND BABIES

Outcomes for mothers are not always positive. During your fieldwork placement you may work with women who experience the death of their baby through stillbirth or neonatal death. This is a devastating experience for the woman and her family. It is important that the woman is given access to support and perhaps counselling and you should also seek support to assist you through this difficult experience. You may find it helpful to read the articles in an issue of *Birth Matters* (Autumn 2009), which was devoted to perinatal loss.

MOTHERS AND BABIES IN THE COMMUNITY

The care of women and babies is passed from their midwives, to the child and family health nurse. The timing of this transfer varies according to the care the woman has received, and where she has spent her postnatal period. The *child and family health nurse*, who works in the community, will often also conduct home visits. The role of this health professional extends from the antenatal period, when the nurse often meets the woman and her family in their home, until the child is aged five years. This scope of practice enables the nurse to establish a relationship with the family so that care can be built on the family's strengths. It is recognised that developing a strong partnership provides the best means of supporting families.

THINK AND LINK 3.2

Chapter 4 discusses working with families and children. This chapter links with this chapter as Chapter 4 discusses the various issues that arise when children have developmental needs and they and their families need support within the community from a variety of health professionals.

SUMMARY

This chapter has provided you with some insights about this specialised area of practice to prepare you for your fieldwork placement working with mothers and babies. Remember to listen when you are on placement and reflect on all that you hear, see and experience about mothers and babies.

This chapter had identified the key aspects of working with mothers and babies as woman-centred care, continuity of care, confidentiality and communication.

A snapshot of Australian mothers and babies has been provided to give you the broader context for your placement. The fieldwork placement areas, such as the maternity unit and the community, have been described, allowing you to gain a better understanding of who you will be working alongside.

References

Cooper, L., Gooding, J., Gallagher, J., Sternesky, L., Ledsky, R. & Berns, S. (2007). 'Impact of a Family-centered Care Initiative on NICU Care, Staff and Families'. *Journal of Perinatology*, 27: S32–S37.

Department of Health and Ageing. (2009). *Improving Maternity Services in Australia: The Report of the Maternity Services Review*. Commonwealth of Australia, Canberra.

Gray, J., Smith, R. & Homer, C. (2009). *Illustrated Dictionary of Midwifery*. Butterworth Heinemann Elsevier, Sydney.

Haggerty, J., Reid, R., Freeman, G., Starfield, B., Adair, C. & McKendry, R. (2003). 'Continuity of Care: A Multidisciplinary Review'. *British Medical Journal*, 327: 1219–21.

Hatem, M., Sandall, J., Devane, D., Soltani, H. & Gates, S. (2008). *Midwife-led Versus Other Models of Care for Childbearing Women*: Cochrane Database of Systematic Reviews, 4.

Laws, P., Abeywardan, S., Walker, J. & Sullivan, E. A. (2007). *Australia's Mothers and Babies 2005*, Australian Institute of Health and Welfare National Perinatal Statistics Unit, Sydney.

Leap, N. (2009). 'Woman-centred or Women-centred Care: Does It Matter?' *British Journal of Midwifery*, 17(1): 12–16.

Further Reading
Birth Matters, Autumn 2009.

CHAPTER 4
WORKING WITH CHILDREN AND FAMILIES

Kelly Powell

LEARNING OUTCOMES

After reading this chapter, you should be able to:
- reflect on several types of paediatric settings
- articulate what makes an effective paediatric clinician
- know what to prepare for when working with children and families
- understand the role of the allied health student in paediatric fieldwork
- articulate how working with children and their families differs from working with an adult
- reflect on the clinical reasoning process.

KEY TERMS

Acute setting
Autism spectrum disorder (ASD)
Clinical reasoning
Consulting therapist
Discipline-specific skills
Family-centred practice
Generic services
Inpatient
Outpatient
Paediatrics
Transdisciplinary team

INTRODUCTION

Health professionals who work in *paediatrics* consider the assessment and treatment of children who have a range of neurological, developmental, genetic and medical conditions that have an impact on their ability to participate in everyday situations. Paediatric settings present you, as a health professional student, with many challenges because the settings are varied—from an acute hospital setting, a community-based early intervention team, or school-based settings, to working in a private practice. The clients and the role of the health professional also vary greatly. This chapter outlines the main issues that you must consider when working with children and families. Your role will vary depending on your year level at university and the setting in which the fieldwork placement is taking place. When working with children and their families, it is important for you to have an understanding in three main areas: family-centred practice (as this model is used in many settings); typical development; and models and frames of reference used to guide intervention. Case Study 4.1 raises important issues that are addressed throughout this chapter.

Case Study 4.1	Sarah

Sarah was a child aged 4 years 6 months who had been given a diagnosis of *autism spectrum disorder (ASD)*. Her parents were extremely distressed about this diagnosis but were keen to assist their daughter to achieve her full potential. Sarah was seen by a multidisciplinary team at a local early intervention agency.

The team assessed Sarah at the clinic as well as attending a session at her local kindergarten. Sarah was found to be nonverbal, constantly mouthing objects, flapping her hands, walking with a wide-based gait and constantly falling over. She required assistance with all self-care activities and was a fussy eater.

Following assessment and several intervention sessions, the team was very concerned that Sarah's mother was not following through on the recommended intervention strategies. Sarah's mother had spoken to her family service coordinator (the early intervention team leader) and expressed concerns that the team's recommendations were 'babyish and pitched at too low a level for Sarah'. The family then withdrew from the early intervention agency and sought services elsewhere. Twelve months later, the family returned to the early intervention agencies requesting ongoing services because of a lack of suitable services in the area. The parents were open to discussion with the staff about the needs of their daughter.

What do you think is happening here? Why did the family withdraw? Could the team have done anything differently to engage with this family? The above case study raises a range of important issues that you may encounter when you undertake a fieldwork placement working with children and their families. These will be discussed throughout this chapter.

TYPES OF FIELDWORK SETTINGS

The type of setting and the clinician's role within each setting will vary. As a result, your role as a student will also vary. The most common types of settings in which you may be required to undertake fieldwork include:

An acute setting

Children can be seen within an *acute hospital setting*, either as an inpatient or on an outpatient basis. An *inpatient* is a child who is staying in hospital and an *outpatient* is a child who lives at home but comes into the hospital for an assessment and/or treatment. Sessions can take place both on the ward and in the hospital departments. Parents may or may not be present during the individual sessions. This is an important issue that needs to be discussed with families prior to the individual sessions. Because assessment, intervention strategies and report-writing guidelines vary from setting to setting, it is important to talk to your fieldwork educator in relation to:

* assessment tools commonly used
* types of reporting required (progress notes, discharge summary)
* specific short-term intervention strategies.

Community settings

Paediatric services in community-based settings are often sometimes limited to children aged 0–6 years because of funding arrangements. Waiting lists are often a major concern within these settings. At times, a child may receive a diagnosis, then remain on a waiting list for a long period. It is important to consider the implications for the child and the family in this situation. Knowledge of the length of waiting times is an important fact that you need to know before seeing the family.

Many community-based settings require health professionals to take on a generic role. A *generic role* often means that a health professional may have to take on the role of *family services coordinator*, the primary person responsible for the organisation of additional services such as seeking funding and organising respite and family meetings. Discipline-specific intervention—assessing and treating in the profession you were trained in—may also occur in multidisciplinary teams, or you may find yourself working in a *transdisciplinary team*, where you carry out treatment suggested by another health professional as well as your fieldwork educator. Many paediatric settings have a number of disciplines working together with the family and child on multidisciplinary teams. In these teams roles can be clearly defined (for example, at some community-based services, physiotherapists do wheelchair prescriptions whereas occupational therapists do this in hospital settings), or generic, such that an early intervention worker is allocated to provide the service to the child and family. It is important to be aware of the role of other team members, so that you know who to refer to in relation to specific issues that may arise. Consult your fieldwork educator if you are unsure about the boundaries of your role or how your role fits into the rest of the team.

Consideration must be given to the environment in which you will be seeing the child: is it in the clinic, the home, daycare or kindergarten? Be mindful that the behaviour you see in one setting may be completely different to another. For example, a young child in a childcare setting may present with increased levels of activity, inattention and distractibility type behaviours because of the amount of noise and stimulation in this setting, but may present as placid in the home environment.

School-based settings

A variety of school settings either employ health professionals directly or contract services for consulting health professionals. For example, allied health professionals are often employed in a special school setting, while nurses can be employed by the government and work in a school district.

Consulting health professionals are very often therapists. The *consulting therapist* is given very limited time to assess and establish recommendations for the child in school settings (often therapists will see children once a month or even once a term). The amount of intervention usually depends on the funding provided for the health service. It is extremely important in these settings to talk with the main caregivers (especially the teacher, integration aide or parent) about their concerns about the needs of the child. A consulting therapist is not necessarily the 'expert' but needs to see him- or herself as part of the school team where common goals can be met. These goals are often outlined in *parent support group (PSG)* meetings, and if the health professional cannot attend (which is often the case because of funding constraints), it is important that he or she gains access to these goals (and where possible contributes to goal-setting before the meeting).

PRIVATE PRACTICE

There are a variety of reasons why a family might seek private services. Often waiting lists for public services are too long, and some parents choose to find a clinician who specialises in a specific field. A student's role within the private practice setting is often limited to observation or conducting assessments under close supervision from the clinician. It is important to be aware that, because of the fee-for-service consideration, many parents prefer the qualified clinician to conduct the sessions but are happy for the student to observe. This opportunity to observe the clinician working directly with the child is an extremely valuable one that may not be always available to you when you graduate. Make sure you take notes about activity ideas and strategies used throughout the session, but remember to maintain confidentiality.

THINK AND LINK 4.1

Private practice

If you find yourself undertaking a placement in a private practice, you may find that you are observing your fieldwork educator interacting with clients more than in other settings. Chapter 9 provides information about working in private practice in more detail, and discusses issues that you need to be aware of if undertaking a fieldwork placement with a private practitioner.

WORKING EFFECTIVELY WITH CHILDREN AND FAMILIES

In order to have a successful fieldwork experience, it is necessary to understand what makes an effective paediatric practitioner. Dunst and Trivette (1996) discussed the elements of effective intervention as:

- technical knowledge and skills
- help-giver behaviours and attributions
- participatory involvement.

Figure 4.1 incorporates these aspects, clearly demonstrating what is required in order to become an effective paediatric practitioner.

Often only after years of experience can a clinician become effective in all four areas: generic skills, discipline-specific skills, interpersonal skills and family-centred practice. However, you can begin to develop these skills during fieldwork placement.

PREPARATION FOR WORKING WITH CHILDREN AND FAMILIES IN A FIELDWORK SETTING

Before you begin the fieldwork, or very early in the fieldwork placement, it is important that you review the following:

- knowledge of typical development
- common assessments and screening tools
- underlying models and frames of references
- knowledge of childhood disabilities and conditions
- knowledge of commonly used intervention strategies.

Review of these areas will help you to begin filling the circles of generic and discipline-specific skills (see Figure 4.1).

Figure 4.1: The effective paediatric practitioner

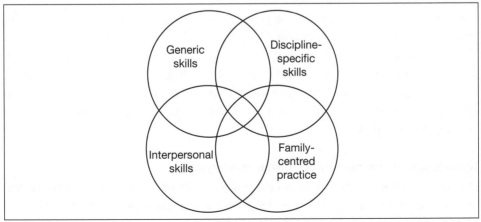

Source: Powell 2009

Knowledge of typical development

It is important to understand at what age typically developing children acquire various skills. Keep in mind that all children vary in their milestones (for example, it is not unusual that a typically developing infant can learn to walk anywhere from 9 months to 18 months of age). You do not necessarily have to memorise all the milestones, as there are many checklists available. Ask your fieldwork educator which are relevant to your profession.

Knowledge of common assessments and screening tools

Assessments and screening tools will vary depending on the facility in which you will be working. If you are required to undertake an assessment with a child, it is a good idea to practise the assessment several times on your partner, parent or another child. If the opportunity presents itself, first observe a qualified professional undertaking the assessment. Where possible (and provided you have parental consent), videotape an assessment session to enable you to review not only the child's skills but also your own. This can be a valuable way to reveal how you interact with the child, the language you use and the structure of the session.

Knowledge of the underlying models and frames of reference

It is important that you understand why you are undertaking a particular task, activity, strategy or technique with a child. Although some models and frames of reference can be applied to all ages, others are specific to working with children. Common ones used by health professionals in paediatrics include developmental, biomechanical, behavioural, psychosocial, neurodevelopment and cognitive frames of reference (Kramer & Hinojosa 1999).

Knowledge of developmental disabilities and childhood illnesses

Before commencing the fieldwork placement (or very early on), it would be useful for you to find out the main diagnoses, disabilities or conditions of children that you may see in the facility you will be going to. For example, some organisations see only children with a specific condition (such as children with physical disabilities). Other organisations see any child who is referred (for example, a community health centre can see children with a wide range of developmental, neurological, genetic and learning difficulties). Before you assess or treat a child, it is helpful to read about the child's condition or diagnosis so that you will have some knowledge before you actually see the child.

Knowledge of common intervention strategies

It is not possible (or practical) here to discuss a range of intervention strategies, as you can only gain such knowledge while on placement. Before going on placement, ask your fieldwork educator what types of intervention strategies are used in the organisation. Prior reading about common strategies related to your profession is recommended.

YOUR ROLE IN A FIELDWORK SETTING WORKING WITH CHILDREN AND FAMILIES

The role of the clinician, and hence the role of the health student, will vary from setting to setting. At times the health professional's role changes, depending on client needs. For example, a physiotherapist may be supporting a child who has cerebral palsy at school on a monthly basis through consultation with the teacher and integration aide, but after that child has tendon release surgery, the physiotherapist may see him weekly for a period of time.

At times, a child may be referred for assessment only. Formal and standardised assessments are often used in these situations. At other times, a health professional may need to see a child in his or her natural environment and undertake an assessment of skills through observation of specific tasks. It is important never to undervalue the observation process as an ongoing assessment. Intervention also varies, and can often be provided through consultation with the caregiver without directly working with the child. For example, it may be important to explain strategies to parents, teachers or integration aides so intervention techniques, such as the Hannen program or sensory processing, can be carried out at home or school by the adult working with the child. Intervention can also take place on a one-on-one basis or within a group setting.

Again, your specific role will depend on the setting and the level of your experience: the year you are in at university and whether you have prior experience in paediatrics. If you are asked to observe the session, use this time to look at a range of important issues. These observations will help you to fill the interpersonal circle outlined in Figure 4.1. Make observations of:

- how the health professional engages with the family or caregiver (through listening, watching and feedback)
- how the health professional engages with the child (language used, behaviour management and physical positioning of the child)
- specific activities and strategies that are used when engaging the child
- what can the child achieve
- the tasks or activities that are difficult for the child.

You may have the opportunity to provide direct assessment or intervention of a child under supervision. It is important not to feel threatened by this experience but to approach it as a valuable learning opportunity. Ask for feedback from your fieldwork educator so that you may know how well you have done or where you can improve. Even experienced health professionals can learn from others!

It is extremely important to consider the environment in which you will be working with the child. This will often be dictated to you by your fieldwork educator, the setting and the time available. Understand that a child can perform differently in different environments. Gathering as much information about the child's performance in each setting is important to your assessment and intervention strategies. For example, if the child is easily distracted in the group setting, but is very placid at home in a quiet setting, you may make recommendations about where he or she could work best on more complex tasks.

HOW IS WORKING WITH CHILDREN AND FAMILIES DIFFERENT FROM WORKING WITH ADULTS?

Case Study 4.1 outlines the importance of understanding the principles of family-centred practice. You may be working with the child, but the family is also your client. Rosenbaum (cited in Rodger & Ziviani 2006) describes three main assumptions of family-centred practice:

1 Parents and family members are the most consistent people in children's lives and the most knowledgeable about their own children
2 Families are different and unique
3 Optimal child functioning occurs within a supportive family and community context

Rodger & Ziviani 2006: 30

The four key interpersonal skills outlined by McBride (1999) are important to develop when working with children and their families regardless of the type of service:
- be positive
- promote family choices and decision-making
- affirm and build on the positive aspects and strengths of the child and family
- honour and respect the diversity and uniqueness of families.

It is important that you ask members of the family about their concerns and the specific areas they would like you to address. All families are different and unique, and therefore their concerns, knowledge and needs will differ. A very experienced health professional said, 'You can only go as fast as the parents allow.' Some families will crave information, knowledge and strategies, and some will only want to hear a small amount of information at a time. How do members of the family like to receive information: through verbal discussion, handouts or books or through practical demonstration? Remember that the Internet has opened up opportunities for families to speak to other families all around the world

(Stagnitti 2005). Many families come to sessions extremely knowledgeable about their child's condition and possible intervention techniques. However, information found on the Internet is often not screened and could be incorrect or not relevant to their child.

In all settings, it is important to realise that members of the family (in particular the parents) are the experts when it comes to their own child. (If there is a child protection issue, you need to discuss this with your fieldwork educator immediately.) In Case Study 4.1, the health professional's opinion about Sarah's skills was very different from that of the family. The health professional needed to discuss her findings with the members of the family and listen to their concerns and needs, finding out where they were in relation to their understanding of Sarah's skills. In Case Study 4.1, intervention strategies recommended by the health professional were not implemented by members of the family, who stopped coming for treatment. Twelve months later, the family requested a program that worked on skills at a much lower level than initially requested.

REFLECTION 4.1

Have you ever been in a situation (either professionally or personally) where someone (who sought your advice initially) has strongly disagreed with your opinion? How did you deal with the situation? How did it make you feel? What were the outcomes?

Consider the family as a whole unit when requesting that strategies be followed up at home. For example, a mother with four young children may not be able to wait for her child who has motor difficulties to dress himself independently in the morning before school. Practice in independent dressing at home in the morning would not be suitable for this family.

It is extremely important to remember that although two children may have been given the same diagnosis, their abilities, needs and skills will be different. A diagnosis does not define the person, but it may give you an idea of difficult areas. For example, in order for a child to receive a diagnosis of autism, he or she would have to have a significant language delay or disorder before the age of three. Therefore you know that the child's language development will be delayed. However, goals and intervention strategies for two children of the same age who have been diagnosed with autism may be completely different.

It is also extremely important to focus on children's strengths as well as their difficulties. Assessments tend to focus on the negatives: the things that a child is not doing rather than what he or she can achieve. Many families may be experiencing a range of emotions in relation to the child's disability or condition. Tell members of a family about what their child can do rather than constantly focusing on what the child cannot do.

REFLECTION 4.2

Think back to Sarah in Case Study 4.1. What emotions do you think Sarah's family experienced when they found out that she was given a diagnosis of autism? Would focusing on Sarah's skills have been helpful to the family at this time? Or do you think the family needed time to come to terms with the diagnosis that had been given to their child?

Even the use of developmental norms may not be appropriate for all children. For example, a child with a severe physical disability may never be able to hold a cup independently, so it is not appropriate to compare that child to other children who can achieve this task. It is important to look at what the child is able to do now, the skill that might be achieved and the best way to do this. The flow chart presented in Figure 4.2 could guide you through this process.

GENERAL SKILLS AND OTHER IMPORTANT CONSIDERATIONS WHEN WORKING WITH CHILDREN

Working with children and families in a fieldwork placement may be the first time you have worked with or even spoken to a young child—since you were a child yourself! Where possible, take time to observe 'typically developing' children, because this provides you with an opportunity to look at how they interact with each other, the language they use and the activities and games they play.

It is important to recognise children's ages and abilities so that you are able to communicate on their level. This does not mean that you need to 'talk in baby language' with children who have receptive language difficulties. However, it does mean that you will keep your language brief, use modelling (show them what to do), gesture, get down on their level (sit on the floor or at the table with them) and give them an opportunity to process the information (wait for a response). At the beginning of your fieldwork placement, use this time to observe how your fieldwork educator engages with a variety of children.

Play is the natural mode for children. Remembering how to play and being playful will help you engage with a child. When you first meet a child, find out about his or her interests so that you can integrate those interests in your intervention sessions. This will assist in developing rapport, and help in engaging a child on more difficult tasks (such as colouring in a picture of a favourite TV character as a way of working on pencil control).

The clinical reasoning process

THINK AND LINK 4.2

How do you know where to start, and what to do with a child that has been referred?

Figure 4.2: Paediatric clinical reasoning process

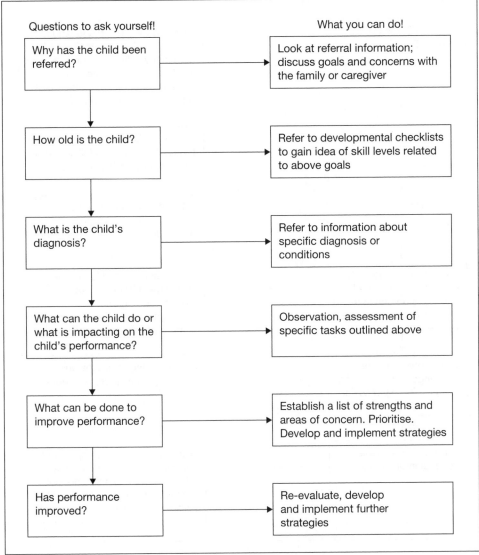

Questions to ask yourself!

What you can do!

Why has the child been referred? → Look at referral information; discuss goals and concerns with the family or caregiver

How old is the child? → Refer to developmental checklists to gain idea of skill levels related to above goals

What is the child's diagnosis? → Refer to information about specific diagnosis or conditions

What can the child do or what is impacting on the child's performance? → Observation, assessment of specific tasks outlined above

What can be done to improve performance? → Establish a list of strengths and areas of concern. Prioritise. Develop and implement strategies

Has performance improved? → Re-evaluate, develop and implement further strategies

Source: Powell 2009

Using Case Study 4.1: Sarah as an example, Figure 4.3 shows you how to think through the paediatric clinical reasoning process.

The system shown in Figure 4.3 will help you as a student to understand the strengths and difficulties of the child. It will help you to work through the intervention process and reevaluate strategies that don't appear to be working. In Case Study 4.1, it would have been worthwhile discussing the parents' goals and concerns in relation to the intervention before the family felt the need to consult the *family service coordinator*. Perhaps this would have led to re-establishing strategies and goals to meet the family's and Sarah's needs.

Figure 4.3: The clinical reasoning process (thinking process) used by the health professional for Sarah

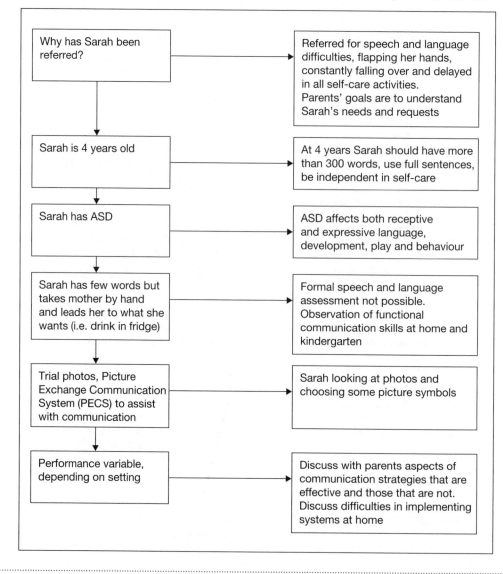

··

SUMMARY

This chapter discussed strategies that will contribute positively to your fieldwork experience. All children and families are different and you need to respect and value them as individuals. Intervention must focus on the areas that are of concern for families and caregivers regardless of setting. Focusing on a child's strengths as well as areas of concern helps you become aware of how you communicate and engage with children and their families. A diagram outlining the clinical reasoning process— important questions to consider when working with children—was presented, and should be referred to during your fieldwork. Given this information, the fieldwork experience should be invaluable to your career regardless of whether or not you choose to work with children and families.

DISCUSSION QUESTIONS

1   List the types of fieldwork settings that you may encounter when working with children.
2   Discuss the four skills required in order to become an effective paediatric practitioner.
3   Discuss why observational skills are important. Outline what information you can gain from observation of a child.
4   How is working with children and families different from working with adults?

References

Dunst, C. J. & Trivette, C. M. (1996). 'Empowerment, Effective Help-Giving Practices and Family Centred Care'. *Pediatric Nursing*, 22(4), 334–7, 343.

Kramer, P. & Hinojosa, J. (1999). *Frames of Reference for Pediatric Occupational Therapy.* Lippincott Williams & Wilkins, Philadelphia.

McBride, S. L. (1999). 'Research in Review: Family-centred Practices'. *Young Children*, 54(3), 62–70.

Rodger, S. & Ziviani, J. (2006). *Occupational Therapy with Children: Understanding Children's Occupations and Enabling Participation*. Blackwell, Melbourne.

Stagnitti, K. (2005). 'The Family as a Unit in Postmodern Society'. In G. Whiteford and V. Wright St Clair (eds). *Occupation and Practice in Context*. Elsevier, Sydney, 213–29.

CHAPTER 5
WORKING IN ACUTE SETTINGS

Jo McDonall

LEARNING OUTCOMES

After reading this chapter, you should be able to:
- identify the types of acute placements and settings
- know how to get organised and prepare for placement
- understand the unique demands of the acute care setting

KEY TERMS

Acute care setting
Arrest trolley
Fieldwork placement
Infection control
On placement
Pace of work
Police Record Check (PRC)
Pre-fieldwork placement
Working With Children Check (WWC)

INTRODUCTION: WHAT DO YOU THINK?

This chapter is designed to provide you with some useful information to assist in your preparation for fieldwork placement in an acute setting. The skills and knowledge you learn in academic classes provide you with the understanding. Fieldwork placement provides you with an opportunity to assess your ability to demonstrate your knowledge and put it into practice. Regardless of the health course you are studying, fieldwork placement is vital to the development of your assessment, diagnosis and treatment skills, as well as providing opportunity to strengthen your professional communication skills. Fieldwork placement is where all the learning comes together and the relevance of the theory becomes evident.

> Placement is where I learnt what it meant to be a nurse ... I had heard all this information in lectures and from my tutors but it only started to make sense when I went on placement and actually saw how the nurse works and what I need to know.
>
> *Second year nursing student, 2008*

Healthcare professionals need to develop the ability to learn and flourish in a wide variety of health settings in order to practise in an everchanging health care environment. While preparing for and completing your fieldwork placement, you may find it beneficial to reflect upon how:

- the theory you learnt relates to this fieldwork placement
- to adapt the learnt psychomotor skills to real-life situations
- to assess and modify assessments depending on the client/patient situation or the healthcare environment
- to interpret patient/client information and its significance and whether you need to adapt your plan of care for the patient or client
- the information collected influences your decisions about interventions or suggested care plans
- to integrate reflective practice into your skill set
- to evaluate the care given.

Critically thinking about these points before and during fieldwork placement will enable you to gain the most from these experiential learning opportunities and be proactive in your professional development. It is important that you are well prepared for fieldwork placement so that the experience is positive, and you take as many opportunities as possible to contribute to client or patient care. The following tips are provided to assist you in your preparation for fieldwork placement in an acute setting. The list is not exhaustive, you may know of other tips, and we encourage you to share these with fellow students.

TYPES OF ACUTE FIELDWORK PLACEMENTS AND SETTINGS

The setting of your acute clinical fieldwork placement will depend on the discipline and the specific course requirements. Sometimes fieldwork placements occur intermittently, such as for one or two days per week over an extended period of time; or in blocks of time of perhaps two weeks to several weeks' duration. Other considerations will be the availability of clinical resources and the degree of supervision required for patient or client safety. Acute fieldwork placements may be in settings such as:

- metropolitan hospital
- private hospitals
- rural or regional hospitals
- medical clinics
- in patients' or clients' home (hospital in the home).

Initially you may have minimal responsibility in terms of patient or client care, as the fieldwork educator may take most of the responsibility. However, as you progress in your course, you assume more accountability for your patients' or clients' care, and

REFLECTION 5.1

An acute setting
You have been assigned to begin in an acute care setting for your fieldwork placement. What are you expecting about the pace of work? What do you understand as the demands on staff on the wards? How do you feel about encountering very ill people? What are your strengths, or areas for improvement?

your interactions with them will also subsequently increase. For instance, in your early placements the emphasis may be on your familiarisation with professional roles and responsibilities of your chosen discipline, the healthcare sector, policies, procedures and services. However, you must always remember that, even though you may not have the majority responsibility for the acute care provided, you do have an obligation for implementing skills and knowledge learnt in your academic program in a safe and competent manner that supports quality patient outcomes and patient safety.

GETTING ORGANISED: PRE-FIELDWORK PLACEMENT

In order to get the most from your acute fieldwork placement it is important that you are prepared. This section will provide some useful tips about what is important for you to know before your fieldwork placement commences.

How do I get there, and now what?
Transport
Preparation for fieldwork placement begins before the commencement of your placement. The better prepared and informed you are about the expectations of the placement—even about where to park the car—the more you will reduce some of the stress that you might otherwise experience. Many acute settings are in large busy hospitals: know where to park or what public transport to take, the building to go to, and how to find the department or ward you will be working in. If you are unfamiliar with the health agency, go for a pre-fieldwork test drive, or take public transport at the same time you will be going on the same sort of day so you can anticipate how long it will take you. This will assure you that you know how to get to the venue and how long the journey may take. Find out the cost of driving or taking public transport, and how far you need to walk from the carpark or bus or train stop, and whether the venue is accessible and safe at night. It is important not to be late when you commence your placement.

THINK AND LINK 5.1

Chapter 1 outlines how to prepare for your fieldwork placement. You might like to review this chapter, then consider the differences between preparing for an acute hospital setting as opposed to preparing for a community-based setting. What is similar? What is different?

Preparation sessions

For some disciplines, you may be required to attend fieldwork placement preparation sessions, which may be tutorials or sessions organised by your university or the host healthcare agency. This session will provide you not only with essential information about the expectations, learning outcomes and key contact personnel, but also those day-to-day bits of knowledge that make the fieldwork experience feel positive, such as lockers for your personal belongings, where to meet on the first day, perhaps the designated area that you will be assigned to for your fieldwork placement and even where the cafeteria is located. Maybe you will have access to a small kitchen to store your meals. If lockers are available, it is advisable not to take any valuables while you are on fieldwork placement, as valuables can be lost or damaged. Alternatively, this type of information may be made available to you via online resources.

It is important that you are familiar with how you will be assessed throughout your fieldwork placement. Therefore not only will you need to make sure you are familiar with any fieldwork placement rules that govern your placement, but also you need to obtain copies of these and any competency assessment tools or competency standards that you will be assessed against throughout the placement.

THINK AND LINK 5.2

Chapter 14 is about assessment within fieldwork placements. Knowing how you will be assessed within an acute setting will assist you to focus on your learning goals. Learning in a fieldwork placement involves more than skills and tasks. What do you want to learn from your fieldwork placement in an acute setting?

The venue

On a pre-fieldwork visit, you may have an opportunity to find out about the ward areas: patient or client profiles, any important pre-reading that may assist you in understanding patient profiles, drugs used and services provided by the institution you will be working in. Other information you may want to obtain on your trial visit to the venue is the emergency numbers or procedures of the venue. Contact your fieldwork educator before your visit to introduce yourself and make arrangements. He or she may request to meet you and accompany you on your orientation.

Specific ward orientation may include the type of ward or area you will be placed on, such as an orthopaedic ward or the physiotherapy department, or reading up on or revising your lecture notes, unit materials, specific ward or venue information. This will refresh your learning and give you confidence about expectations and an ability to answer questions that the fieldwork educator will pose to you. Depending on your discipline, before placement it may also be important for you to revise information about common drugs and procedures or surgeries that will be used on that ward. This information may be available at the pre-fieldwork placement information sessions. If this information is not given before placement, ask questions of your lecturers or fieldwork educator.

Goals and objectives for placement

Often students arrive on the first day of fieldwork placement unsure of the learning objectives for the placement or what they want to achieve. Valuable time can be lost if you need to discuss at length your goals and objectives with the fieldwork educator. It is also very frustrating for fieldwork educators, as it can distract them from meeting their own responsibilities. It might appear that you are not interested in the placement because you have come ill prepared. Therefore, in order to get the most out of your placement, consider before placement what your specific goals and objectives are and how your theoretical program relates to these objectives and goals. The learning outcomes, objectives and goals will often be derived from current units of study or overall course objectives and aims, such as being able to perform a particular complex task or to develop an understanding of specific conditions or situations.

Be prepared with the right documentation

As you are a health professional, it is important that your immunisations and any other health department requirements are up to date and that you have documentary evidence of your health status. Each state and territory will have individual requirements, so it is important to note that if you cross state and territory borders you are familiar with the requirements of all jurisdictions.

This may vary slightly between acute care settings, so you need to check with your university clinical coordinator to make sure you are aware of any additional immunisations you may require. The Victorian Government provides a list of the common vaccines you will require (see the website <http://www.health.vic.gov.au/immunisation/factsheets/guide_hcw>). You will need documentation that you have had these vaccines with you during the placement. The acute care staff can ask at any time to make sure that you have been immunised. If you have had your immunisations but do not have a record of them, you will need to speak to your academic clinical coordinator or campus nurse/doctor to discuss alternatives (such as a blood test).

In Victoria, the Department of Health also requires you to provide a Victoria *Police Record Check (PRC)*. This can be obtained via: <http://www.police.vic.gov.au/content.asp?Document_ID=274>.

You must have a current PRC at the commencement of every year of your course. Agencies can refuse to take you for placement if you cannot produce a current PRC.

The Justice Department requires that you also provide a *Working With Children Check (WWC)*. This check is required for any student who may come into contact with children while on clinical placement. The WWC is free as you are not being paid for your placement, and will last for five years. The following link takes you to the WWC site <http://www.justice.vic.gov.au/workingwithchildren>.

You may also be required to provide your school with consent forms or other documentation prior to an acute clinical fieldwork placement, so please check with your clinical coordinator or administrative staff at the commencement of the trimester.

THINK AND LINK 5.3

Chapter 21 also discusses your responsibilities for your fieldwork placement. More information on police checks and working with children checks are given in this chapter. Why do you think a police check or a working with children check is necessary?

Looking good

All students must maintain a professional appearance while on fieldwork placement. You will need to make sure you have the appropriate uniform, as approved by the university. You will also need a student identification card that clearly states what university you are from and that you are a student. If a particular acute placement requires alterations to dress, students will be notified prior to the commencement of that placement. In line with Occupational Health and Safety policies, no jewellery is to be worn, except for small ear studs, and fingernails are to be short, clean and free from nail polish.

REFLECTION 5.2

I'm getting nerv ous now ... checklist
Take time to go through the information below. Tick off what you have prepared, and note what you need to prepare, before you begin your acute care placement.

Table 5.1: Preparation list before beginning an acute care placement

Information required for placement	Tick	Notes
Agency/facility: Name/address/contact details Transport/parking/cafeteria Ward/unit name/location/contact details Look at website/emergency procedures		
Type of acute placement (e.g. hospital/community/rural)		
Duration of placement		
Shift times/your roster/work times		
Uniform requirements		
Pre-reading of agency requirements		
Review university objectives and rules for placement		
Objectives for placement		
Review unit material relevant to ward or placement area		
Clinical facilitator/teacher's name/contact details		
Place to meet (orientation) on day 1		
What I need to take: Uniform Identification badge Pen/watch/stethoscope/calculator Other items advised by agency Clinical assessment tool Other relevant assessment tasks Learning objectives Any other documents as advised by your school		

ON PLACEMENT … HELP

It is normal to feel a little nervous or apprehensive on your first day. Understanding what is expected from you as a student on your first acute care placement will go a long way to help relieve some of the anxiety.

Emma, a second year Nursing student, recalls her first acute care placement:

I remember having to wait in the foyer for the clinical teacher … I was so early because I didn't want to be late on my first day, but waiting around made me a little more nervous. I remember thinking: what is my clinical teacher like? Will she think I'm okay? What will the ward be like that I'm going onto? Will I know enough to look after the patients there?

It is important you arrive a little early for your first day of fieldwork placement. You will be expected to meet your fieldwork educator or hospital representative at a designated place, or you may be directed to go straight to the ward or unit or department you will be working on.

In acute care settings, you need to be prepared for the following:

- the pace of work
- strict adherence to infection control
- patient stress
- communication.

Pace of work

Things move fast in the acute setting. Patient or client movements are happening all the time. Some patients may be arriving back to the ward after procedures; some are being discharged; and as you discharge one, another is waiting for you to clean the space so they can be admitted. Often there are many tasks that need to be done: for example, medication administration, preparing a patient for operations or admission reports.

As a student this can lead to you feeling a little lost at times. Remember to allow yourself to be a student: it is okay to sit and read a patient's or client's notes, watch procedures being performed and take the time to talk to your patients or clients. Always be on the lookout for learning opportunities. If you see something that you would like to do, for example, complex wound management, take the initiative! Go home that night and read all you can about complex wounds. The next day you can ask if you can undertake the dressing with supervision.

Work intensity

The past decade has seen increasing patient acuity and shortening lengths of stays in acute care hospitals. This has intensified the work for the staff in acute hospitals. You will be confronted with varying degrees of illnesses, from major traumas or illnesses to minor procedures. With the reduction in patients' length of stay in acute care facilities, the stress for the health care staff has increased, as they seek to ensure that patients are provided with appropriate learning opportunities and information regarding how to care for themselves when they are discharged home. To assist you in preparation for your fieldwork placement in an acute setting, learn about common conditions specific to the area you are going to, and understand how to manage them. This will enable you to keep up with what is going on in the ward.

Infection control

You will learn a lot about infection control. Just remember that infection control protects both your patients and you! Patients are at risk of acquiring infections in the healthcare environment because of lower resistance to infectious agents and an increased exposure to disease-causing microorganisms. Ensure you protect yourself and your patients by wearing gloves when coming into contact with body fluids. Wear goggles when there is a risk of splashing. Personal hygiene practices are necessary to ensure you do not transmit infections: handwashing between patients is crucial in ensuring you do not transmit infectious agents. Make sure you are familiar with the occupational health and safety guidelines for infection control in the area you are working in.

Communication

Talk to all the staff in your team. Relating to the interdisciplinary team (doctors, physiotherapists, nurses, dietitians and occupational therapists) can be daunting.

Case Study 5.1	What a day!

Jill was in her final year. She was confident and organised. She had worked in community-based settings, a private practice and an aged care facility. This placement was her first acute setting in a large busy hospital. She had made a pre-fieldwork placement visit and was on time with all her documentation. She had planned out her first day in her head. However, when she arrived at her placement, there was a Code Blue being called out over the speakers and staff were rushing everywhere. She was ushered into a room and told to stay there and wait and the door was closed. She waited for over an hour! Eventually, someone came and took her out of the room to orientate her to the ward where she was going to stay for the duration of her placement. She was annoyed that one hour had been wasted of her time but also frightened about the events that had just occurred. She said so to her fieldwork educator. The day didn't go as planned. Events moved quickly; tasks had to be completed without the time for preparation she was used to. She felt as if she were drowning.

Questions

1   What had Jill not understood about an acute care setting? What had she not prepared for?
2   How could her fieldwork educator help her understand the demands of this particular setting?

Knowing who to talk to about specific questions is one key aspect of learning in the clinical environment. Observing how your fieldwork educator interacts with this team will enable you to learn how to communicate in various situations. Effective communication is a skill that you will develop with experience. Use your fieldwork placement time to improve how you communicate with colleagues and the interdisciplinary team, and with patients and their families. Don't forget to smile; this not only helps your patients feel better but also others in the team.

What to do if you are absent

If you find you are unable to attend placement for any reason, such as illness, you must let the relevant persons know as soon as you are feeling unwell, preferably before your expected arrival. You will need to contact the university representative (such as the clinical administrative coordinator) and your fieldwork educator and the contact person on the ward, unit or department you are working on. You may also be required to provide a medical certificate or statutory declaration when you return. (You will need to check the clinical rules relevant to your course.)

If you are leaving the ward for any reason (such as taking a meal break or transferring patients), it is common courtesy to inform the person in charge that you are off the ward. This is not only as a courtesy, but also so that the person in charge knows where the staff are at all times in case of an emergency. It is not recommended that you transfer or accompany any patient off the ward without direct supervision or written approval.

Emergencies ... what do I do?

At times you may be involved with unexpected events or emergencies, such as a cardiac arrest or patient fall. You must be familiar with the emergency codes and procedures of the agency where you are on placement. The emergency codes will be explained to you on the first day. However, it is your responsibility to ensure you know the different codes and what they refer to. If there is an emergency on your ward you may be expected to assist where necessary.

Emergency codes can vary between organisations. It is imperative that you familiarise yourself with the codes used in the organisation where you are on placement. Some common codes you are likely to hear in the acute setting are:

- Code Red: fire or smoke discovered
- Code Orange: evacuation procedure when instructed to do so
- Code Purple: bomb threat
- Code Black: personal threat (police assistance required)
- Code Grey: patient threat (patient-initiated violence)
- Code Blue: medical emergency
- Code Yellow: internal emergency
- Code Brown: external emergency.

Case Study 5.2 — It's all in a day

David was placed in a day surgery ward on his first day. That's where he would be working for the whole of his time on placement. Patients came in at 7 a.m. in the morning, had surgery and were discharged at noon. The second group of patients would come in at 12 noon, have surgery and be discharged at 5 p.m. the same day. He was not used to such a large turnover of patients, and sometimes felt that his patient care was dictated by the institution and not by the needs of the patients. In his course he had been taught about patient-centred care and always working with patients or clients and their needs. But here, in this placement, people went in and out. He hardly had a conversation with any of them, let alone knowing their goals, needs and who they were, and whether they required any other services, such as community-based care. They were just conditions that came through the door, and four to five hours later left through the same door.

Questions

1   In such a setting, how do you combine patient-centred care with the pace of work? Is it possible?
2   How do you cope with the clash of cultures; that is, the culture you were taught to work in and culture of the actual workplace?

REFLECTION 5.3

An emergency
What are you like in an emergency? How do you behave? If you are not comfortable with dealing with emergencies, what are some strategies to help you to cope?

You will need to know the emergency telephone numbers to call and what to say. You will also be expected to know the evacuation procedures of the agency or ward, and the location of your nearest evacuation assembly areas. It would be expected that you are also familiar with the emergency procedures and equipment on the ward you are working on, so always check at the commencement of each shift where the *arrest trolley* is placed. Check individual medical emergency equipment, such as oxygen and suction equipment, at the back of the patients' beds.

SUMMARY

This chapter has provided you with some useful tips to help you get ready and survive your first acute fieldwork placement. Pre-planning is important for fieldwork placements in large metropolitan or rural hospitals, and pre-fieldwork visits will help you to orientate yourself to the geographical location, the wards or departments you will be working on, and how to get around the physical setting. Undertaking a placement in an acute setting, you will learn about infection control, adjusting to a faster pace of work, coping with emergencies and communication with other staff. Acute care can include hospital in the home, day surgery and in-patient wards. You need to be well prepared and open to learning.

DISCUSSION QUESTIONS

1   How would you best prepare for your first acute fieldwork placement?
2   What are your expectations when undertaking placement in an acute care setting?
3   What would your learning goals be in an acute hospital setting?

CHAPTER 6
WORKING WITH OLDER PEOPLE

Jennifer Nitz

LEARNING OUTCOMES

After reading this chapter, you should be able to:
- know where older clients will be encountered, and about the interdisciplinary team that manages older people
- understand the importance of a person-centred approach to client management
- know your role as a student when participating in fieldwork placement with older people
- understand the importance of communication, interpersonal skills and body language in clinical practice
- discuss the framework for practice
- discuss the impact of age-related changes on all aspects of geriatric practice and the depth of knowledge needed to practise effectively
- articulate where health promotion and preventive interventions fit.

KEY TERMS

Communication
Chronic condition self-management program (CCSM)
Geriatric care
Health promotion
Work-integrated learning

INTRODUCTION

Geriatrics is 'a branch of medicine or social science dealing with the health and care of old people' (*Australian Oxford Dictionary*). A common misconception of working with older people (*geriatric care*) is that the experience will be encapsulated into a single placement. In fact, you will encounter older patients or clients in most of your fieldwork placements, not just during a defined geriatric placement. Most students will experience fieldwork placements in an institution or community. Figure 6.1 illustrates the scope of fieldwork placements when working with older people.

When working with older people during your fieldwork placement you will be part of an interdisciplinary team that includes patients, their significant others, doctors, nurses and a combination of allied health professionals. The team members will be determined by the condition of the patients, and will vary across the time

Figure 6.1: Scope of fieldwork settings when working with older people

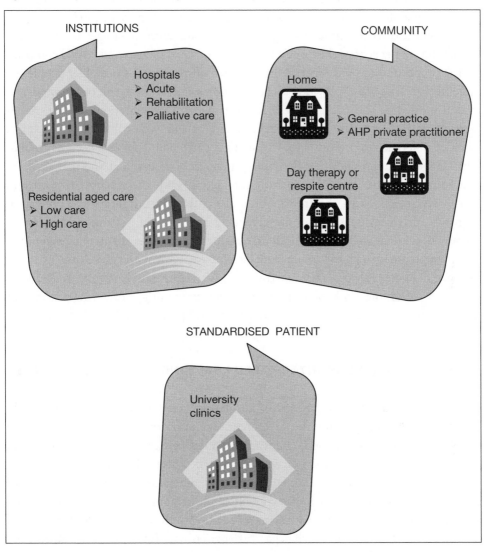

frame as the needs of patients are likely to change with their medical status. The most crucial aspect of team efficacy is communication among the team members and ensuring that the health professional who is most suited to attend a particular aspect of treatment provides that treatment. For example, treatment of pneumonia with assisted secretion removal is provided by the physiotherapist who has specific training in the techniques required for that treatment, as well as the capacity to evaluate and modify interventions as indicated by the patient's condition. This skill is profession specific, just as changing wound dressings is a nursing skill and treating speech problems is speech pathology specific.

Irrespective of the environment in which you experience fieldwork placement with older people, the same broad expectations of you will apply. In 2007, 1.6 per cent of the population of Australia was aged over 85 years, with those aged over 65 years comprising 13 per cent of the population. Working with older people could comprise a large proportion of your practice, irrespective of profession since older people are more likely to need care provided by health professionals as a result of acquired age-related morbidity and pathology. This complexity of presentation is what makes working with older people exciting and challenging. No two adults will be the same, so strict adherence to protocols for managing a particular diagnosis become fraught with danger. Having said that, there are principles of assessment and management that form a framework for therapeutic interaction with the elderly that you will morph and colour with the information you gather during interviews, physical, cognitive and social assessments, problem identification, goal-setting and treatment, thereby developing an individualised management plan. This chapter endeavours to assist you to broaden your horizons and develop excitement and commitment to the care of older people through demonstration of work-integrated learning in fieldwork placement. Working with older people is very rewarding, presenting a constant challenge to your inventive initiative and continued professional development.

PREPARING FOR WORK-INTEGRATED LEARNING WITH OLDER PEOPLE

Older patients encountered in hospitals, residential care and community commonly have multiple, complex and chronic conditions, and what you learn from these encounters is priceless. If the content and context of exposure to geriatric clients during fieldwork placement is not well supported by clear learning objectives and your fieldwork educator does not facilitate your understanding of the relevance of information and experiences in the context of professional practice, it is likely that this will discourage you from working in settings with older people. Powers and colleagues (2005) found that such negative experiences led students to avoid working with older people after graduation.

Flexibility and being able to respond to the guidance provided by individual patient responses is vitally important for practice with older people. Remember every person is different. This is why the clinical reasoning processes you utilise during your interactions must be patient centred and patient driven. This means that the patient's presentation and presenting problems will be the guide to your assessment and treatment approach, together with the patient or patient's carer suggestions about their own goals.

Preparing for fieldwork placement where older people will be encountered depends on the year of your studies you have reached. Most placements will demand a variety of levels of knowledge expectation and education objectives and goals commensurate with theoretical knowledge preparation. If you are lucky, you will undertake fieldwork with older people in every year of your study program. This will enable you to develop your skills in communication, assessment and intervention as you learn and acquire these attributes. If your fieldwork exposure is limited to the final years of your study, then expectations for participation in practice will be greater. You will be expected to achieve basic practitioner competency by the completion of the placement. The basic competencies for practice should be found on your professional association website. You are encouraged to consult this information in conjunction with your course outcome expectations to map how you are acquiring the profession-specific skills for independent practice.

Fieldwork contract

When you arrive at your fieldwork placement you will usually draw up a contract with your fieldwork educator. It will identify the necessary, desirable and wish-list experiences you should achieve by the end of the fieldwork placement. If such a contract is not formally made, it is a good idea to itemise all the aspects of work with geriatric or older clients that you would like to encounter. Negotiate with your fieldwork educator opportunities to participate in the experiences you have identified. Remember that you might have to fulfil your wish list over a few fieldwork placements. For example, if acute condition management is not available in the facility where you are undertaking your geriatric fieldwork, you could arrange a visit to another facility, or consider this aspect of working with older persons if available in another placement.

Framework of fieldwork placement

To gain most from your fieldwork placement with the older person, it is essential that you have a thorough understanding of the framework for geriatric practice. This framework includes:

1 *Communication:* Primary communication is between you and the patient. Additional information might be gained by sharing information regarding the patient with other team members via patient medical files and by talking with the patient's family or carer. The information from family and carers is often needed to validate the information gained during patient interview when cognitive decline is suspected or known.

2 *A broad knowledge base of 'normal' ageing and pathologies* (Nitz & Hourigan 2004) likely to be encountered should have been included in your pre-fieldwork preparation. If not, you will find it beneficial to access normal age-related data from the literature regarding outcome measures that are pertinent to your field of practice: for example, normal performances for clinical balance measures as provided by Isles and colleagues (2004). Ideally this theoretical knowledge would include palliative care and information regarding advanced health care directives otherwise known as living wills or end-of-life directives.

3 *Competency in application and interpretation of profession-specific skills:*
  (a) ability to assess the older person (using, for example, balance tests and body system assessments) and interpret the results
  (b) ability to develop treatments specific to the condition and the person.
4 Utilisation of clinical reasoning skills to enable effective patient-centred problem-solving and goal-setting.
5 Empowerment of patients to gain or retain self-determination through goal-setting, and full participation in and implementation of their treatment plan.
6 Effective measurement of outcomes through re-evaluation of older people, at intervals appropriate to the acuity of their problems.
7 Consideration of health promotion and prevention of age-related decline or complications of current morbidities to ensure preservation of independence and quality of life for the patient and carers.
8 A willingness to investigate and learn independently, as indicated by an openness to exposure to medical conditions not previously encountered, new social attitudes and expectations and the ability to adapt intervention strategies to the cultural, physical and cognitive abilities encountered in older people.

Successful learning and professional development in the field of geriatric practice requires you to integrate many theoretical and practical skills that will have been or will be addressed during your student training.

REFLECTION 6.1

Preparing to work with older persons
What are the important steps you should take in preparing for a fieldwork experience where older people will be encountered? Do you need to prepare for a geriatric fieldwork placement in an acute hospital ward any differently than you would prepare for acute ambulatory care or residential aged care?

COMMUNICATION IS MORE THAN JUST TALKING

Communication may take the form of spoken words, written words or drawings, gestures, demonstrations or sign language. It might take place through face-to-face contact, through videoconferencing, or telephone, email or mail hookup.

Form of address
A respectful form of address when working with the older people, their families and carers is mandatory. On initial contact, and during subsequent meetings, until and unless the patient or family member has sanctioned change, you should address your patient as Mr Jones or Mrs Jones, not Bill or Jill. Verbal interaction during interview,

social discourse and treatment or intervention should not use complex medical terminology or phrases. Ask your patient if they understand what you have said or whether they need more explanation. If you are still concerned about whether they understand, ask your patients to tell you what you have been discussing with them.

Types of contact

Get down to eye level when talking with your patients. Nonverbal communication is very useful in enhancing understanding and retention of the spoken word. This might take the form of written instructions, drawings or gestures as a way of demonstrating what you want your patient to do. This is particularly important when working with people with receptive problems caused by stroke and aphasia or dementia.

Body language indicates whether you are interested or uninterested in what is happening with older people. Poor or uninterested body language is a common reason why patients lose interest and motivation to participate in their treatment. Similarly, patients' body language tells you a lot about how they feel. If they are depressed or in pain their demeanour will lack affect and motivation, and sometimes your patient may cry. Therefore listen to your patients and their families and carers. Patients will tell you what their problems are, which in general will indicate the goal for treatment. If you disregard this information it is very unlikely that patients will comply with your treatment.

Communication interference

A number of factors might interfere with communication between you and your patients. Impaired hearing is very common in the elderly. Find out if the patient has a hearing aid, then encourage its use. Make sure the patient can see your face clearly, so lip reading, facial expression and gesture can be used to augment what is heard. Where English is not a patient's first language, he or she may not understand complex questions or instructions, or you will fail to find out important assessment facts, and will achieve only poor treatment outcomes. Always avoid excessive use of medical jargon, for the same reason.

Client and carer education comprises a major part of your work with older people. When you are treating the patient, it is pertinent to educate clients and carers as to the reason for the treatment. Education on preventive health components is especially important for carers in order to prevent them becoming injured or sick, which could stop them continuing as carers.

THINK AND LINK 6.1

Sometimes when English is not the person's first language, a translator may be included in the assessment and/or treatment sessions with older people and their carers. Chapter 2 gives details of what to consider when working with translators and diverse populations.

REFLECTION 6.2

Communicating is more than verbal
Try instructing one of your family members or friends who is not a health professional to do a task that is novel for them. How do they respond? How could you clarify the instructions so they understand more readily what you want them to do. Feedback from this exercise will greatly benefit your fieldwork practice.

Body language

Some elderly patients are affected by medical conditions that interfere with their capacity to understand the spoken word. People who have suffered a stroke that has caused right side hemiplegia often have aphasia, which interferes with understanding what has been said. People with dementia or delirium might also have difficulty in interpreting the meaning of words, and so respond to instructions in ways that are not anticipated. An example of this is when a person with dementia is asked to step backwards before sitting in a chair. 'Backwards' is a concept that has been lost, so the person will likely step forwards, as the only word understood is 'step'. You will succeed if you stand beside the person, then step back while gently guiding the patient back and saying 'step back'.

Engagement with the elderly patient is communicated through facial expression and other caring actions. Boredom and lack of interest is quite evident to older people, who will respond in like manner by not wanting to help themselves or participate in their treatment. You need to show that you are enthusiastic and happy in order for your patient to benefit. Such behaviour will enhance your own learning capacity, so you will start to become a more independent learner and a much better practitioner.

Confidentiality and consent

Members of the care team must consider respect for privacy and confidentiality of personal information when caring for older people. You need to always be aware of how and where you discuss patient information. It is best practice to keep case discussions to non-public areas so that this aspect of privacy is respected. Gaining informed consent regarding treatment is mandatory, and hinges on good communication between the treating team and the patient. Consent may need to be sought from a patient's guardian when cognitive impairment or unconsciousness is present and renders the patient unable to provide personal consent. Only the person who has been given the legal right is permitted to provide proxy consent. You are encouraged to undertake independent enquiry into this topic.

THINK AND LINK 6.2

Chapter 20 discusses the ethical issues health professionals encounter when working with vulnerable populations. As people age and become frailer and/or have cognitive decline, they become more vulnerable to being misled or abused. When reflecting on ethical practice with older persons, don't forget to read Chapter 20.

INSTITUTIONAL SETTINGS FOR FIELDWORK PLACEMENTS WITH OLDER PEOPLE

Acute hospital wards

Older people encountered in adult orthopaedic, surgical and medical wards comprise two main groups: those who are well and admitted for elective procedures, and those who are more or less dependent and admitted with injuries or illness. They are therefore optimally well or quite unwell, which is the basis, in addition to their age and current morbidity and medical, social and behavioural history, for developing treatment goals. Thus patients must be seen and managed as individuals, where their present condition needs to be considered in the framework of their health, social and behavioural environment. In acute hospital wards, older people may be admitted to one of the following wards:

- *Orthopaedic wards*: the well elderly who present for elective surgery commonly are admitted for hip or knee joint replacement or laminectomy. Older patients who are often quite unwell and dependent are admitted for non-elective surgery, which frequently includes treatment of proximal femoral fractures after falls.
- *Surgical wards*: patients who could be considered reasonably well might be undergoing elective surgery for cancer treatment, which could include bowel resection, lung resection, neck resections or arterial bypass surgery. Conversely, surgery might be required to correct a life-threatening situation such as bowel obstruction or rupture, ruptured aortic aneurysm or arterial embolectomy, and the patient is acutely ill.
- *Medical wards*: in most instances patients admitted to medical wards will be dependent in some aspect. Many are admitted to hospital because they need their medical conditions investigated and optimal management initiated. These patients often will be frail and fall frequently. These patients require specific ward management if they are to be safe. Other elderly patients admitted to the medical wards will have had acute cardiac events, stroke, or chest or other infections, and will be dependent.

Rehabilitation or transitional care hospital wards

In rehabilitation or transitional wards the elderly patients that you will encounter are normally still recovering from an acute illness. Although their condition has improved, they are still not sufficiently independent to return home safely. They might also be waiting for home modifications to be undertaken to enable them to function at home, so there is no other option but to stay in hospital. Others will be waiting for nursing home bed availability.

Palliative care wards

Some patients will be admitted at the end of life, when they can no longer be managed at home, and hospice accommodation is not an available option. You might also participate in a fieldwork placement in a hospice where all inpatients will be receiving palliative care. The focus in these experiences is not curative but palliative. In palliative care, minimising the experience of symptoms is the primary issue in treatment, especially prevention of undesirable complications, such as pressure ulcers caused by difficulty in moving. Enabling the best quality of life during a patient's final days is the main aim of palliative care.

DISCHARGE PLANNING OCCURS AT ADMISSION

There are a number of similar aspects relating to each case (see Case Study 6.1). Each woman is having similar right hip replacement surgery, lives in the community, is cognitively capable and should expect to return to her previous situation on discharge from hospital.

What might confound the expected outcome of returning home, especially for Mrs Falls, is a preconceived expectation of failure to achieve independence in activities of daily living. This attitude might be fuelled by her confused state on admission, which was a result of her hip trauma and inability to move. Her age

Case Study 6.1	Comparison of management for elective hip replacement surgery between a well and a frail elderly person

Patient 1

Anna Arthritis, 68 years old, has been admitted to the orthopaedic ward for right total hip replacement surgery tomorrow. She has a long history of osteoarthritis, and the pain in her right hip has persuaded her to have surgery so that she can get back to unrestricted participation in family, leisure and part-time work activities. She has no additional medical conditions, has never fallen, lives independently in her own highset home with her husband, who is well.

Patient 2

Flora Falls, 84 years old, has been admitted to the orthopaedic ward via the hospital Accident and Emergency Department. She was brought there by ambulance after being found on the floor of her bedroom by the person delivering Meals on Wheels to her home. Mrs Falls lives alone in a lowset home. In addition to receiving community assistance from Meals on Wheels three days per week she also has home help come in once a week to assist with house cleaning. Her niece, who takes her shopping weekly, is her only relative living locally. Mrs Falls has controlled left ventricular failure and hypertension, diet-controlled type 2 diabetes and osteoporosis. She has a BMI of 20, and very good vision since her cataract operation last year.

Mrs Falls had fallen returning from the bathroom some time during the night before she was found. This meant she has been lying on the floor for about 10 hours and was quite confused due to hypothermia and hypoglycaemia, and shock as a result of these conditions and her fractured right hip, which was confirmed in hospital. The planned management of her hip fracture was to surgically replace the femoral head tomorrow after her medical state has become stable.

---

of 84 years might also confound the appropriate diagnosis of delirium with a misdiagnosis of dementia, which, when written in a patient's record, changes the approach of health professionals to planning discharge because of the expectation of dependency. In some instances, access to appropriate rehabilitation might also be denied by a diagnosis of dementia, so all health professionals working with Mrs Falls should realise their responsibility to ensure equity of access to services.

Ageism should not contribute to any disparity between the post-operative rehabilitation of Anna Arthritis and Flora Falls, since both were successful community dwellers before hospital admission. Having said this, a study by Ubachs-Moust and colleagues (2008) has shown that the patient's age has an impact on every phase of decision-making, and is a factor in every component of the clinical reasoning process when clinical cases involving octogenarians were evaluated. Ubachs-Moust and colleagues suggest that, ethically, age should not predominate when the clinical pathway for each patient is determined by the team and each team member should question decisions made from an ageist perspective rather than from the clinical evidence.

The approach taken when planning the discharge of these women should include the patient's desires and needs with consideration to physical, spiritual, social and behavioural aspects, such as:

- the patient's current living situation and how supportive and successful this was before the event
- the family support and support from other parties

- the patient's financial situation and ability to pay should additional assistance be required on discharge.

Mrs Falls might have a slower path to recovery because of her pre-admission complications caused by the circumstances of her fracture. This might require her to undertake inpatient rehabilitation for a few days longer than the usual five to seven days required post total hip replacement, such as that in the case of Anna Arthritis.

REFLECTION 6.3

Post-operative management of Mrs Arthritis and Mrs Falls

1 Should the usual post-operative management of the patient after this type of surgery be modified from the 'procedures manual directions' to accommodate for the individual differences encountered in each woman?

2 What prevention interventions need to be instituted to prevent complications related to the surgery or age so that the planned outcome eventuates? Examples of prevention interventions might include prevention of pressure areas and further falls.

COMMUNITY GERIATRIC FIELDWORK PLACEMENTS

Fieldwork placement in the community encompasses the management of clients in their place of residence (see Case Study 6.2). This will include home visiting to the client's private residence, as well as residential aged care, including hostel (low-care) and nursing home (high-care) residence.

Case Study 6.2	Comparison between two frail older persons who both have complex and chronic conditions

Client 1 (lives in community)

Miss Heart lives alone in a retirement village. She has controlled left ventricular failure, chronic obstructive pulmonary disease (COPD), chronic low back pain and urinary stress incontinence. She manages without any home services, but has a very poor exercise tolerance and most activity leaves her short of breath. Cognitively she has no problems.

Client 2 (low-care residential aged care)

Mr Chester lives in a hostel (low care residential aged care facility). He has COPD, controlled hypertension, painful osteoarthritic knees, urinary urge incontinence since prostate surgery three years ago and early-stage dementia.

Clients' goals direct care

Neither of these clients requires acute medical or health professional care at present. Each would, however, benefit from preemptive intervention to maximise his or her current functional ability for easier participation in lifestyle activities. Both these clients' goals are to remain in their current living situation for as long as possible and with optimal quality of life. Health professionals work with these clients to empower them to achieve this goal. This might be in various ways, and through provision of specific treatments or advice, but of most importance is the development of self-management ability by the clients. One way to achieve this would be to enable these clients to participate in a *chronic condition self-management (CCSM)* program run by community-based teams specifically trained to deliver this education program. As part of your training and as part of your fieldwork placement you might participate in a program such as this, either as leader or observer. The CCSM program teaches participants how to better manage their chronic medical conditions, helps them make informed decisions regarding their health and reduces the reliance on direct health care until needed. This type of program addresses preventative health and health promotion issues, and your role as a health professional might be to provide information to the client regarding where to access physical activity programs or social programs in the community.

CLINICAL REASONING 6.1   Optimal treatment outcomes

Optimal treatment outcomes will be variable, and depend on the individual elder person. In all instances a clinical reasoning approach to management should be used. Basic requirements for this reasoning process include:
- a comprehensive understanding of the patient's ageing process and morbidities
- an assessment that considers all aspects of the individual as well as the physical and social environment he or she lives in
- identification of primary problems:
  - all potential confounders to treatment efficacy, contraindications or special precautions that need to be taken
  - secondary problems of lesser importance for the patient
- short-term goal-setting that is determined in conjunction with the patient and agreed upon by all involved parties
- use of suitable outcome measures that will enable change in patient status to be tracked and for informed decision making to be made regarding satisfactory progress or need for a change in intervention strategies or referral to another specialist practitioner such as a physiotherapist or podiatrist for example.

REFLECTION 6.4

The individual older person

It is very easy to be overwhelmed by the complexities of patients' medical or surgical diagnoses and to lose sight of the elderly patient as a person. Think about why it is important to find out about the social, behavioural and spiritual aspects of your patient. To assist in understanding how these aspects might shape your decision making ask yourself the question: 'If this were my grandparent, how would I approach this patient's management?' This is how you should approach all clinical encounters.

SUMMARY

Older patients will be encountered in institutions and the community. Every elderly patient or client is an individual and must be considered as such. Most older people will present with multiple comorbidities that will need to be assessed for how these will impact on mobility and function and any chosen interventions. Assessment and treatment will be determined by the medical status of the individual elder, their social situation of living, their behaviour and their expectations. In addition to managing the presenting problems, holistic management should include pre-emptive preventive intervention to enable optimal quality of life to be attained or maintained.

DISCUSSION QUESTIONS

1   Think about the cases provided earlier. Identify specific assessment, problem identification and clinical reasoning processes and possible treatment interventions that might be indicated for your profession-specific team contribution to the patient's management. Jot this information down, as well as your rationale for the decisions you have made. Discuss your thoughts with your fieldwork educator. You might find this very useful in developing your professional skills for the field of practice (institutional or community).

2   On completion of the fieldwork placement, you need to reflect back on your expectations and activities undertaken. Did this work-integrated learning experience eventuate as you expected? Did it mirror your life experiences with older people you have encountered in everyday life away from study? How and why was it different?

3   If you have been lucky enough to do a fieldwork placement working with the older person in year 1 or 2 of your program, how might you use the lessons learnt and clinical skills attained to enhance your performance in all aspects of practice, including subsequent placements or when a graduate health professional?

References

Alford, C. L., Miles, T., Palmer, R., & Espino, D. (2001). 'An Introduction to Geriatrics for First-Year Medical Students'. *Journal of the American Geriatric Society*, 49(6): 782–7.

Isles, R. C., Nitz, J. C., & Low Choy, N. L. (2004). 'Normative Data for Clinical Balance Measures in Women Aged 20 to 80'. *Journal of the American Geriatric Society*, 52(8): 1367–72.

Nitz, J. C. & Hourigan, S. R. (2004). 'Physiological Changes With Ageing'. In J. C. Nitz & S. R. Hourigan (eds) *Physiotherapy Practice in Residential Aged Care*. Butterworth Heinemann, Edinburgh.

Powers, C. L., Allen, R. M., Johnson, V. A., & Cooper-Witt, C. M. (2005). 'Evaluating Immediate and Long-Range Effect of a Geriatric Clerkship Using Reflections and Ratings from Participants as Students and as Residents'. *Journal of the American Geriatric Society*, 53(2): 331–5.

Ubachs-Moust, J., Houtepen, R., Vos, R., & ter Meulen, R. (2008). 'Value Judgements in the Decision-Making Process for the Elderly Patient'. *Journal of Medical Ethics*, 34: 863–8.

Useful Website

Australian Bureau of Statistics, *Population Projections, Australia, 2006 to 2101* <www.abs.gov.au/AUSSTATS/abs@.nsf/Lookup/3222.0Main+Features12006 to 2101?OpenDocument> accessed 28 April 2009.

CHAPTER 7
WORKING IN MENTAL HEALTH

Geneviève Pépin

LEARNING OUTCOMES

After reading this chapter, you should be able to:
- define mental health
- reflect about individual perception of mental health and mental illnesses
- discuss challenges in mental health practice
- develop strategies to be better prepared.

KEY TERMS

Mental health
Stigma/stigmata
Stress
Teamwork

INTRODUCTION

Working in a mental health setting can be challenging, surprising, rewarding and confronting. As you start a placement or a new position in a mental health setting, you might be confronted with stigma and discrimination. You might have your own opinions and beliefs about mental health-related issues, and you can be influenced by the opinions and beliefs of others. Also, your profession might have helped you develop certain skills and attitudes with respect to mental health practice and mental health-related issues. But how prepared are you to deal with the reactions and behaviours of clients, family members and the wider community? How prepared are you to be part of a mental health team? How comfortable are you with overlapping of roles, tasks and responsibilities?

This chapter will address mental health practice from an interdisciplinary perspective. Various aspects of mental health practice will be presented and discussed. Remember that each health profession has theoretical frameworks, and specific tools and strategies to provide services to a person with a mental health condition. This chapter will identify aspects of mental health practice that can be challenging, and strategies will be provided to cope with these challenges. You will also be encouraged to reflect on your own beliefs and attitudes toward mental health and mental illnesses.

WHAT IS MENTAL HEALTH?

First, it is important to define mental health. However, defining mental health can be problematic, as it may be understood differently by different groups of people and in a wide range of contexts (Blair et al. 2007). What someone from West Africa considers as an appropriate definition of mental health may very well differ from what someone in Eastern Europe would say. This implies that the concept of mental health varies according to cultural and contextual factors. As a result, the community in which a person lives may be welcoming and ready to support someone with a mental health issue or it may alienate and isolate this person.

REFLECTION 7.1

What is mental health?
1 Based on your personal experiences, training and professional expertise, what is your own definition of mental health? What would be the important components of your definition of mental health?
2 When you have developed your own definition of mental health, ask three people to come up with their own definition and compare theirs to yours. What are the similarities and the differences?

The World Health Organization (WHO) defines mental health as 'a state of well-being in which every individual realizes his or her own potential, can cope with the normal stresses of life, can work productively and fruitfully, and is able to make a contribution to her or his community' (WHO 2009). Other authors have described mental health as: 'the successful performance of mental functions, in terms of thought, mood and behaviour that results in productive activities, fulfilling relationships with others, and the ability to adapt to change and to cope with adversity' (Sadock & Sadock 2007: 12). The Scottish Public Mental Health Alliance (SPMHA 2002) has developed the concept of positive mental health. It identified attributes such as the ability to (1) communicate and do things; (2) express oneself; (3) develop a sense of autonomy; and (4) form and maintain relationships with others. These attributes are believed to provide the base for positive mental health and promote wellbeing (SPMHA 2002).

These definitions highlight some very interesting concepts such as wellbeing, adaptation and ability to cope, participation, engaging in fulfilling relationships, communication and self expression and autonomy—all of which relate to the health professions.

STIGMA, LABELS, MYTHS AND MENTAL HEALTH

Movies such as *One Flew Over the Cuckoo's Nest* (1975) depict a brutal view of mental illness and related interventions. Realistically, not all individuals with a mental illness behave like the characters portrayed in some movies and television series. However, sometimes what you see in movies is very close to reality, but much more needs to be known to fully understand mental health and mental illnesses. In the meantime, incorrect information and misconceptions are common in society.

The *Australian Oxford Dictionary* defines 'stigma' as 'a mark or sign of disgrace or discredit' (Moore 2004: 1269). Stigma labels a person as not being 'normal', not 'fitting' in the broader community (Department of Veterans Affairs 2008a). Stigmata often arise from myths about mental health and people with a mental health condition, and contribute to portraying a negative image of these persons. Our own beliefs can contribute to maintaining stigmata about mental health.

You might have personal beliefs or have heard incorrect information and myths about mental health and mental illnesses. You may have specific opinions about the settings in which a mental health professional works or about the behaviour or appearance of individuals with a mental health condition. Myths can arise from a variety of sources. They can be a result of a lack of understanding about a particular situation, incomplete knowledge or incorrect information, or they may be the result of a fear or unpleasant past experience.

The Department of Veterans Affairs of Australia (2008b) has published a fact sheet about myths and mental health specifically addressing the circumstances of war veterans. Consider some of the following myths:

- People with mental health problems are violent and dangerous.
- Mental health problems are caused by personal weakness.
- Mental health problems are hereditary.
- People with mental health problems are 'crazy'.
- People with mental health problems never get better.

REFLECTION 7.2

Identifying your myths
Think about your personal views about mental health and mental health-related conditions. What are your myths?

KNOWING YOURSELF

Before starting your fieldwork in a mental health setting, it is important to take the time to reflect on yourself and your perception of mental health. You probably have hopes and desires to reach specific goals during your fieldwork experience. You may strive to increase your knowledge and skills in mental health practice and grow as a health professional and you most probably want to pass this fieldwork placement.

During your fieldwork placement in a mental health setting you may see clients with acute manifestations and severe mental illnesses. You may meet family members and carers who are scared, don't understand and are seeking answers. You may also work with clients who look perfectly 'normal' to you, and you may not understand why they are receiving service from your organisation. You may meet clients who are eager to recover and will engage in their recovery process easily, although other clients may challenge and resist you or even refuse interventions.

It is important for you to address your personal beliefs, views and concerns about mental health and mental health-related conditions. Knowing yourself, identifying your strengths and areas to improve will help you identify who to talk to, the training or information you should obtain and where to get it. It will help you deal with fears or concerns and will assist you in your learning experience. Sladyk (2002) has developed a few tools to help students know themselves better. One of these tools is a list of fears expressed by students. Reflection 7.3 is an adapted version of this list. Look at some of these fears and add your own concerns.

REFLECTION 7.3

Knowing yourself
I will be stressed, uncomfortable or scared if I...
- see an aggressive client
- see someone who looks really strange
- find myself alone with clients
- have to find something to say to clients
- say something wrong and get the client upset, aggressive or sicker
- see someone I know
- have to comfort parents
- have to interact with individuals whose values are different from mine.

What about you? What are your concerns? _____

_____

Reflecting honestly on your thoughts about mental health and identifying areas of concern are important. It should lead to strategies to deal with these concerns to facilitate your fieldwork experience. One way is to develop a proactive plan.

Sladyk (2002: 49) defines proactive plan as 'a way to prevent problems on fieldwork. It begins with a positive attitude about fieldwork and your approach to learning'. This plan aims to identify your strengths and areas for improvement and come up with strategies to address these areas. The implementation of your plan also rests upon your ability to discuss issues and strategies with your fieldwork educator.

THINK AND LINK 7.1

A proactive plan to prevent problems on fieldwork can result in a surprising amount of enjoyment of a fieldwork placement. It can also help you face potential problems that could have otherwise led to failure. Chapter 17 discusses learning from failure on a fieldwork placement. In particular, two case studies explore two students' different reactions to failure.

These questions will help you develop your proactive plan:

REFLECTION 7.4

My proactive plan

Table 7.1: My proactive plan

What are my skills and knowledge? *Determine your strengths with regards to mental health practice.*	In which areas are there room for improvement? *Identify your limits with regards to mental health practice.*	What will I do? How will I do it? *Identify actions/strategies to maintain your strengths and to address your limits.*

This plan should be developed in collaboration with your fieldwork educator. It could also be an interesting exercise to do with students from other disciplines. When writing up your plan, keep the following questions in mind (Sladyk 2002):
- In which areas of your profession's theoretical foundations are you comfortable?
- Which type of assessments and interventions are you familiar with?
- What feedback did you get from previous fieldwork, and how can it be useful in a mental health setting?
- How would you rate your skills and knowledge about interaction and communication skills?

MENTAL HEALTH PRACTICE: THE SETTINGS

Mental health practitioners can work in very different settings. Some work in a more traditional context, such as a psychiatric hospital or a psychiatric ward, interacting with clients presenting acute symptoms of a wide variety of mental illnesses.

Other practitioners, who work in outpatient settings, will support clients in their journey from the hospital to their home and community. They will work with clients who probably won't present acute manifestations of their mental health-related condition. There will be residual symptoms, and the impact on the person's level of functioning will vary greatly. Your main goals may be orientated toward housing and community living skills.

You can also find mental health professionals in community settings, not-for-profit organisations, mental health associations or private practice. Again, clients receiving services in any of these settings will have different needs, and present with a wide variety of mental health-related issues. As a result, practitioners may focus their interventions on symptom reduction, using specific approaches and interventions, or they may address issues related to return to work and vocational rehabilitation or psychosocial rehabilitation. Remember that these are just a few examples of mental health settings.

Depending on the region, state or country where you live and work, the focus of your interventions, your tasks and responsibilities may vary greatly. Knowing about the setting where you will be doing a placement will help you understand what is expected of you and what you can expect from the placement.

MENTAL HEALTH PRACTICE: A FEW ROADBLOCKS

Despite some important differences between settings, common features of mental health practice have been highlighted in the literature, especially stress, teamwork and role blurring (Lloyd et al. 2005).

Stress

Stress experienced by health professionals in relation to mental health practice has been discussed in the literature for several years (Lloyd et al. 2005; Peck & Norman 1999). The main causes of stress reported by health professionals working in mental health settings are workload, poor job satisfaction, lack of skilled staff, and inadequate training and supervision (Lloyd et al. 2005).

These findings are very helpful, as they provide you with guidelines to become a better mental health professional. Increasing your skills and knowledge about mental health conditions and clinical manifestations of different psychological and psychiatric disorders will target the issue of insufficient skills identified in the literature. *The Diagnostic and Statistical Manual of Mental Disorders*, which is now available in a revised version (the 4th edition: DSM-IV-TR), covers mental illnesses in detail. It is widely used throughout the different health professions. There might be other textbooks that you have used in your own course that will provide you with the information about mental health conditions. There are several books and papers on therapeutic relationship, client-centred practice and interviewing techniques and skills that will help you build your skills and consolidate your knowledge. These resources may be generic, or profession specific. Also, revisiting the intervention process related to your profession will give you a structure to develop your intervention plan.

Clinical reasoning is another powerful tool for you to use. Using clinical reasoning when making decisions about and with a client will contribute to the implementation of a thorough intervention plan. It will enable you to justify your decisions and interventions. Clinical reasoning brings theory and practice together. It helps you make a decision based on evidence (Higgs & Jones 2000).

As a health student you will be supervised by an experienced mental health professional. Although these persons' roles, functions and titles may vary according to each profession, they are there to help you through your fieldwork placement (Healey & Spencer 2008). By making the most of the relationship you have with your fieldwork educator, you can maximise your fieldwork supervision with her or him by setting goals, revisiting these goals and discussing your perceptions and the challenges you are facing. Other examples of supervision activities are brainstorming to identify intervention strategies, then justifying your decisions.

Teamwork and role blurring

The importance of working as a team goes without question, but role blurring is an issue that should be considered (Lloyd et al. 2005). When you start your fieldwork placement you will probably join a team. In this team, each person plays a role and performs certain tasks. When thinking about teamwork, ask yourself a few questions. How specific is each role? Which tasks are common to more than one member of the team, and which ones are profession specific? How easy is it to identify, understand and deal with each other's role? How do you understand your role as part of a mental health team? How comfortable are you with the boundaries that define your role? How comfortable are you with a possible blurring of the roles among the team members?

You might have a precise idea about the different categories, roles and functions of health professionals who are part of a mental health team. Reflection 7.5 addresses some of these questions.

REFLECTION 7.5

Me as part of a team

Table 7.2: Me as part of a team

Think about your practice as a member of a mental health team. Reflect on your training and think about what you have learnt about your profession. What distinguishes you from other members of the mental health team?
Answers:

Hint: Have you thought about consulting the documentation from your professional association? Textbooks on foundations of your profession can also help you in your reflection. Discuss these questions with your fieldwork educator and other health professionals and students.

Case Study 7.1 | John Doe

John Doe is a 39-year-old IT technician in a secondary school. He has been married for 15 years. His wife is a stay-at-home mother who takes care of their four children. Recent budget cuts and restructure in the education system have meant that now John needs to travel between three different schools. He has been feeling anxious and has had trouble sleeping for the last four to five weeks. Originally, John seemed a bit depressed and tired, but over the past few weeks his mood has changed. He is very enthusiastic about his work, has several major IT projects for the different schools, and even plans a trip overseas to promote his projects to other schools. He can get a bit aggressive when his wife tells him that his plans are not realistic, and that he might have to tone down his ambitions a bit. He has been spending money irresponsibly, and John's wife is seriously concerned about his behaviour.

Recently, John has bought a brand new and very expensive car with every possible gadget. One afternoon, he picked up his children from school and took them for a ride to test the new car. He was arrested on the freeway after being chased by the police for over 45 minutes. John was driving 50 kilometres over the speed limit. When the police finally stopped him, he was disorganised, overexcited and irrational. He was saying he had been hired by a major car company to test the new IT technology on their latest cars.

The police officers contacted John's wife, and they took him to the nearest hospital. John was admitted to the psychiatric ward after a bipolar disorder was diagnosed at the

(continued)

emergency department by the consultant psychiatrist. John wants to leave the hospital and go back to work and to his family. He says he values his work and that his role as a father means everything to him. John's employer is concerned about John's capacity to return to work and John's wife is afraid he will put the children's lives and his own in danger again. She is also concerned about loss of income.

You are part of the mental health team. The team is made up of a psychiatrist, a nurse, an occupational therapist, a social worker and a psychologist. Here are a few concerns the team members have identified.

Your first task is to match each concern with one (or more) member of the team and to provide one justification for each choice.

Return to work	
Medication management	
Living arrangement	
Family interactions	
Role as a father and a husband	
Cognitive skills	
Expression and management of emotions	
Meaningful activities	
Parental capacity	
Social interactions	
Others:	

Once you have completed the first part, compare your results with other health students or professionals. Discuss your choices and justifications and decide if any adjustment should be made.

Feel free to add ideas about any other areas of John's level of function and match them to ideas presented by other members of the team.

> **Something to think about**
>
> 1   How did you find this exercise?
> 2   How well did you know the different roles of the team members?
> 3   Was there role blurring?
> 4   How can you maintain your specificity and be part of a team?

Knowing and understanding each other's role and responsibilities within the team is important because it decreases professional self-doubt, limits conflicts and adherence to uniprofessional culture, promotes continuity of care and of services and increases job satisfaction (Lloyd et al. 2005; Peck & Norman 1999).

SUMMARY

This chapter aimed at exploring the field of mental health. The very nature of mental health and mental illnesses may contribute to some of the feelings and perceptions individuals have towards them. Stigma and myths about mental health are common among members of the general public, and we are all exposed to them. It was important to take time to acknowledge individual concerns and perceptions, as you are getting ready to start a placement in mental health.

Reflecting on your own perceptions and beliefs about mental health helps you to face any resistance you might have to undertaking the placement. Discussing these beliefs with your fieldwork educator or with other health students that are in a similar situation can help you identify strategies and actions. This chapter was also aimed at identifying strategies and actions to prepare you for some of the challenges reported in the literature about mental health. However, remember that specific theoretical foundations, intervention procedures and other aspects of your work in mental health will be influenced by your professional background and training. Instead, it was meant as an introduction to mental health practice and aimed at demystifying the possible concerns or fears you might have toward this field of health care services.

DISCUSSION QUESTIONS

1   Reflect on a past or current situation where you felt particularly stressed, sad or anxious. How did your emotions have an impact on your daily life? How did you deal with the situation? What sort of support did you get?

2   Think about a person with a mental health issue that you might have met or worked with in a fieldwork placement. What were your first thoughts and reactions then? Have they evolved? In what way?

3   What are the aspects of mental health practice, services and resources that affect you the most? What surprises you? What makes you feel uncomfortable? What should change? How can you, as an individual and as a mental health professional, contribute to these changes?

References

American Psychiatric Association (2002). *Diagnostic and Statistical Manual of Mental Disorders* (4th edn) Text Revision, American Psychiatric Association, Washington, DC.

Blair, S., Hume, C. & Creek, J. (2007). 'Occupational Perspectives on Mental Health and Well-being'. In J. Creek & L. Lougher (eds) *Occupational Therapy and Mental Health*. Churchill Livingstone Elsevier, Philadelphia, PA.

Department of Veterans Affairs (2008a). *Stigma*. <http://at-ease.dva.gov.au/www/html/88-stigma.asp> accessed 30 January 2009.

Department of Veterans Affairs (2008b). *Debunking the Myths*. <http://at-ease.dva.gov.au/www/html/87-debunking-the-myths.asp> accessed 30 January 2009.

Healey, J. & Spencer, M. (2008). *Surviving Your Placement in Health and Social Care: A Student Handbook*. McGraw Hill, New York.

Higgs, J. & Jones, M. (2000). *Clinical Reasoning in the Health Professions*. Butterworth Heinemann, Boston, MA.

Lloyd, C., McKenna, K. & King, R. (2005). 'Sources of Stress Experienced by Occupational Therapists and Social Workers in Mental Health Settings'. *Occupational Therapy International*, 12(2), 81–94.

Moore, B. (2004). *Australian Oxford Dictionary* (2nd edn). Oxford University Press, Melbourne.

Peck, E. & Norman, I. (1999). 'Working Together in Adult Community Mental Health Services: Exploring Inter-Professional Role Relations'. *Journal of Mental Health*, 8(3): 231–42.

Sadock, B. J. & Sadock, V. A. (2007). *Kaplan and Sadock's Synopsis of Psychiatry: Behavioral Sciences/Clinical Psychiatry* (10th edn). Wolters Kluwer Health/Lippincott Williams & Wilkins, Philadelphia, PA.

Scottish Public Mental Health Alliance (2002). *With Health in Mind: Improving Mental Health and Wellbeing in Scotland: A Document to Support Discussion and Action*. Scottish Development Centre for Mental Health, Edinburgh.

Sladyk, K. (2002). *The Successful Occupational Therapy Fieldwork Student*. Slack Incorporated, Thorofare, NJ.

World Health Organization (WHO) (2009). *Mental Health*. <http://www.who.int/topics/mental_health/en/> accessed 30 January 2009.

CHAPTER 8
WORKING IN WORKPLACE PRACTICE

Michelle Conlan

LEARNING OUTCOMES

After reading this chapter, you should be able to:
- provide an overview of areas of work practice for health professionals
- describe the aims and processes of occupational and vocational rehabilitation
- locate resources and references to enable further information gathering
- discuss the behaviour expected of students on fieldwork placements in work practice
- reflect on how to approach a particular problem when practising in the field of work practice

KEY TERMS

Injured worker
Job seeking
Negotiation
Occupational rehabilitation
Rehabilitation provider
Return-to-work plan
Vocational rehabilitation
Work practice

INTRODUCTION

In case you are not familiar with what is involved in workplace practice, this chapter begins with an explanation of what workplace practice is and what is involved. Health professionals are employed in a wide variety of areas within the health care sector, including rehabilitation consultants, injury management advisers and rehabilitation coordinators, or clinicians, such as occupational therapists, physiotherapists, psychologists, podiatrists or social workers.

In this chapter, work practice refers to workplace-based or work-related services to employers, insurers and other stakeholders. It also refers to services provided to an individual seeking employment or currently working.

Areas of employment for health professionals in work practice include but are not limited to the following:
- rehabilitation providers
- insurance companies

- private and public companies
- private practice
- training organisations
- government authorities, such as Comcare (federal workers compensation authority), state workers compensation and occupational health and safety bodies
- hospitals and community health centres
- medical equipment supply companies.

Health professionals employed in work practice areas provide a wide range of services, such as health treatment and examinations, educational programs and consulting.

Health treatment services include, for instance, counselling, physical manipulation and treatment, exercise, massage services to injured workers, immunisation programs or pre-employment medical examinations. Other services include the management of occupational health and safety within the company or return-to-work programs offered to injured workers.

Health professionals may consult to industry on a range of issues, including developing policies and procedures to improve health and safety of employees, change management strategies and mediation services. Educational services may involve providing training to employers, employees and service providers, or in providing employee assistance programs to staff. Health professionals employed in these areas of work practice are also often members of multidisciplinary teams providing services to assist individuals to manage their injuries or disabilities and to return to or enter the workforce.

OCCUPATIONAL REHABILITATION

Health professionals employed in occupational rehabilitation agencies aim to 'return injured workers to appropriate work in a timely and sustainable way' (Worksafe, 2008). Within Australia, workers' rights are protected by state and federal workers compensation legislation. Rehabilitation consultants work within the guidelines of the relevant Acts to assist individuals to return to the workforce following a work

REFLECTION 8.1

Your work habits
Have you or do you work in paid employment? Under what conditions and awards do you work? Are you aware of safety procedures at your paid employment? What are these? Do you adhere to them?

related injury. Rehabilitation consultants may also assist those individuals to return to work if they are covered by legislation such as compulsory third party, motor vehicle and military compensation schemes. Figure 8.1 shows the stakeholders in the occupational rehabilitation process.

In occupational rehabilitation, unlike many other areas of health practice, the customer is usually the insurance agent. It is the insurer who approves the services to be provided and payment for services, and dictates the timelines for meeting specific milestones.

Although the rehabilitation consultants' aim is to assist the worker to return to work and address any identified barriers, this is performed in the context of claims management and under the guidelines of what is and is not allowed under the relevant Act. The insurer will decide whether or not a rehabilitation provider can continue to provide services. At times rehabilitation consultants will be asked to withdraw from a case before they have achieved all that they wanted to or believed they could achieve.

As occupational rehabilitation is provided at most workplaces, you can expect to visit a variety of workplaces while on fieldwork. The purpose of these visits may be to meet with injured workers, the workers' supervisor and/or the return-to-work coordinator for the company. During these meetings information is gathered regarding:

• the injury
• current work capacity

Figure 8.1: Stakeholders in the occupational rehabilitation process

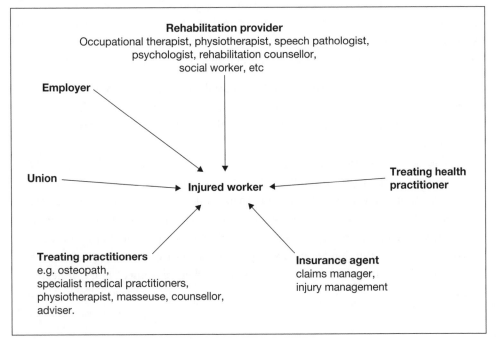

- medical restrictions
- planned treatment
- social and psychological status
- usual work performed
- opportunity to provide or perform alternative duties at the workplace.

Often a worksite assessment is conducted following such meetings to gain an understanding of the specific physical, cognitive and environmental requirements of the usual and/or alternative job options for the injured worker. Following an initial assessment visit, the rehabilitation consultant will write reports and prepare return-to-work plans. At this time, contact is made with other stakeholders, including treating health practitioners and the insurer. Depending on your course year level, this may be an area that you observe, but may be unable to undertake independently, or will have to complete under supervision.

You may have limited opportunity for direct involvement in a case, because of current or potential legal claims.

Through observation you can begin to understand the processes involved and can identify skills required to facilitate a successful return to work. Although it may not always be possible to conduct an assessment or provide counselling to a client, you may be able to practise this with your fieldwork educator or peers.

VOCATIONAL REHABILITATION

Vocational rehabilitation services in Australia are generally provided to people with disabilities who receive government benefits, including unemployed people and single parents. The scheme is currently managed by the Commonwealth Department of Education, Employment, and Workplace Relations (DEEWR).

> Vocational Rehabilitation Services (VRS) provide a comprehensive intervention, combining vocational rehabilitation with employment assistance. VRS assists people who have an injury, disability or health condition to work independently in the open labour market.
>
> The focus of the intervention is to assist the job seeker to understand, compensate for or manage their injury, disability or health condition, or the resulting limitations or restrictions they may face. It helps them build work capacity and/or avoid re-injury, find and/or retain employment. Vocational Rehabilitation providers work closely with employers to ensure safe and sustainable employment opportunities. Vocational Rehabilitation Services also provide assistance for existing employees who may be in danger of losing their job due to their disability, injury or health condition.

<workplace.gov.au> 2009

Case Study 8.1   A referral from the DVA

Joe, a 42-year-old ex-serviceman, was referred by the Department of Veterans Affairs (DVA) for assistance to return to meaningful employment. He presents with the following problems:

Medical history

- Psoriasis
- Hearing loss
- Anxiety
- Depression
- Bilateral hip arthritis
- Alcohol abuse.

Additional issues

- Recent marriage breakup, property settlement pending, limited access to children, living in temporary accommodation
- Withdrawal from social network, few interests, working part-time in a job he doesn't enjoy
- Has applied for 80 jobs over 2 years; has had 18 interviews but has been unsuccessful
- Sensitivity to products containing formaldehyde, such as photocopiers, chipboard, new carpets.

You have been observing your fieldwork educator interviewing Joe, and feel overwhelmed by all the issues that need to be considered to keep Joe at work. After Joe has left, your fieldwork educator turns to you and asks you:

- 'What are the barriers facing Joe?'
- 'How do they have an impact on his ability to work?'
- 'What interventions could you recommend to address these?'
- 'How do you ensure all key stakeholders remain connected and aim for the same outcome?'
- 'What strategies would you put into place to try to keep this man at work?'

You feel a little stunned, because you are still coping with all the issues that confront Joe. Your fieldwork educator recognises that you are not sure where to start, so she begins to discuss some of the actions that may be taken by a health professional in this scenario.

(continued)

These include:

- liaison with the treating health practitioner and other treatment providers—such as counsellor to establish the prognosis for each of his medical conditions—and to seek information relating to suitable work guidelines and restrictions
- monitoring the effectiveness of current strategies in place to deal with Joe's social problems; referring Joe on to other qualified service providers to address some of these issues if necessary, such as alcohol rehabilitation, personal counselling, involvement in social activity (community or support groups) and legal consultation
- preparation for *job seeking*: clarify suitable work areas, write new resumé, provide interview practice, provide education and/or counselling re disclosing details of his disability to potential employers, and answering questions related to his personal life in a way that doesn't create emotional distress during a job interview situation
- providing job-seeking assistance: identify job vacancies, review job application letters, investigate and apply for employment incentives and specific employment-related programs if available
- supporting and monitoring the client throughout the rehabilitation process and once employment is obtained
- maintaining regular communication (verbal and written) with all stakeholders, and ensuring all parties are in agreement and aware of this man's rehabilitation goals.

REFLECTION 8.2

Joe

Did you think about the questions on Joe's plan before you read some solutions? How would you implement the solutions suggested by the fieldwork educator? Joe will require ongoing case management. Ongoing case management tasks would include writing progress reports, liaising with key parties to seek or provide information to progress the case, checking that funding is available and planning timelines are still valid to ensure the rehabilitation provider will be paid for the services provided. Record the time spent on the case, and invoice DVA monthly.

Case Study 8.2   Workplace safety

You visit a car-manufacturing factory with a psychologist and an occupational therapist to consult with management as part of a plan to improve workplace safety and integrate a second factory into the operations. You have been informed that the second group of workers (from the second factory) is unhappy about moving locations and being asked to take a pay cut to work at a lower classification.

The psychologist aims to advise management about how to introduce the second group of workers to head off issues of job uncertainty, competition, poor communication and poor morale.

The occupational therapist has been asked to undertake a workplace assessment to evaluate the work currently performed and the working environment, and to make recommendations to improve workplace safety and minimise the risk of injury.

As you move around the factory with the health professionals, you notice what appears to be a worker removing a guard from one of the process lines. Before you have time to investigate further, you are taken into an office to meet with representatives of management.

Immediately you feel tense in the stomach. Several questions arise about your role as a student in this situation:

1   What should you do about what you have seen?
2   Is it your place to mention the apparent tampering with equipment and resultant safety hazard?
3   If you do raise the issue, who should you talk to and when?

REFLECTION 8.3

Uncertainty

Have you ever had an experience where you were not sure about the boundaries of your role—how you should act, if you have the authority to speak out and the scope of your responsibility? Have you ever experienced conflict between your professional, moral, ethical, and legal responsibilities? Should there ever be a conflict between these four responsibilities?

In a situation such as Case Study 8.2, it is important that you are reasonably certain about what you have seen and not jump to conclusions. It would not be appropriate to interrupt the meeting and state your suspicions or speak in an accusatory manner in front of management. It would, however, be appropriate to mention to the health professionals privately, and as soon as possible, what you saw or thought you had seen. This would ensure you act professionally and are meeting your duty of care obligations to do what you can to facilitate safety in the workplace.

If after investigation you conclude that there was no risk to workers, the worst thing that could happen is that you have increased your knowledge of workplace safety and the method of assessing potential hazards.

You should be encouraged to raise your observations and uncertainties with the fieldwork educator; however this needs to be done in a non-judgmental way and at an appropriate time and place.

Case Study 8.3   The negotiation

You have accompanied a rehabilitation consultant to a workplace and are sitting in a boardroom observing the negotiations taking place between the employer and an injured worker. The negotiation is being facilitated by the rehabilitation consultant, who has recommended what she believes to be suitable hours and duties for a return-to-work plan. It is apparent that the worker is resistant to returning to work, and the employer is prescribing the limited options available. The employer is only interested in returning the injured worker to his pre-injury duties, and will not consider flexible work hours.

When the group breaks for coffee, the worker begins talking to you. He reveals that he is planning to sue the employer for negligence. He plans to exaggerate his incapacity in the hope of getting a larger sum awarded to him.

REFLECTION 8.4

Dilemma

The worker has just informed you of his intentions to sue and exaggerate his incapacity (see Case Study 8.3). You try to stay calm and composed. What should you do in this situation? Should you mention to the injured worker's supervisor what has just been said? What should your immediate response be to the injured worker?

An appropriate response

It is important that the rehabilitation consultant knows about the information given to you, as this could have a serious impact on the return-to-work program. It also gives an insight into the reason behind the hostilities between employer and employee. You should discuss this with your fieldwork educator; however, do this privately and at an appropriate time and place.

You need to remain professional at all times and not be drawn into the worker's plans. As you must remain objective and impartial, an appropriate response to the worker might be, 'It is important that the rehabilitation consultant knows this. Would you talk to her about this after the meeting?' You could then politely excuse yourself from the conversation, thereby limiting the opportunity for further dialogue when the rehabilitation consultant is not present.

SKILLS REQUIRED FOR WORKING IN WORKPLACE PRACTICE

Health professionals require a range of skills to be effective providers of vocational and occupational rehabilitation, and to provide services in the area of work practice.

You can offer many skills because of the depth of your education and personal development as well as because of family and community interactions. These skills include:

- communication (written and verbal)
- negotiation and mediation
- observation
- computer proficiency
- time management and organisation
- problem-solving ability
- leadership (ability to facilitate progress and drive the process)
- ability to motivate clients
- ability to manage a budget
- customer focus
- awareness of the importance of outcomes
- task analysis and assessment
- knowledge of health and disability benefits (Mitchell 2008)
- understanding of numerous health conditions: their functional, psychological and social implications and likely treatments
- knowledge of the accident compensation and occupational health and safety Acts (both state and federal)
- knowledge of the service requirements and procedures required of health professionals working in various compensation systems, such as the ability to work to specific requirements; for example, specific forms, time lines and key performance indicators.

The health professional's role in vocational and occupational rehabilitation and work practice areas is to provide expertise to facilitate the return-to-work process. Comcare (2008) states that an approved rehabilitation provider is required to:

- provide expert, objective advice to the case manager to assist the timely, safe and durable return to work of an injured employee
- engage the injured employee, treating doctor and supervisor in the development and implementation of a tailored return-to-work plan
- monitor the return-to-work plan and communicate regularly with all parties to ensure the goals are achieved.

You will observe specific activities during a workplace fieldwork placement. Although they will vary according to the nature of the injury and individual circumstances, these activities could include:

- assessments of such matters as initial needs, vocational and functional capacity, and worksite, physical and cognitive abilities
- counselling
- job analysis to identify the nature and physical requirements of the job tasks (Mitchell 2008)

- negotiation of return-to-work plans
- career counselling
- stress management
- conflict resolution
- coaching and training
- work conditioning
- case management, including managing a program, seeking funding, invoicing and liaising with all stakeholders
- report writing
- provision of job-seeking assistance; for example, preparing resumés, conducting interviews, and providing education to clients about job seeking and helping them to acquire or improve the required skills.

FIELDWORK PLACEMENT AREAS

You may attend a number of different fieldwork placements to expose you to the area of work practice and to apply and consolidate your knowledge and skills in these areas. Placements may be alongside other health professionals in a hospital or with a vocational rehabilitation provider, or you may be placed in a workplace where you observe a variety of work operations, practices and environments. Traditional health placements, such as hospitals and community health settings, can provide you with the opportunity to assess and provide interventions for an individual of working age who requires assistance to keep or return to his or her job.

Preparation for fieldwork

You will gain a great deal from your fieldwork placement if you are willing to observe and understand the work area you are observing. When undertaking a placement in the area of work practice, it is recommended that you prepare the following:
- research the workplace or industry being visited to gain an understanding of the scope of the work undertaken, workplace hazards and types of injuries that are prevalent in the industry. This information can generally be found on the Internet, through company annual reports and from occupational health and safety/workers compensation authorities; for example, Worksafe Victoria (injury hotspots)
- become familiar with assessment checklists used by health professionals
- become familiar with the relevant legislation; this will assist your understanding of the purpose of the referral and what is expected to be achieved. In particular, look at the rights and responsibilities of employers and employees, as this will help you gain an understanding of the requirements and motivations of these key stakeholders

- read client files before an appointment in order to understand the background to the case, and question your fieldwork educator if it is not clear what is taking place
- familiarise yourself with the current labour market, including where current job vacancies appear and areas of skill shortage.

Student behaviour

As in any other area of fieldwork, you are expected to display professional and appropriate behaviour at all times while on placement. It is important that you consider the environment, and dress appropriately. For example, if you are visiting a refrigerated meat-processing plant, dress for cold conditions and wear appropriate footwear and clothing. You should also consider the mix of workers (male and female) and the culture of the workplace, and ensure your clothing is appropriate.

You must protect the privacy and confidentiality of your clients, and carefully store and, where necessary, destroy all written materials, notes and assessment forms according to the agency policy. You must be mindful of commercial confidences and not publish or talk freely about the practices of the workplace you have visited. In addition, you must consider the sensitivity of the information received, and communicate information with sensitivity and professionalism.

THINK AND LINK 8.1

Chapters 21 and 22 go into more depth about your responsibilities as a student on placement. Protecting privacy and confidentiality of clients in all placements is a vital part of your professional behaviour.

When writing reports and case notes, be careful to ensure that what is written is accurate and objective. In the area of work practice, the likelihood of a health professional being subpoenaed to court is increased because of the high levels of legal action taken by injured workers, employers and insurers.

Familiarise yourself with the workplaces you are visiting, and comply with the site-specific occupational health and safety requirements. For example, if hard hats, hearing protection and high visibility vests are required, you must comply for your own and others' safety.

Gobelet and colleagues (2007) state that there are financial costs in vocational rehabilitation that are borne by state organisations and by employers and private insurers. You need to be aware that each interaction with an individual will attract a fee, and therefore you need to be well prepared and attempt to provide a service of the highest possible quality.

THINK AND LINK 8.2

Undertaking fieldwork placement in services where fees are charged changes the relationship between the client and the student. Chapter 9 discusses fieldwork placements in private practice, highlighting what is different about this context of fieldwork experience.

SUMMARY

Undertaking a fieldwork placement in workplace practice will expose you to the development of many skills and a different type of health service. When working with individual clients (that is, injured workers or job seekers) you will be learning about the health conditions suffered by clients, including likely prognoses and treatments. You will learn about which legislative system (if any) the client is covered by, such as workers compensation, transport or accident. You will be undertaking a placement where customers are usually insurance agents who have asked rehabilitation providers to provide a certain service. In workplace practice, you will need to discuss with your fieldwork educator whether there are any conflicts between stakeholders. These stakeholders are the worker and employer, and worker and insurance company. You will learn the format of writing case notes or reports, and you should welcome your fieldwork educator's comments on your writing so that you learn to be objective in your written and verbal communication and not make assumptions. You will learn about negotiation, and how not to make promises to workers or employers, as you are a student on placement. You will, however, discuss with your fieldwork educator the scope of your job. In these situations, you should be keenly aware of your professional boundaries, which means that you do not advise on areas outside of your area of expertise. For example, an occupational therapist providing occupational rehabilitation services should not give advice on claims management areas, such as entitlement to benefits.

DISCUSSION QUESTIONS

Set up a role play between an injured worker and an employer. The injured worker wants to talk to you about his or her dislike of the employer, and starts to make accusations about the employer.

1   How do you professionally keep a distance between yourself and the injured worker?
2   What would you say to the injured worker?
3   Discuss several ways to keep your professional boundaries when in conflict situations and under pressure.

References

Australian Bureau of Statistics (2007). *Work-Related Injuries*. Commonwealth of Australia, Canberra, 2005–06.

Gobelet, C., Luthi, F., Al-Khodairy, A. T. & Chamberlain, M. A. (2007). 'Vocational Rehabilitation: A Multidisciplinary Intervention'. *Disability and Rehabilitation*, 29(17): 1405–10.

Mitchell, T. (2008). 'Utilization of the Functional Capacity Evaluation in Vocational Rehabilitation'. *Journal of Vocational Rehabilitation*, 28: 21–8.

Worksafe Victoria (2008). *Annual Report 2008* <worksafe.vic.gov.au> accessed 24 January 2009.

Useful Websites

Australian Psychological Society: www.psychology.org.au

Comcare: www.comcare.gov.au

CRS Australia: www.crsaustralia.gov.au

MyCareer: www.mycareer.com.au

OT Australia (Australian Association of Occupational Therapists): www.ausot.com.au

CHAPTER 9
WORKING IN PRIVATE PRACTICE

Tim Kauffman, Phoebe Maloney and Adrian Schoo

LEARNING OUTCOMES

After reading this chapter, you should be able to:
- discuss how private practice settings differ from traditional placements
- recognise the importance of private practices as treatment centres
- appreciate the transition from an academic to a clinical education
- understand the challenges to you as a student in a private practice setting
- understand the opportunities for students and practitioners in the private practice setting.

KEY TERMS

Entrepreneur
Private practice
Private practitioner

INTRODUCTION

Fieldwork placements are crucial to your professional development as health professional student. At present, one expanding area of health education is the delivery of physical and occupational therapy programs that explore the use of the private practice settings as learning opportunities for students. In general, private practice is autonomous, entrepreneurial and possibly lucrative; but it is also challenging, litigious, and takes the capital and resources of the private practitioner to establish it, with some of them going into debt as they build up their private practice. These factors make work-integrated learning in a private practice different from a hospital or clinic setting. Also, the privately owned practice is not identical to the hospital established outpatient clinic, the physician-owned practice or the corporate-owned franchise. Such settings reduce or mitigate the autonomous and entrepreneurial nature of practice, and reduce the personal risks to capital and resources. This chapter will introduce you to some of the similarities of and differences between fieldwork placement experiences in private practice settings compared with the more traditional hospital, clinic or ward settings.

Private practice is international, and is growing as a therapy and health service area. The World Federation of Occupational Therapists recognises private practice as an important expanding area for the delivery of patient care services. The World

Confederation of Physical Therapy's specific declaration of principle states, 'there should be no impediment to physical therapists entering into private practice in which physical therapists deliver services to patients or clients in accordance with government laws, rules and/or regulations'. The worldwide importance of private practice is evidenced by the International Private Practitioner Association (IPPA), which is a subgroup of the World Confederation of Physical Therapy. There are 21 member countries in the IPPA, and numerous other countries are involved with it (Jerry Klug, President of IPPA, personal communication 2008). It is difficult to estimate how many health professionals work in private settings worldwide, because some work full-time, others work part-time and others see only an occasional patient. Also, private practice may not be defined the same in all countries.

WORK-INTEGRATED LEARNING AND THE STUDENT

Regardless of the setting, the fundamentals of work-integrated learning are the same. These include the interactions between patients and you and your fieldwork educator (Paschal 2002). One major difference between hospital and non-hospital settings is the patient. Especially in the United States, hospitals are largely acute care facilities, and the goals of health care are to stabilise the patient as quickly as possible and discharge him or her to another setting. In community or non-hospital care, the patient or client is usually not in acute distress or in a medical emergency. As a result, you see a different stage and a wider range of rehabilitation, and thus intervention and goals of care are different. Clients have other daily needs, such as school, work, sport, health, fitness and recreation, and hence their decision to seek care and their desired outcomes are not identical to those of hospitalised patients. The client's health needs usually do not warrant daily care, and treatments may extend for long periods, possibly even for months.

Perhaps a greater issue for you is to recognise the fundamental difference between academic and work-integrated learning. This difference applies to both hospital and private practice settings. As Gandy (2002) indicates, academic education occurs within a higher education setting, with its purpose to teach core knowledge, skills and behaviours. Work-integrated learning takes place within a practice environment that is focused on providing cost-effective, high-quality care, as well as education for patients and their families. One very important factor to recognise is that fieldwork educators usually are not paid for teaching students, and this can influence the decision of the private practitioner to accept or refuse students. In 2009, a survey of allied health professionals in rural settings was undertaken to gather data on the challenges and opportunities of supervising students in a private practice (Maloney 2009). The majority of the respondents were aged 50–54 years, and there were 45 females and 27 males in the sample. Seventy-two private practitioners returned their surveys; of these 53 had experience supervising students. Seventeen respondents did not supervise students. Of these respondents, 16.7 per cent indicated that practice profitability influenced their decision not to supervise students and 61.1 per cent of private practitioners reported that financial recognition for supervising students would encourage them to supervise in the future (Maloney 2009). Nonetheless, fieldwork educators in all settings have the responsibility for assisting you to make a transition between academic learning and clinical skills with real patients or clients. Work-integrated learning is not a university laboratory practice session.

As Paschal stated, 'the clinical education experience belongs to the student, despite the fact that it occurs in the CI's clinic' (2002). In other words, you must be actively engaged in fieldwork learning; and this includes setting specific learning objectives with your fieldwork educator. On placement in a private practice, it is important for you to have a reasonable level of personal autonomy and independence. Working in private practice involves varying amounts of client contact time and time spent fulfilling other administrative and business responsibilities. To make the most of your private practice placement, it is important for you to be willing to accept fluctuating levels of client–contact time, and be prepared to use your 'down time' productively. The end result is you becoming a graduate who can undertake clinical decision-making based upon knowledge and clinical skills, and also able to demonstrate professional demeanour, interpersonal communication and self-directed learning.

THINK AND LINK 9.1

Undertaking a placement in a private practice setting will introduce you to a range of new skills. Chapter 13 provides information and some reflections on how to capitalise on your learning opportunities.

CHALLENGES AND OPPORTUNITIES

The skills required to provide care to clients in a private practice setting are similar to those in other settings, but also include financial requirements that are often not experienced in other healthcare settings by health professionals. The financial considerations are similar to the business skills required by the manager of a clinic in a hospital setting. In a private practice experience, you may have more opportunity to be exposed to business issues, including fees, target revenues, costs for labour, taxes, equipment, supplies, overhead, medico-legal concerns and marketing. The concepts can be invaluable for later career decisions about going into one's own practice or moving into management.

Often in the private practice setting, there is a reluctance to accept students because of a sense of greater liability (Doubt et al. 2004); but this may be illusory, because there are fewer layers of management than in large health centres. As Jette and colleagues (2007) indicated, safety is a crucial issue in health settings. Maloney (2009) found that the top three reasons given by private practitioners to supervise students were: the level of clinical skills and experience of students (23.6 per cent); benefits to the professional's own clinical skills and experience (20.8 per cent); and their past experience supervising students (18.1 per cent).

In many countries, clients can now enjoy direct access to therapy and other health services without a physician's referral. This is becoming more common; a World Confederation of Physical Therapy (2003) report indicated that the outcomes of educational programs in Australia, Brazil, Canada, Jamaica, Norway and South Africa are intended for graduates to work autonomously and/or in primary care (Takahashi et al. 2003). Forty-four states of the United States of America, the District of Columbia and the entire military system permit direct access to physical therapists who have received special training and licensure.

But this access to direct primary therapy care increases risk, especially in a litigious society like the United States. This is more of a concern in private practice, which does not have the protection given to large hospital or national health systems. Private practitioners also must pay their own insurance, which is often high. On the other hand, a large study involving direct access by 50,799 patients in US military healthcare facilities showed no adverse events for patients or therapists. There were no licence, credential, litigation or disciplinary actions for the physiotherapists working in military facilities (Moore et al. 2005).

Other challenges that you may encounter in the private practice setting include the difficulty of supervision at all times and the patient paying for service. In the United States in particular, some insurance companies and specifically Medicare, the national health insurance system for most persons over the age of 65 years in the United States, clearly state that students may not treat Medicare beneficiaries and bill for those services unless they are directly supervised in the room by a licensed practitioner. This requirement has had an adverse effect on the training of students in private practice in the care of older persons. Similar concerns were found among private practice physiotherapists and occupational therapists in Canada (Doubt et al. 2004).

The requirement for you to be supervised at all times when treating patients or clients in private practice presents time constraints for the fieldwork educator, and may discourage private practitioners from working with students. In the 2009 survey (Maloney 2009), the top three reasons given by private practitioners for deciding not to supervise students were: time taken from productive work directly with clients (43.1 per cent); concern with client satisfaction in being seen by a student (27.8 per cent); and practice productivity (22.2 per cent). When the concerns of all 72 professionals were taken into consideration, time taken to supervise a student (72.2 per cent); the client's willingness to be treated by a student (51.4 per cent); and workplace productivity (43.1 per cent) were cited as the top three barriers in supervision of students. These findings agree with Doubt and colleagues (2004) that 'time is money'.

Also, some private practices have concerns about their reputation in the patient population and among their referral sources; thus they do not want students to treat their patients. This may become more problematic when the patient does not get fully refunded from a health fund. For example, 10 years ago for physiotherapy the patient only paid $5–15 in Northeast United States. Now it is $10–50. Do patients feel they are 'getting their money's worth' when they are treated by a student? This may become more problematic, as health insurance companies or possibly health funds require patients to make a payment for each date of care.

Case Study 9.1   Be quick in private practice

A physiotherapy student, who was in her final year, was asked to evaluate a client with multiple sclerosis. The student prepared for this responsibility, but failed to realise the importance of time that pertains to the clinic's schedule for the treating therapist and for the client who may need to return to work. The student in this case performed a comprehensive but not fully focused evaluation that lasted 3½ hours and could have gone longer. The student was doing everything she was taught in the academic setting, and the client, in this case, was enjoying the personal attention. However, the fieldwork educator had to stop the session because it was unrealistic for an evaluation to take so long. The student still did not focus on any specific problem and plan of care. Most importantly, the client was also exhausted and the student failed to recognise it. In this circumstance an inordinate amount of therapist's time was spent on this one case and student. Despite the length of time, the clinic was going to be paid a set fee for an initial assessment, not for the full 3½ hours.

Questions
1. What are three reasons why the fieldwork educator intervened in the evaluation being conducted by the student?
2. Why is time a crucial factor in private practice?
3. How could the student prepare for the session to be more time efficient?

In the private practice setting, you usually have to deal with the requisite issues concerning time spent and charges: 'billable units'. This, however, can be an opportunity instead of a challenge, since you have a chance to learn some business skills and financial management.

Another opportunity for you during fieldwork placement in a private practice is the increased exposure to skilled and reputable practitioners, which may lead to future opportunities, including employment in that private practice. The same may be true in other fieldwork placement settings. However, the challenge may be to acknowledge that not all clients are comfortable with students, especially when the client is seeking and expecting care from an experienced and recognised therapist. Usually, this can be surmounted by you working together with the therapist, which allows you to demonstrate knowledge. Often clients are pleased to get extra attention from two persons. Having said that, whether you are on placement in a public or a private setting, client privacy and confidentiality should be at the core of all good therapeutic practice.

Case Study 9.2	Pleasing the client

A middle-aged woman with osteopaenia researched the Internet and the community to find a specialist to evaluate her risks and abilities and to establish a plan of intervention. The client was quite pleased because she found a therapist in her community who had spoken internationally and has published work on the subject of osteoporosis and bone health. Before proceeding with the evaluation, the specialist asked the client if she would permit a student to observe and participate. The client consented. During evaluation, many questions were asked by the client, and the specialist answered by speaking to the client and the student. Also, the physical findings, as well as palpation, were shared with the student. The specialist and the student felt the session went well.

Three weeks later, when the client returned for a review and to advance the intervention program she complained that she was frustrated with the time and focus that she felt was taken from her and spent teaching the student. From the specialist's perspective, the time spent explaining, answering and teaching was aimed at the patient and the student, and was beneficial to both. In this case, despite asking the client's permission to allow the student to participate, it presented a challenge.

Question

How would you deal with this situation? What factors need to be considered for the best interests of:

- the client?
- the student?
- the practitioner?
- the private practice?

It is a good idea to ask your clinical supervisor about client–practitioner confidentiality policies before commencing any work pertaining to clients.

You may have the opportunity to observe and learn entrepreneurial skills and autonomy of practice when undertaking a placement in a private practice. In the future you may establish your own private practice. Observing a successful private practitioner is one of the best learning experiences for establishing one's own private practice.

One serious professional issue in any fieldwork education setting is the possibility of losing the focus of work-integrated learning. Some practitioners and managers may purposely understaff their clinics with licensed and expensive personnel in order to reduce their costs or to maximise their profits. Students can be used in this setting to offset those expenses. From an ethical perspective, this is improper.

SUMMARY

Fieldwork education is a crucial stage in the development of a profession. Private practice settings offer you experience in working in a business where fees, time spent with clients and quality of client care become a high consideration in practice. These considerations make fieldwork placements in private practice distinctive compared to other settings. In private practice settings you will be more closely supervised and may find that you observe more often than interact directly with clients.

DISCUSSION QUESTIONS

1   What do you think you would learn in a fieldwork placement in a private practice compared to a hospital setting?
2   How would you balance learning from the client and fieldwork educator with the pressure of time and time as money?

References

Doubt, L., Paterson, M. & O'Riordan, A. (2004). 'Clinical Education in Private Practice: An Interdisciplinary Project'. *Journal of Allied Health*, 33, 47–50.

Gandy, J. S. (2002). Preparation for Teaching Students in Clinical Settings. In K. F. Shepard, & G. M. Jensen (eds). *Handbook of Teaching for Physical Therapists* (2nd edn). Butterworth Heinemann, New Jersey: 211–53.

Jette, D. U., Bertoni, A., Coots, R., Johnson, H., McLaughlin, C. & Weisbach, C. (2007). 'Clinical Instructors' Perceptions of Behaviors that Comprise Entry Level Clinical Performance in Physical Therapy Students: A Qualitative Study'. *Physical Therapy*, 87: 833–43.

Maloney, P. (2009). Barriers and enablers to clinical placement in rural public and private practice. Unpublished honours thesis. Deakin University, Geelong.

Moore, J., McMillan, D., Rosenthal, M. & Weishaar, M. (2005). 'Risk Determination for Patients with Direct Access to Physical Therapy in Military Health Care Facilities.' *Journal of Orthopedic Sports Physical Therapy*, 35, 674–8.

Paschal, K. A. (2002). 'Techniques for Teaching Students in Clinical Settings'. In K. F. Shepard & G. M. Jensen (eds). *Handbook of Teaching for Physical Therapists* (2nd edn). Butterworth Heinemann, New Jersey: 255–85.

Takahashi, S., Killette, D. & Eftekari, T. (2003). *Exploring Issues Related to the Qualifications Recognition of Physical Therapists*. World Confederation of Physical Therapy, London.

CHAPTER 10
WORKING IN RURAL AND REMOTE SETTINGS

Paul Tinley

LEARNING OUTCOMES

After reading this chapter, you should be able to:
- discuss and contrast health issues in rural, regional, remote and metropolitan areas
- prepare for a fieldwork placement in a rural or remote setting
- discuss professional behaviours while on fieldwork placement.

KEY TERMS

Accommodation
Indigenous health settings
Professional standards and image
Remote and rural health settings
Royal Flying Doctor Service

INTRODUCTION: THE LIE OF THE LAND IN RURAL AND REMOTE AUSTRALIA

There are currently many government initiatives to promote practice in rural health settings, as this is seen as a 'priority area'. As a health professional student, you will be asked to attend a fieldwork placement in a regional, rural or remote setting as part of your professional entry level course. These fieldwork placements can appear exciting and challenging, but if not carefully managed, they can become problematic. With the correct preparation and flexibility, these placements can be very rewarding, with lots to be learnt and experienced. The rural experience may throw you out of your comfort zone, so knowing how to adapt will be an important part of success in these environments.

Before giving some useful hints and tips to surviving and getting the best out of your rural experience, it is important to discuss the issues and problems of life and health in rural practice. Perhaps this chapter should be called 'Don't Get Sick in Rural Areas'. The framework presented in this chapter, together with the suggested background reading, needs to be considered before you take part in a rural or regional fieldwork placement.

It is important to understand the lie of the land before you can fully appreciate why things happen differently in the rural and regional environment. Below are some useful data on rural health problems, access and numbers of rural health professionals in Australia. It is important to understand that these data are based on the Australian experience, and may not apply to other countries. For other countries, please check the relevant population demographics to give you the required snapshot of the population in which you will be working.

Australia has one of the most urbanised populations in the world. With 70 per cent of the population living in capital cities and major metropolitan areas, most of the population lives within 80 kilometres of the sea, making vast areas of inland Australia sparsely populated. Fifteen per cent of the population lives in or around major regional centres and 14 per cent lives near country or coastal towns surrounded by agricultural areas. Only 1 per cent of the Australian population lives in remote areas.

While city populations are increasing relatively fast, rural and remote populations are showing growth of less than 5 per cent per annum, and in many cases there is even a decline in growth. This means that populations are leaving rural and remote areas for cities and regional centres. Reasons for this include job accessibility, improvement in lifestyle and greater access to medical and social activity.

When we look at the 1 per cent of the population living in very remote areas, 40 per cent of this population is Indigenous. This compares with 5–25 per cent of the population in rural and remote areas being Indigenous, with less than 5 per cent in metropolitan centres. Rural populations also have greater numbers of children, but lower numbers of young adults. Younger adults form the population group most likely to be moving away from their rural townships and communities.

Other differences between rural and metropolitan areas are educational standards. Rural areas have generally lower educational standards than metropolitan centres. This may be a result of access issues, and in areas with high Indigenous populations perhaps lack of attendance. Rural areas have lower employment levels (less work available) and lower family incomes.

In general, food prices in rural and remote areas are 10 to 23 per cent higher because of transport costs, which means that there are fewer healthy food choices. Unhealthy food is generally cheaper than healthy foods, and use of tobacco and alcohol an accepted part of life.

Rural populations are involved in lower levels of physical activity, have greater levels of obesity, smoke more, drink more alcohol, have higher blood pressure and are more likely to have poor nutrition than city populations.

Hospital admission rates for remote populations are higher than in the city, with 1.5 to 1.8 times the rate of metropolitan populations. Factors that contribute to this may be distance from hospital or a greater incidence of accidents (farm and manual labour injury)—the true reason is unclear.

Death rates are 10 to 20 per cent higher in rural and regional areas than in metropolitan areas. This statistic, alarming in its own right, is mainly a result of increased overall Indigenous death rates, which are very high compared to those in metropolitan areas of Australia. The Indigenous median age is 20 years, whereas the Australian population median age is 34 years. The average life expectancy of the Indigenous population is 19–20 years lower than the rest of the population, with 2003 census data showing Indigenous males on average dying at 56 years, compared with the national average of 76 years. Indigenous females die at an average of 63 years, compared with the national average of 82 years (Australian Bureau of Statistics 2006). Indigenous populations are four times more likely to have type II diabetes, and have greater levels of respiratory and heart disease. They are more likely to have physical injury or suffer poisoning, and have a greater incidence of digestive disorders, kidney disease and renal failure. They also have a higher percentage of mental and behavioural disorders. We can clearly see that Australian Indigenous populations suffer a much greater health risk than metropolitan-based populations.

THINK AND LINK 10.1

Working in Indigenous communities can be a large part of fieldwork placement if your placement is in a rural or remote area. Chapter 11 is about working in Indigenous communities, and what you need to prepare for and understand when working in an environment that may be culturally different from your own. The second half of Chapter 2 also discusses working with people who come from backgrounds different from your own.

SO WHO CARES FOR THE RURAL AND REMOTE COMMUNITIES?

Another aspect of rural and remote settings is the number of health professionals per head of the population.

Table 10.1 is a snapshot of the ratio of health professionals to populations in rural and remote areas compared with metropolitan areas in Australia.

The good news is that some health professions show greater numbers in rural and remote areas compared with metropolitan areas. Community Health Service workers in metropolitan areas are 216:100,000, compared with 320:100,000 in remote areas. Ambulance services are generally better in regional and remote areas, with a ratio of 54:100,000 compared with 36:100,000. However, in very remote communities this decreases to 31:100,000.

The other significant factor is that distance is the major obstacle, with perhaps 100,000 people being spread very thinly across remote areas, with hundreds of kilometres between centres.

Table 10.1: Ratio of health professionals to population

	Ratio metropolitan areas	Ratio rural/remote areas
Non-psychiatric hospital health workers	1147:100,000	601:100,000
Nursing home staff	334:100,000	71:100,000
General practitioners	351:100,000	109:100,000
Specialist medical services	93:100,000	11:100,000
Optometrists	53:100,000	1.7:100,000
Physiotherapists	48:100,000	7.2:100,000
Child care services	311:100,000	199:100,000

Source: Australia's Health (2002). Australian Institute of Health and Welfare, Canberra. AIHW Cat. No. Aus 25.

So what does this all mean for rural populations? We have in broad terms a sicker, less educated population with poorer nutrition. This means that what works in the city may not be applicable in rural and remote conditions. There are fewer specialised rural health professionals, although they may have a broader set of generic skills than their urban-based colleagues. Despite having multiple skilled workers in rural and remote centres, access to health services is diminished, and we need to persuade more health professionals to move to rural and remote positions to improve the health of these populations.

PREPARING FOR RURAL PLACEMENT

The better prepared you are, the more you will gain from your fieldwork placement. Obtain background information from a number of sources to see which Indigenous group you will meet in your fieldwork placement, and the cultural differences and current clinical themes most commonly seen in the area. Is the Indigenous population matrilineal or patrilineal? Which tribe or clan is predominant in the area you are about to work in? Ensure that you are culturally prepared by reading a relevant text about the group you are about to meet. If you know of another student who has worked in this area before, talk with him or her: how did that student prepare? What advice can he or she offer you?

Consider the type and level of practice you will be expected to work in, and the background your fieldwork educators have. Are you working with a fieldwork educator who comes from the same discipline as you, or from another discipline but within a multidiscipline team? In many remote areas you may find that there is only a general health worker (possibly an Indigenous health worker), and no one from your discipline to lead and direct you, so you must be clear what it is you want to get out of the placement. Some flexibility will be expected, as often it's 'all hands on deck'. Have a clear understanding of why you are there.

It is also critical that you have a clear idea of the objectives of the fieldwork placement. Is it purely observational? Are you supposed to be learning a practical skill and become competent at it, or will you be working at a novice level?

THINK AND LINK 10.2

Health workers in Indigenous communities have a complex role to play in their community. Chapter 11 explains the health system within Indigenous communities and the roles of the workers within these communities.

FIND OUT FIRST (FOF)

Some critical issues you must address in preparation:
- What are the uniform requirements of the fieldwork placement? Should you be in a uniform? What does the university require of you? What does the placement require of you? Do you understand the placement standards? (Are there any?) Ask your fieldwork educator.
- How will your performance be assessed while on fieldwork placement? Is this a competency-based assessment? How do you meet the competency?
- How many hours are you expected to be engaged in the fieldwork placement? Often in remote situations you can have a feeling that you should be engaged all the time. Is this realistic, expected and appropriate? How will you get the best from this fieldwork placement?
- What are the start and finish dates for the fieldwork placement? Is travel time included? Who is providing the transport? Is it your responsibility to get to the rural centre and then be transported out to the remote centre? Is there a road trip or a flight on a transport plane? (FOF).
- Do you need a driver's licence?
- What time do you need to start on day one? (FOF)
- Can you confirm your accommodation? What type? What cost is the room, dormitory or tent?
- Where do you get food and drinks while on fieldwork placement?
- What are you going to do in the evenings: read a good book, listen to an iPod, play computer games or DVDs?

- What are the options for playing your sport? Many young people review their sport as a major part of their life. Can you still participate to a greater or lesser extent? Is it safe to do so?
- Will you be involved with the flying doctor service?

PROFESSIONAL BEHAVIOUR AND SURVIVING

Your *professional standards and image* will form an important part of how you will be evaluated by your fellow health professionals and others. First impressions do count, so your enthusiasm and flexibility for your fieldwork placement will be paramount. Your knowledge base should be of the correct standard. Saying 'I'm sorry I do not know' is just as important as having all the right answers. Remember that health theory and concepts often have a 25-year life span, so current clinical thinking may not be well accepted by longstanding health professionals, or may not be appropriate to the situation you are in. How you manage this may well have an impact on your enjoyment of your fieldwork placement. Be aware that even though your first impression might be 'I do not think I would do it like that!', the ability to use critical thinking within the environment in which the health care is being provided may be of much greater significance overall than best practice.

Issues of access, health and nutrition are all compromised in rural and remote environments. As a health professional, you may have to struggle long and hard to reach an effective compromise with your patients. Do not be too hasty with any criticism you have of technique and protocols used by local practitioners, as you may not be aware of the history of practice. Remember that communication is the key: ask the 'silly question', 'Why do you do it like that?' For support, you may need to stay in contact with your university placement officer, who may be able to advise you how to proceed in difficult situations.

Getting to know the team and the professional hierarchy is important. As a student, you are often way down the list in terms of role. Know who is in charge formally and informally: perhaps the reception staff or Indigenous health worker have a clearer understanding of the way the centre functions than the fly-in, fly-out specialist. Without local knowledge and a close relationship with the local community, remote centres cannot function. For example, often the janitor is also the security guard, the radiographic technician and plaster cast technical person. Show respect to everyone, as everyone is a cog in the complete machine.

A student's reflection on rural placement in Broken Hill
I have really enjoyed my stay in Broken Hill. I have been exploring, bushwalking in Mutawintji National Park, camel riding and bike riding, and visiting numerous art galleries. My time with the Royal Flying Doctor Service is one I will cherish forever. It is an experience few get to see, and I loved it!!! The health worker was a fantastic supervisor who guided me to become a better practitioner. I will continue to learn and use the skills she has shared with me. An experience that I will never forget ...

Question
What can a rural fieldwork placement offer that a metropolitan fieldwork placement cannot?

Working towards a particular competency assessment may be the objective of the placement, so what are these competencies and how will they be evaluated? Make sure your fieldwork educator has time to do the required assessments. Sometimes this is difficult, particularly during a crisis, when patient care overrides everything else. Try not to ask for your evaluation at the end of the day when everyone has gone to the pub. Make sure time is set aside for feedback and review of your fieldwork placement competencies.

In rural and remote settings you may work with several health professionals. Ensure you are *very* clear about your scope of practice, and stay within the bounds of your own discipline. You may be able to assist another professional from another health field, but never work independently outside your discipline.

THINK AND LINK 10.3

Working with others outside your discipline is discussed in more depth in Chapter 15. Chapter 15 considers fieldwork placements when you might be supervised by someone outside your discipline-specific area. In these situations you will often need to explain your profession and what your profession does. The same may occur when working in a rural or remote setting.

A positive aspect of this type of placement is that government agencies are currently trying to breach the workforce shortage in rural and remote areas, so you may be eligible for substantial scholarships or grants, to assist you with travel and living costs, for undertaking a rural or remote placement. Ask your university placement officer for more information about these schemes.

ACCOMMODATION AND LEISURE

The lack of 'quality' accommodation is often complained about while on fieldwork placement. Look around you. What is the local standard? Maybe your accommodation is the best there is in this particular setting. How much are you paying for it? Is it subsidised? If this is the case, can you really complain? Is it clean, with access to water and sanitation? It may lack air-conditioning and computer access, but it could be the only choice available.

If you are using shared facilities, ensure that you care for others. Is there a nightshift worker or nurse who is also in the accommodation? Can you really steal 'just a drop' of milk for your tea from the shared fridge? Many disputes have occurred from taking liberties in shared accommodation. It's just not worth it, so go get your own! Or ask.

What do you do in the evenings? When you are away from home, the status quo may not be possible; access to a TV may be limited, wireless access for your laptop or even power may be limited; so be flexible. Reading your study text might have seemed a good idea before you went on fieldwork placement, but relaxing with a trashy novel may just be the release you need after a busy day. Whatever you plan to do while you are away you will be lucky to get half of it finished. You may not get that essay written, or those ten chapters reviewed before the end of the fieldwork placement.

Enjoy the whole rural experience. Talk to the locals, go along to the dance on Saturday night, do the camel ride or enjoy the rodeo or whatever is on offer. Remember that pub culture is strong in rural communities, be it the football (footie) club bar or town pub. These are often the centre of all social and community functions. Make sure you have control of yourself; you need to uphold your self-control and drink sensibly, and stay in control. Excessive alcohol drinking will dehydrate you the next day, and may make you unfit to see patients. You must be able to function at your best while on fieldwork placement. One less drink is better than one more. For international students, or students whose background does not condone alcohol consumption, the best bet is to stay clear of the environment altogether. If you do attend, drink soft drinks and do not be pressured into alcohol consumption.

An important issue is: 'Where do I get food from?' Many fieldwork placements go out of their way to help and assist visiting students, as they want to give you the best experience possible. Often these special considerations have been hard fought for, so don't complain about what you have been given. Many placement sites in rural and remote centres have extremely limited resources, and food costs can be very high because of transport costs and lack of competition among providers. Basic food items are often two to three times more expensive than in the city. You may well be getting the best available, but not what you are used to. If you have special dietary needs, these must be known ahead of time, as access to specialist food items may not be possible or may be too costly. This may even be the reason for not going on placement in remote areas.

Other factors that you may not have thought about include fatigue from long working days and relative lack of sleep. Hot sun, hot days, hot nights, no sleep, dehydration (alcohol induced or otherwise) or acclimatisation issues will all add to your fatigue. Even small trips away can give you travel lag or jet lag. All these factors may take a toll on you and will affect your performance. Recognise your limitations: go to bed when *you* need to. Do not compromise yourself.

ROYAL FLYING DOCTOR SERVICE (RFDS)

The Royal Flying Doctor Service (RFDS) is an organisation you could become involved with, because of the distances involved on some placements. Remember, first, to minimise the stuff you want to bring. Take only a small bag with your essentials. If you do not like small planes, take a sick bag and nausea pills. If you really cannot cope with flying in a small aircraft, do not apply for this type of placement. If you cannot fly, you become a liability for those around you, with dehydration and anxiety a real issue in the bush. Staff have enough to do without having to cope with your sickness.

You could easily find that you are 'dumped or dropped' from a flight. Missing out on a trip is unfortunate, but you must remember that you are there at the invitation of the fieldwork placement staff, so emergencies will take priority over your education needs. You need to see the big picture when lives may be at risk.

Some of you will read this chapter and wonder why they would want to put up with so much change and disruption. Why bother with a rural fieldwork placement? The rewards are there for those with an open mind, a give-it-a-go attitude will give you an experience never to be forgotten and never repeated. The intention of this information is to encourage you to become part of the regional, rural or remote health care team in the future. It's not for everyone, but you will *make a difference*.

Case Study 10.1	My first week

My first week consisted of working with a number of visiting practitioners. We went up with the Royal Flying Doctor Service twice, once to Ivanhoe and once to White Cliffs. I got to ride in the cockpit both times! They made us homemade scones at White Cliffs. I love country hospitality!

I also went out to a remote centre with a large Aboriginal population. Our clientele was 80% Aboriginal, which was a good cultural experience for me. The diabetes centre provides free care to all patients with diabetes and they do a terrific job. They have excellent, culturally sensitive education and follow-up care, which is maybe why there is a reduction in the problems seen in this population. Many of the clients are high risk, which is directly linked to the high level of obesity and the number of people in the area with diabetes.

For this week and next week my fieldwork educator has returned to Sydney, so I am spending time with different disciplines around the local hospital. I went out with the ambulance officers for a ride on Monday, which was an awesome experience, an intense and rewarding day. I have seen knee replacement surgery and took part in falls classes with the physios, which was really interesting. It has broadened my knowledge of rehabilitation, including muscle building and strengthening before and after surgery.

I also spent a day with the OTs (occupational therapists) and did a house assessment for a patient who they were trying to get home. Very interesting; it involved a lot of measuring and risk analysis. I think that I now understand what OTs do! I will spend my last two weeks with the podiatrist again. I'm off to the Royal Flying Doctor Ball tonight with a bunch of other students. The Ball is their major fundraiser for the year. This fieldwork placement has certainly been keeping me busy.

Questions

1   Do you think the attitude of the student in the case study helped or hindered his or her experience?
2   Discuss what this student learnt about working in teams.
3   Would this student's experience extend beyond his or her professional learning? If so, how?

SUMMARY

Undertaking a rural and remote placement can take you out of your comfort zone. You need to prepare well in order to get the most of your placement. For example, you need to check the time to start and the time spent on placement, transport (how to get there and how you get around when you are there), accommodation, food (particularly if you have special dietary needs) and what you do after work (how you relax and spend your evenings).

You may encounter situations that you have never come across before, and this may be challenging but also extend your professional skills. You will work with a range of health professionals, and may be involved in delivering health services to Aboriginal communities.

DISCUSSION QUESTIONS

1   Is there anything that would stop you from undertaking a rural and remote placement?
2   Are you prepared to step out of your comfort zone?
3   In a rural setting, you are likely to see a variety of clients or patients. Are you prepared for that?
4   What would you want to get out of your rural and remote fieldwork placement?

References

Australian Bureau of Statistics (2006). *Deaths, Australia, 2005.* ABS Catalogue No 3302.0. Commonwealth of Australia, Canberra.

Australian Institute of Health and Welfare (2002). *Australia's Health.* Canberra. AIHW Cat. No. Aus 25.

Further Reading

Australian Institute of Health and Welfare (2001). *Health and Community Services Labour Force.* Cat. No. HWL 27. AIHW, Canberra.

Eckermann, A., Dowd, T., Chong, E., Nixon, L., Gray, R. & Johnson, S. (2006). *Bridging Cultures in Aboriginal Health* (2nd edn). Elsevier, Marrickville, NSW.

Levett-Jones, T. & Bourgeois, S. (2007). *The Clinical Placement. An Essential Guide for Nursing Students.* Elsevier, Edinburgh.

Reynolds, F. (2005). *Communication and Clinical Effectiveness in Rehabilitation.* Elsevier, Edinburgh.

Useful Website

Australian Institute of Health and Welfare (AIHW)—Publications: www.aihw.gov.au/publications

CHAPTER 11
WORKING IN INDIGENOUS HEALTH SETTINGS

Deirdre Whitford, Angela Russell, Judy Taylor and Kym Thomas

LEARNING OUTCOMES

After reading this chapter, you should be:
- knowledgeable of fieldwork placement at an Indigenous health setting
- able to discuss Indigenous health issues
- able to give a critique of the state of Indigenous health outcomes
- able to reflect on your own attitudes towards Indigenous culture.

KEY TERMS

Aboriginal and Torres Strait Islander (ATSI) people
Aboriginal community-controlled health service
Aboriginal health workers (AHWs)
Determinants of health
Exclusion
Indigenous health
Indigenous health settings
Multiple language groups

INTRODUCTION

Student fieldwork placements in *Indigenous health settings* aim to increase the capacity of non-Indigenous students to improve Indigenous health outcomes, contribute to service delivery to the Australian Aboriginal people and develop partnerships between Indigenous and non-Indigenous organisations and universities. These aims are of particular importance because the health outcomes for the Australian Aboriginal population are markedly worse than for the mainstream population (ABS/AIHW 2008).

While the Australian health care system is recognised globally for its solidarity and quality, it must be said that in general it has not met the needs of the Indigenous population well, particularly in terms of its appropriateness, equity of access and cultural safety. It has been suggested that barriers to improving Indigenous health include the funding of medical services; the nature of the early contact between Indigenous people and early European settlers; and the complex nature of Indigenous cultures (Hayes 2002).

The social, economic, environmental and biological determinants of health differ between cultural groups, and result in differences in context, case mix, care and care delivery needs. These differences are most obvious between Indigenous and non-Indigenous cultures, but they also occur between different Aboriginal and Torres Strait Islander groups. It is essential that you learn to deliver care differently to different cultural groups to meet their needs equitably and appropriately, and recognise that working in Indigenous health requires you to work collaboratively across disciplines and sectorial boundaries.

In Indigenous health care settings, the health problems encountered are very complex, with ill-defined boundaries and multilayered causal links. Further complexity is added when the health service provides services to multiple language groups. *Multiple language groups* within the overall consumer group will mean a variety of group histories, beliefs, practices and needs, and while adding diversity to fieldwork placements, may limit the extent to which you can become immersed in any one particular Indigenous culture.

Issues such as exclusion, poor education system outcomes, unstable housing, unemployment, relatively high levels of domestic and child abuse, and drug and alcohol abuse have an impact on the health outcomes of many Indigenous Australians (Carson et al. 2007). Many of these risk factors are the responsibility of the wider community; however, Indigenous Australians will continue to require care in the health care system until the causes of their poorer health outcomes are addressed. It is therefore the responsibility of all health professionals to provide care to Indigenous Australians in the most effective and appropriate manner possible, whether at the bedside or in the community, and participate in bringing about social and political change to improve Indigenous health outcomes.

GUIDING PRINCIPLES OF STUDENT FIELDWORK PLACEMENTS IN INDIGENOUS HEALTH CARE SETTINGS

The Australian Rural Health Education Network (2008), the peak body of the University Departments of Rural Health (UDRH) lists on its website <http://www.arhen.org.au/network/network-isn.htm> the principles that should guide student placements in Indigenous health care settings:

> Student placements within Indigenous organisations need to be seen as a privilege, not a right, and need to be guided by the following principles:
> * The right of the Indigenous community to decline to take students on fieldwork placement.
> * That adequate payment should be made available to organisations which participate in the process.
> * The community should determine access within the program.

- There should be collaborative business planning within the community in relation to student fieldwork placements, which may involve a revisiting of current Memoranda of Understanding or other agreements with Aboriginal health bodies and other Aboriginal bodies.
- Aboriginal Health Workers should be included in negotiations prior to student placements.
- At the placement site, all members of the organisation e.g. AHWs, bus drivers and other Indigenous staff, should be briefed; and agreed commitments should be developed regarding the program.
- UDRH Indigenous staff should be included and consulted prior to placement of health students in communities or organisations.
- Cultural protocol training sessions should be provided for students before they go into communities.
- Assessment of students' performance from the fieldwork placement should be recognised as part of their overall assessment.
- Where appropriate and available, mentoring programs should be utilised.
- There should be separate debriefing sessions with students and communities at the end of the placement.

The context of Indigenous health

The multicultural Australian population generally enjoys high living standards and health outcomes. The determinants of these health outcomes are debated; however, factors such as the relatively robust economy and high standards of public infrastructure, education, housing, and healthcare are recognised contributors.

The Australian Indigenous population does not enjoy the same health or wellbeing outcomes as the population as a whole. The factors affecting Indigenous health and wellbeing are also debated; but are thought to be based in historical, social, language and cultural issues affecting social inclusion. Poor social inclusion touches all aspects of physical and emotional life.

While individual members of the Indigenous population are spread across all strata of the Australian economic, academic, sporting, music, art, business and entrepreneurial scenes, Indigenous people are overrepresented in the lower strata for income stream, education achievement, health and wellbeing measures, unemployment, unstable housing and imprisonment. Some Indigenous individuals are achieving high levels of attainment in politics, law, science and arts, and enabling change for greater social inclusion of Indigenous people generally. Indigenous people are diverse in their health care needs.

Traditional Aboriginal cultures developed over many thousands of years in sympathy with the Australian land. Traditional cultures had well-developed systems for the maintenance of tribal laws, family structures and health and wellbeing. All Indigenous Australians share the history and heritage of the impact of colonisation. Colonisation and settlement of Australia by Europeans in the 1700s led to a period of conflict between the traditional Indigenous owners of the land and the colonisers. Colonial and postcolonial governments denied Indigenous Australians' land ownership and the inherent Indigenous cultural significance of the land; as well as Indigenous citizenship rights. Disastrous experiments with 'assimilation' policies were imposed, including the removal of half-caste children from their Indigenous families (the lost generation), a policy that persisted into the mid 1900s. These actions added to the pain, grief and loss experienced by Aboriginal people as a result of the settlement of Australia by non-Indigenous Australians.

Since the settlement of European populations, generations of Indigenous Australians have experienced social disharmony and dysfunction, marginalisation and disadvantage, loss of culture and identity and lack of social inclusion into the wider Australian population. The impact of this shared history is variable, with some members of the Indigenous population continuing to live more or less as Indigenous people have for thousands of years (traditional lifestyle) while integrating aspects of contemporary lifestyles. This balancing of social life to incorporate cultural components while living as integral members of the broader Australian society poses significant challenges for all Indigenous peoples.

Progress has been made to reinstate traditional land ownership and the citizenship rights of Indigenous people within the changing Australian social landscape. 'Sorry Day' (26 May) sees many thousands of mainstream Australians expressing the sorrow these actions caused for the current generation of Australians. The apology to the members of the stolen generation made by Prime Minister Kevin Rudd in 2008 went some way toward repairing the relationship between the Indigenous Australian population and the mainstream Australian population. Much work remains to ensure Indigenous Australians enjoy the benefits of their unique place in Australian society. The challenge is to develop an environment in which Indigenous–mainstream relationships and partnerships can further improve, and in which Indigenous people can retain their connection with their cultural identities, while also enjoying the opportunities available through full participation and inclusion in the wider Australian society and beyond.

Indigenous health outcomes

Queensland, Western Australia, the Northern Territory and South Australia are the only jurisdictions that have data of sufficient quality to compare health and welfare outcomes for the Indigenous population compared with that of the Australian population as a whole. In July 2009, Kevin Rudd, the current Prime Minister, acknowledged that statistics on Indigenous Australians were inadequate, and has given a commitment to the task of collating accurate statistics. The health status of

Indigenous Australians has shown little improvement in recent years, and remains considerably below that of non-Indigenous Australians:

- Indigenous adults are twice as likely as non-Indigenous adults to report their health as fair or poor
- hospitalisation rates are higher for Indigenous Australians, particularly for conditions that are potentially preventable, such as diabetes type II and kidney disease
- the mortality rates of Indigenous people in 2001–2005 were almost three times the rate for non-Indigenous people in Queensland, Western Australia, South Australia and the Northern Territory, the only jurisdictions for which coverage of Indigenous deaths was deemed sufficient to report.

Other findings from the most recent report on Aboriginal and Torres Strait Islander health and welfare outcomes (Australian Bureau of Statistics /Australian Institute of Health and Welfare 2008) include:

- Indigenous people were half as likely to complete Year 12 as non-Indigenous people
- Indigenous adults were more than twice as likely as non-Indigenous adults to smoke regularly
- more than half of Indigenous people were overweight or obese
- Indigenous people face barriers in accessing health services, in particular primary health care.

REFLECTION 11.1

1   What factors contribute to poorer health outcomes for Indigenous Australians?
2   What could your health profession do to improve health outcomes for Indigenous Australians?

Indigenous health strategies

In order to overcome health disparities between Indigenous peoples and Australians as a whole, state and federal governments have put in place national targets. These health targets are contained in the 'Close the Gap' targets set by COAG at the National Indigenous Health Equality Summit in March 2008 <http://www.hreoc.gov.au/social_Justice/health/targets/index.html>. A section of the summit targets outline is:

> The Council of Australian Governments has agreed to a partnership between all levels of government to work with Indigenous Australian communities to achieve the target of closing the gap on Indigenous disadvantage. COAG committed to:
> - closing the life expectancy gap within a generation;
> - halving the mortality gap for children under five within a decade; and
> - halving the gap in reading, writing and numeracy within a decade.

The aim of these targets is to achieve the three COAG goals, and particularly the two health goals. Hence they address:

- the main components of excess child mortality—low birth weight, respiratory and other infections, and injuries;
- the main components of life expectancy gap—chronic disease (cardiovascular disease (CVD), renal, diabetes), injuries and respiratory infections account for 75% of the gap. CVD is the largest component and a major driver of the life expectancy gap (~1/3); and
- mental health and social and emotional wellbeing, which are central to the achievement of better health.

In the Department of Health and Ageing 2008 Budget Papers, Indigenous health outcomes are stated as:

> The Australian Government is committed to closing the 17-year gap in life expectancy between Indigenous and non-Indigenous Australians within a generation, and to halving the gap in mortality rates between Indigenous and non-Indigenous children within a decade. Through Outcome 8, the Government aims to ensure that Aboriginal and Torres Strait Islander people have access to health care services essential to improving health and life expectancy. The Government aims to achieve this outcome by working in partnership with Aboriginal and Torres Strait Islander people and organisations, and through collaboration with State and Territory governments. Including initiatives announced since being elected, the Australian Government will invest around $3.1 billion in Indigenous health over the next four years, compared with around $2.2 billion provided over the last four years.

The key strategic directions in Indigenous health are listed as:

- improving access to effective primary health care, substance use and social and emotional wellbeing services for Aboriginal and Torres Strait Islander people
- improving child and maternal health
- working with other governments and the broader health sector to improve health outcomes for Aboriginal and Torres Strait Islander people.

ABORIGINAL HEALTH SERVICES

Community-controlled health services

An *Aboriginal community-controlled health service* is a primary health care service initiated and controlled by the local Aboriginal community to deliver holistic, comprehensive and locally appropriate health care. While services differ markedly with regards to governance, extent of service delivery and availability of different types of health professionals, they are initiated and operated by the local community.

Although referred to as Aboriginal community controlled-health services, the term is understood to include both Aboriginal and Torres Strait Islander people.

The first services commenced with minimal government funding, and relied heavily on donations. However, there is now an expanding and more established network of over 140 services in every state and territory, and in rural, remote, regional and urban locations. The National Aboriginal Community Controlled Health Organisation (NACCHO) provides a national voice and mandate to speak on health issues for Aboriginal communities throughout Australia. Each state and territory has a regional body affiliated with NACCHO (Hunter 1999).

As many Indigenous health fieldwork placements take place in an Aboriginal community-controlled health service, it is important to understand the differences between Aboriginal-controlled and mainstream health services. Most importantly, Aboriginal community-controlled health services are a living embodiment of the aspirations of Aboriginal communities and their struggle for self-determination (NACCHO <http://www.naccho.org.au/>). They have come about because of strong community interest in improving health, and as an alternative to mainstream health services, which for various reasons have been, and to some extent still are, inaccessible or inappropriate for Aboriginal and Torres Strait Islander people.

Aboriginal health services are highly participative, having been built through community control and community participation, particularly in their establishment (Wakerman et al. 2000). Participation occurs in board membership, through the process of defining needs and priorities, and by providing feedback about service delivery. The health service usually plays an important role in the community, and therefore has a knowledge base about Indigenous affairs and an infrastructure from which to develop programs and services. Because of the holistic nature of service delivery, and because Aboriginal health services are community controlled, they are an effective platform for the community to develop related initiatives to promote socioemotional wellbeing. Often, Indigenous staff working in these organisations take leadership positions in planning and advising governments and other agencies on Indigenous health and wellbeing issues.

Because the organisations have a cultural orientation, it is inevitable that there is some overlap between organisational and social and family affairs as part of health service delivery. This is usually considered a strength, leading to an indepth understanding of how programs need to be developed in order to make them accessible by those who most need to use them. However, community obligations and responsibilities from time to time may come into conflict with, as well as complement, the functions that the organisation performs in delivering services. There are always challenges in balancing sectional interests and family and organisational demands, and Aboriginal and Torres Strait Islander health managers use high-level management skills.

Aboriginal-controlled health services cover many different language and *first nation groups*. Attitudes toward having you as a student on fieldwork placement may vary. Many ATSIHS would regard you as Indigenous health advocates for the future, and work to provide lifelong changes in attitudes and effective cross-cultural skills to improve Indigenous health and patient outcomes.

Rural and remote settings

Placements in rural and remote Indigenous health care settings have an added layer of complexity when compared with fieldwork placements in urban Indigenous health care settings. Bourke and colleagues (2004: 181) described five concepts that distinguish rural and remote from urban placements: rural–urban health differentials, access, confidentiality, cultural safety and team practice. These factors have an impact on access to services and care delivery, because there are 'fewer services, greater distances, smaller populations, less choice of services and smaller workforce'. Students need to be prepared for the positive and negative aspects of placement in rural and remote locations, and for a diversity of practice, potentially extended roles and opportunities for bringing about change (Bourke et al. 2004).

THINK AND LINK 11.1

Rural and remote settings can provide an interesting and challenging experience for your fieldwork placement. Chapter 10 discusses how to prepare for these settings, and provides other useful information to consider.

Other Indigenous health settings

You may be placed in health care settings that are not community controlled. These placements may include Indigenous health units within tertiary hospitals, or field trips to health services within Aboriginal communities. You will be better able to provide appropriate care and deal with the difficulties of providing care to Indigenous people in tertiary care services, who are far from home and in the alien hospital with predominantly Western culture, if you have had a prior placement in a community-controlled service, undertaken a field trip to an Aboriginal community or undertaken extensive cultural training. You may also be placed in non-health settings; however, their learning objectives will generally be health related.

Case Study 11.1	Nancy and Geoff

Nancy and Geoff undertook an occupational therapy placement in a small regional Indigenous school where, among the 200-plus students, there was only one non-Indigenous student: the son of one of the teachers. The school was proactive in encouraging students' attendance and participation, providing buses to collect children from wherever they were spending the night, provided that the school was notified during the previous day. Attendance varied between 85 and 95 per cent on most days, and children were given awards for attendance at school. The learning objective for Nancy and Geoff was to create a do-able intervention to address at least one of the determinants of ill health in this population of Indigenous children.

Geoff and Nancy noted that the children did not always have adequate food provided for them at lunch time: inadequate in terms of quantity as well as nutritional value. Nancy and Geoff decided to address the issues involved in the children's lunchtime nutrition. They noted that interventions that had previously been used in non-Indigenous schools to improve lunchtime nutrition had focused on education programs for parents. In this case, Geoff and Nancy decided to focus on educating the parents about nutrition through the students themselves.

Nancy and Geoff devised a series of lessons in food preparation, value and handling for the children, with a focus on food suitable for lunchboxes. The children also wrote a play about good lunches, and practised the play during the term, as well as making some large collage posters about good lunches in their art lessons. At the end of term the parents were invited to the school to see the play and the posters, and to have a healthy packed lunch prepared by the children.

The short-term outcomes for Nancy and Geoff, the children and the parents were evident on the day, so the school decided to include these activities in the curriculum. An unforeseen outcome was that a number of Indigenous students began to ask questions about how they could study occupational therapy in the future. In turn, this highlighted the problem that students leaving the school to attend the local high school were not finishing year 12, because the same support was not available at the local high school as at the school, and VET opportunities were not available as an alternative pathway for Indigenous students interested in taking up health-related careers. These observations led to a local collaboration between the schools and the TAFE sector.

This student placement provided Nancy and Geoff with a feeling that they could have an impact on Indigenous health, and they reported high levels of satisfaction with the placement. The school has since continued to seek to have students on placement.

Questions

1   Are there many Indigenous Australians in your course?
2   What would you have done if you were Nancy or Geoff?

REFLECTION 11.2

1   Aboriginal Australians have a holistic view of health involving their relationship with their land and community. How does this differ from your own view of health?
2   How would you anticipate that an Aboriginal Australian who felt well and had good community connections would perceive a diagnosis of illness based on a pathology test result?
3   Why is respect the most important element in cross-cultural communication?
4   Why is cultural safety in Aboriginal health services very important in improving Aboriginal Australian health outcomes?
5   How can students on placement have an impact on Indigenous health outcomes?

INDIGENOUS HEALTH WORKFORCE

In 2006, it was reported in the *Medical Journal of Australia* that 34 per cent of the Australian population lived outside major cities, along with 70 per cent of the Indigenous population. The percentage of health professionals who lived outside urban areas represented a shortfall at 23 per cent of medical specialists; 27 per cent of general practitioners; 34 per cent of nurses and 25 per cent of physiotherapists. The extended roles of these health professionals, as well as the unpredictability of their availability to the Aboriginal and Torres Strait Islander (ATSI) population, were also noted (Murray & Wronski 2006).

Murray and Wronski (2006) noted that rural student fieldwork placements were effective in increasing the rural workforce. It is likely that these findings are generalisable to the Indigenous healthcare setting, and that positive student fieldwork experiences in Indigenous health will provide the same success in recruitment to Indigenous health professional careers. There is also a need for the extension of roles, particularly those of *Aboriginal health workers (AHWs)*, through supervised delegation; improved Indigenous entry to health professional programs and improved training and recognition of AHWs (Murray & Wronski 2006).

Development of the role and training of Aboriginal health workers (AHWs) was a strategy to improve access to health care for Indigenous people, particularly in remote areas. However, the designation of the title AHW includes people with no clinical training, as well as those providing advanced clinical care in emerging areas of need such as haemodialysis and midwifery. National competency standards have been developed and now need to be incorporated into human resourcing processes and education pathways.

In spite of favourable selection processes, few Indigenous people gain university places in health professional training courses. The underlying cause is educational disadvantage as a result of isolation, remoteness, poverty and negative primary and secondary school experiences resulting in poor literacy achievement (Adams et al. 2005). In the short term, meeting the workforce needs of Indigenous people cannot be achieved through the training of Indigenous health care professionals alone. Current strategies indicate the need for widespread training of non-Indigenous health care professionals in Indigenous health and cultural issues to improve Indigenous health outcomes and the appropriateness and effectiveness of health care delivery. The Indigenous Allied Health Australia Network has also been set up to encourage and support Indigenous Australians to take up an allied health profession.

CURRICULUM AND LEARNING OBJECTIVES FOR STUDENT PLACEMENTS IN INDIGENOUS SETTINGS

You will discover that the learning objectives of student fieldwork placements in Indigenous health settings are broad-ranging. They include practical and conceptual preparation for providing culturally safe and effective care to Indigenous patients in all healthcare settings, including mainstream and Indigenous healthcare settings.

These objectives are best served by a broad curriculum encompassing:
- public health, including the social determinants of health (Baum 2002)
- epidemiology: the incidence and prevalence of risk factors and disease in Indigenous populations
- Indigenous people's histories
- discipline-specific skills, including cross-cultural consultation skills
- evidence-based care in Indigenous health (Couzos & Murray 1999)
- social determinants of Indigenous health and their impact on care delivery (Carson et al. 2007)
- personal and professional development, including capacity for self-awareness and reflection on practice
- immersion in delivery settings and service delivery, including frequent patient and supervisor feedback and mentoring
- understanding Aboriginal and Torres Strait Islander community life (Taylor et al. 2008).

REFLECTION 11.3

You are about to embark on your first Indigenous Health fieldwork placement. Reflect on what you know about Indigenous health and cultural practices, and your attitude to Indigenous Australians.

Personal development

You will find it helpful to reflect on the attitudes you have developed over your lifetime to all minority and marginalised groups, including Australia's Indigenous people. In doing this, you need to develop an awareness of what you bring to your interactions with Indigenous people, and how what you bring influences the outcomes of your interaction. Your effectiveness as a health professional in Indigenous health care will depend on your capacity to develop and engender trust and mutual respect with the Indigenous patients you treat.

The context of all cross-cultural interactions is multilayered, and includes historical, cultural and spiritual differences and mismatches. These mismatches affect all aspects of verbal and nonverbal communication within the interaction, and can have a serious impact on the desired outcomes of the interaction.

While academic teaching around cultural differences, historical events and context raise your awareness of Indigenous health issues; immersion in the Indigenous healthcare setting provides richness of understanding, as indicated by these comments from students following fieldwork placements in an Indigenous community setting.

'Getting the opportunity to speak to the native inhabitants of the Coorong region was moving—and having their struggle from a first-hand personal account ...'

'I am more interested in working with Indigenous people after this week. Definitely got me thinking about Indigenous health issues and understanding that everyone is responsible and needs to start doing something ... will definitely now try to raise awareness and look into future Indigenous placements and ways to make some sort of difference.'

'Made me realise that there is much to learn about Indigenous culture if you were to work in a career with such interactions. It has helped me realise how important such understanding is for them. I would be motivated to learn about appropriate and significant issues before considering myself fit to pursue such a career.'

'I never knew that people could be living in such conditions so close to a major centre.'

'I didn't realise the impacts of grief and loss, and how close the bond was between extended families.'

'I didn't know there was so much nitpicking and racist attitude.'

'I hadn't looked at Australia's history through others' eyes.'

With even these beginning understandings, students are more able to contribute to improving Indigenous health outcomes: the ultimate aim of student placements in Indigenous health care settings.

WHAT HAPPENS ON PLACEMENT IN AN INDIGENOUS HEALTH SETTING?

Some Aboriginal-controlled health services provide health care to many different Aboriginal language and 'first nation' groups. In these services you will usually be assigned an ATSI mentor, and undertake cultural awareness training to engender the showing of respect, tolerance of being corrected, overcoming language obstacles, avoiding eye contact, male–female protocols, relating information to a third party in a consultation, how the communities served will read body language, getting used to what is considered humorous, personal space issues, and being questioned about your background, marital status and other personal details.

You can contribute in many practical ways to Indigenous health outcomes at the time of the placement. If you are in the earlier years of your course, you can undertake clinical audits, pharmacy reviews, health promotion projects and health checks, as appropriate to your discipline. If you are more experienced, you can undertake history and examinations, and commence supervised practice.

You will need to be prepared for the increased complexities of the underlying causes of the presentations to an Indigenous health service, including housing, poverty and social and emotional wellbeing issues. You also need to understand that clients may present late (or even at a critical stage) in the disease process, as a result of believing the condition should just be tolerated or 'put up with'.

Each university develops its fieldwork placements in collaboration with the hosting Aboriginal health service. Even though each university has different learning objectives, you will need to embrace a multidisciplinary—preferably an interdisciplinary—approach to your learning.

THINK AND LINK 11.2

Chapter 16 considers fieldwork placements where you spend your time with students from a different discipline to your own. Working in Indigenous health settings requires you to take a multidisciplinary or interdisciplinary approach. Chapter 16 will guide you through what would be involved when working with students from other disciplines.

You should also be aware that the Aboriginal health service is granting a privilege to you to learn within the service. It is strongly advised that you are provided with preparatory teaching to develop cultural awareness for the geographic areas and predominant Indigenous language group(s) of that area. Preparatory work might also include instruction in the history of European settlement and the impact of European settlement on Indigenous people; the history of the health service and how it contributes to Indigenous health; the predominant health risk factors and healthcare needs of the health service's catchment area; and how the healthcare service differs from a mainstream service. The health service may provide outreach to many Aboriginal communities over a wide area; so be prepared for the long distances to be travelled, and basic rural/remote survival.

You also need preparation for the possible impact of fieldwork placement, in terms of having your family or fellow students failing to understand the changes you have undergone or the experiences you have had while on placement. As for all fieldwork placements, you need to be provided with appropriate counselling services for support in the rare event of a traumatic experience.

Field trips

On field trips to an Aboriginal community you will be exposed to local culture and health-related issues such as the distances that need to be covered by the inhabitants of these communities to access services in large centres; living conditions; and lack of access to support services such as pharmacies, and primary health care in general, within Aboriginal communities. Field trips provide an opportunity for you to develop skills and knowledge, and acquire cultural understanding, relevant to working with Aboriginal people in varied locations and environments. It also promotes more effective ways for you and the professionals and agencies working within health to initiate contacts with individuals, communities and organisations to develop and enhance programs, research activities and collaborative activities. This knowledge will assist you to provide appropriate care and discharge arrangements for Indigenous people. Field trips also inspire and assist you to advocate for change on behalf of Indigenous people, and provide the exposure that will influence your decision-making. You have the opportunity to interact with Aboriginal people, witness environments and social determinants that play a vital role in the health status of Aboriginal people and delivery of health services. The field trips also allow Aboriginal health workers to share knowledge about health issues, unwritten cultural protocols and community concerns. Field trips expose the relationship between ill health and direct causative and underlying factors. Also, social and economic factors need to be acknowledged, and are non-negotiable in understanding the health of Aboriginal people. Some quotes from participants:

> 'Seeing the situation firsthand in communities has made it all real for me, instead of just media reports or lectures or readings.'

'I liked the way that we were shown things and told about how things worked and were given time to digest that and think on it. It was a safe environment to ask questions and think through things.'

'I learnt an enormous amount and was inspired by some of the people I met. I will use what I have learnt to make a difference.'

SUCCESS IN YOUR PLACEMENT

Success in assessment of your performance during the fieldwork placement will generally reflect that you have grasped the principles of working with Aboriginal people and families: you now understand how Aboriginal health services work and what makes them successful in improving Aboriginal health; and you now know how to participate successfully in providing health services, education, research and/or project work.

Research has demonstrated the benefits of rural and community-based education (Gibbs 2004; Worley et al. 2004). It is likely that these findings are generalisable to health professional education in Indigenous rural and community health settings. Student feedback from placements in Indigenous health settings demonstrates improved knowledge of health issues and Indigenous health services, awareness of gaps and development of positive attitudes and advocacy intentions. Students report that they feel they were able to make a real difference to the lives of Indigenous Australians, and that they have 'learned a lot':

'Personally, it wasn't until I spent time at —— that I was able to see firsthand many of the problems as well as some of the programs used to target and improve quality of life in Indigenous communities.'

SUPPORT FOR STUDENT PLACEMENTS IN INDIGENOUS HEALTH SETTINGS

In order to encourage students in the health professions to undertake rural placements, the Department of Health and Ageing (DoHA) has developed and funded a number of schemes for the placement and support of health students in rural and Indigenous healthcare settings. You can access information about these schemes on the DoHA website. Under these schemes DoHA contracts with the university, or a collaboration of universities or an agency to provide: Undergraduate Departments of Rural Health (UDRH), Rural Clinical Schools (RCS), Medical Rural Bonded Support Scheme (MRBSS); Rural Australian Medical Undergraduate Scholarships (RAMUS); Commonwealth Undergraduate Remote and Rural Nursing

Scholarship Scheme (CURRNSS); John Flynn Scholarship Scheme (JFSS); and the university student Rural Health Clubs (RHCs) programs. There are also a number of state-based initiatives, including the Queensland Health Rural Scholarship Scheme, the NSW Rural Resident Medical Officer Cadetship and the South Australian Allied Health Scholarship Scheme. Each scheme is funded on the basis of key performance areas in terms of the quantity and quality (student satisfaction) of rural or rural Indigenous placements, scholarships or cadetships undertaken.

WHAT ARE THE CHALLENGES AND BENEFITS OF STUDENT PLACEMENTS IN THE INDIGENOUS HEALTH CARE SETTING?

As a result of inadequate numbers and maldistribution of the health workforce, and therefore a lack of suitable fieldwork educators, student fieldwork placements in underserved care settings are not always available. This is a challenge to finding you a placement in such a setting.

You may often feel poorly prepared for the greater levels of acuity and urgency of the cases you see, and for the extended practice roles often needed in Indigenous health care settings, where in some cases conditions may more closely resemble a Third World healthcare setting than a mainstream Australian healthcare setting. In very remote settings, the paucity of resources can challenge you: colleagues to call on for help, family and friends; and professional development.

Similarly, health professionals in better-resourced mainstream settings can feel professionally and personally inadequate and poorly prepared to provide for the needs of Indigenous patients who require their care in these settings, which are often very strange and unfamiliar.

Learning to communicate across cultures continues for a lifetime. While greater understanding can be achieved during your fieldwork placements, culturally based organisations need a high level of cultural sensitivity, which takes time to learn. You will become aware of the challenge of achieving high levels of sensitivity, and may perceive this as a barrier to effective practice in Indigenous health, rather than an opportunity for lifelong learning. You will develop a healthy sense of 'becoming' rather than 'being' culturally competent.

SUMMARY

Student placements in Indigenous health settings accrue benefits to student learning and personal and professional growth as well as to Indigenous health outcomes. Students require preparation for Indigenous health placements in terms of their knowledge, attitudes and cross-cultural skills.

Placements in rural and remote Indigenous health care settings have added value as well as added complexity.

The knowledge base for what works for student placements in Indigenous settings is based on learning to communicate across cultures and becoming sensitive to the worldview and circumstance of Indigenous peoples.

Student placements in Indigenous health settings are supported by government policy and strategies.

DISCUSSION QUESTIONS

1   On deep reflection, what are your assumptions about Australian Aboriginal and Torres Strait Islander peoples?
2   What would be your expectations for a placement in a rural or remote Indigenous healthcare setting?
3   What could you bring to such a placement?

References

Adams, M., Aylward, P., Heyne, N., Hull, C., Misan, G., Taylor, J. & Walker-Jeffreys, M. (2005). Integrated Support for Aboriginal Tertiary Students in Health-Related Courses: The Pika Wiya Learning Centre. *Australian Health Review*, 29(4): 482–8.

Australian Bureau of Statistics/Australian Institute of Health and Welfare (2008). *The Health and Welfare of Aboriginal and Torres Strait Islander Peoples*. ABS Cat. No 4704.0, Australian Bureau of Statistics, Canberra.

Baum, F. (2002). *The New Public Health*. Oxford University Press, Melbourne.

Bourke, L., Sheridan, C. M., Russell, U., Jones, G. I., Dewitt Talbot, D. & Liaw, S. (2004). 'Developing a Conceptual Understanding of Rural Health Practice'. *Australian Journal of Rural Health*, 12(5): 181–6.

Carson, B., Dunbar, T., Chenall, R. D. & Bailie, R. (2007). *Social Determinants of Indigenous Health*. Allen & Unwin, Sydney.

Couzos, S. & Murray, R. (1999). *Aboriginal Primary Health Care: An Evidence-Based Approach*. Oxford University Press, South Melbourne.

Gibbs, T. (2004). 'Community-based or Tertiary-based Medical Education: So What Is the Question?' *Medical Teaching*, 26(7): 589–90.

Hayes, R. (2002). 'One Approach to Improving Indigenous Health Care Is through Medical Education'. *Australian Journal of Rural Health*, 10(6): 285–7.

Hunter, P. (1999). Aboriginal Community Controlled Health Services (ACCHS): Keynote address, 5th National Rural Health Conference, Adelaide.

Murray, R. B. & Wronski, I. (2006). 'When the Tide Goes Out: Health Workforce in Rural, Remote and Indigenous Communities'. *Medical Journal of Australia*, 185(1): 37–8.

Taylor, J., Wilkinson, D. & Cheers, B. (2008). *Working with Communities in Health and Human Services*. Oxford University Press, South Melbourne.

Wakerman, J., Matthews, S., Hill, P. & Gibson, O. (2000). 'Beyond Charcoal Lane. Aboriginal and Torres Strait Islander health managers: issues and strategies to assist recruitment, retention and professional development'. Menzies School of Health Research and Indigenous Health Program. University of Queensland, Alice Springs.

Worley, P., Prideaux D., Strasser, R., March, R. & Worley, E. (2004). 'What Do Medical Students Actually Do On Clinical Rotations?' *Medical Teaching*, 26(7): 594–8.

Useful Websites

National Aboriginal Community Controlled Health Organisation, *Annual Report 2007–2008*: www.naccho.org.au/Files/Documents/NACCHO_AR08_final_press.pdf

National Indigenous Health Equality Summit in March 2008: www.hreoc.gov.au/social_Justice/health/targets/index.html

PART 1 CHECKLIST
PREPARING FOR PLACEMENT

The following points have been collated from Part 1 of the book. They are a quick reference for you when you undertake placement in different settings.

PREPARING FOR PLACEMENT

☐ I have found out the geographical location of my placement and know how to get there.

☐ I have completed all of the program administration needed to organise my placement.

☐ I have applied for my Police Check.

☐ I have applied for my Working with Children Check.

☐ I have compiled my curriculum vitae to take to my placement agency.

☐ I have accessed the agency annual report and/or information about the services of the agency where I will be going on placement.

☐ I understand the dress code for my placement agency and have appropriate clothing to wear during the practicum.

☐ I have a good idea of four or five learning objectives I hope to address on placement.

☐ I have discussed with my family and/or flatmates the extra work obligations and time commitments I need to meet while being on placement.

WORKING WITH DIVERSITY

☐ I can state the difference between public and private hospitals in Australia.

☐ I can define what the PBS is, and the two different categories in it.

☐ I can state other healthcare settings outside the hospital setting.

☐ I can identify five strategies that could potentially be used to aid in my orientation to my placement site.

☐ I can name five potential members of an interdisciplinary healthcare team and define their roles.

☐ I can define cultural competence in my own words.

☐ I can identify four visual aspects of a person's culture and five invisible ones.

☐ I can name four things that I need to consider when working with an interpreter.

WORKING WITH MOTHERS AND BABIES

☐ The language used when working with mothers and babies differs from other areas of work. Am I familiar with the terms used? Do I use woman-centred language?

☐ Have I prepared or thought through how I will cope with a stillbirth while on placement? Where do I seek assistance to help me cope with this?

WORKING WITH CHILDREN AND FAMILIES

☐ I have a grasp of typical development from 0 to 5 years.

☐ In my discipline area, I know some paediatric assessments.

☐ In my discipline area, I know some intervention strategies.

☐ I have looked up the service that I will be working in during my fieldwork placement and understand:

☐ the age range of children they service and any specific diagnoses

☐ the types of families they serve

☐ the range of services that are provided.

☐ When I observe a session working with a child and family, things to note are:

☐ how the health professional engages with the family or caregiver (including listening, communicating, feedback)

☐ how the health professional engages with the child (including language used, behaviour management and physical positioning of the child)

☐ specific activities and strategies to be used when engaging the child

☐ what the child can achieve

☐ what tasks or activities were difficult for the child.

WORKING IN ACUTE CARE SETTINGS

☐ Do I know where I am going and how to get to the acute care setting?

☐ Will I be driving or taking public transport?

☐ Do I know where to go (such as ward or department) within the acute care setting?

☐ What time do I start? Will I be on placement at night?

☐ Do I have my health immunisations up to date?

☐ I know I need to take the documentation on my immunisations with me to placement.

☐ Do I need to wear my uniform? If not, what is the dress code where I will be working?

☐ I have my student identification card ready for placement.

☐ I realise I can't wear jewellery to my placement except for small ear studs, and fingernails should be short, clean and free from nail polish.

☐ I have prepared for the following:

   ☐ the pace of work: it is going to be fast

   ☐ strict adherence to infection control: have I washed my hands? should I wear gloves?

   ☐ acuity of patients: am I familiar with the patients' conditions I will encounter?

   ☐ communication: who is on the interdisciplinary team

   ☐ the emergency codes.

WORKING WITH OLDER PERSONS

☐ I have prepared for my placement by understanding conditions of older persons.

☐ I have read up on normal age-related data, so have an idea of what normal ageing entails.

☐ I understand that every person is different, and that I need to consider:

   ☐ communication

   ☐ normal ageing

   ☐ the person's condition

   ☐ the setting

   ☐ the types of assessment that would be suitable for the setting, including reassessment

   ☐ the types of treatment interventions

   ☐ working in a way that empowers the older person

   ☐ health promotion and prevention activities that would assist the older person.

☐ I understand that communication is more than verbal explanation, and that I might need to use demonstration, drawings, gestures and body language to communicate.

☐ I understand that I am respectful of the person and call each person by his or her formal name: Mr [name] or Mrs/Ms [name].

☐ Some older people may have a hearing aid, so I will make sure patients can see my face clearly, so lip reading and facial expression and gesture can be used to augment what is heard

☐ When explaining treatment, I don't use jargon.

☐ I am aware that with older persons there may be comorbidities, and that I need to consider these when assessing and planning treatments, including preventative care.

WORKING IN MENTAL HEALTH

☐ Before I begin my placement, it will help me if I reflect on my understanding of mental health and whether I hold any misbeliefs about people with a mental illness.

☐ I have made a list of my fears about this placement.

☐ I have found out about the mental health service I will be going to.

☐ I know about the range of mental illnesses that people may present with in this setting.

WORKING IN WORKPLACE PRACTICE

☐ I understand that I may be required to do a lot of observing on this type of placement because of legal restrictions.

☐ I understand that insurance companies are often the clients in this type of practice.

☐ I am prepared because I know I need to:

  ☐ wear appropriate clothing and footwear to workplace sites

  ☐ take a pen, paper and enclosed document holder for storing notes and checklists

  ☐ have knowledge of the workplace I am visiting: the type of industry, work undertaken, hazards and history of injuries

  ☐ be aware of site-specific Occupational Health and Safety (OH&S) procedures: wear required safety gear

  ☐ maintain confidentiality in what I say and write

  ☐ keep a resource list.

WORKING IN PRIVATE PRACTICE

☐ I am prepared to use my downtime productively; for example, I have prepared readings in areas I need to increase my knowledge.

☐ I am prepared to work quickly, as 'time is money' in private practice. Therefore, I have prepared for what I need to get done in the time I have with my client.

WORKING IN RURAL AND REMOTE SETTINGS

☐ I have inquired about the local Indigenous community and whether I will be working with individuals from that community.

☐ I have asked about the uniform requirements of the fieldwork placement.

☐ I have asked about the placement standards (are there any?).

☐ I have asked about my performance assessment while on fieldwork placement.

☐ I have checked the following:

  ☐ What are the number of hours I am expected to be engaged in during the fieldwork placement? I will remember that often in remote situations I can have a feeling that I should be engaged every day 24 hours a day. I know that this is unrealistic.

  ☐ What are the start and finish dates for the fieldwork placement? Is travel time included? Who is providing the transport? Is it my responsibility to get to the rural centre, then be transported out to the remote centre? Is there a road trip or a flight on a transport plane? What time do I need to start on day one?

☐ Do I need a driver's licence?

☐ What is my accommodation like? What is the cost of room, dormitory or tent?

☐ Where do I get food and drinks while on fieldwork placement?

☐ If I have special dietary needs, are these available where I am going?

☐ What am I going to do in the evenings: good book, iPod, computer games, DVDs?

☐ What are the options for playing sport?

☐ Will I be involved with the Royal Flying Doctor Service?

WORKING IN INDIGENOUS HEALTH SETTINGS

☐ I have reflected on my attitudes to Indigenous Australians. Have I tried to be truthful in reflecting whether I am influenced by media reports? Do I know any Indigenous Australians personally?

☐ Before starting my Indigenous health setting placement, I need to prepare. This is a helpful list of suggested preparatory work:

  ☐ the history of European settlement and the impact of European settlement on Indigenous people

  ☐ the history of the health service and how it contributes to Indigenous health

- the predominant health risk factors, and health care needs of the health service catchment area
- how the health care service differs from a mainstream service.

I also checked out:

- the distances I be travelling
- who I go to for counselling if I encounter a traumatic event
- whether my attitudes will change greatly, and if they do, whether they will be in conflict with my family's views on Indigenous Australians

PART 2

MAKING THE MOST OF YOUR FIELDWORK PLACEMENT

Chapter 12:   Models of Supervision   145

Chapter 13:   Making the Most of Your Fieldwork
              Learning Opportunity   159

Chapter 14:   Assessment of Clinical Learning   171

Chapter 15:   A Model for Alternative Fieldwork   186

Chapter 16:   Interprofessional Learning: Working
              in Teams   199

Chapter 17:   Learning from Failure   218

Chapter 18:   Using Online Technology   231

This section teases out in more detail issues directly related to you on fieldwork. Issues covered in this section include: making the most of your fieldwork experience; supervision; assessment; failing; alternative types of fieldwork; and online technology.

CHAPTER 12
MODELS OF SUPERVISION

Ronnie Egan and Doris Testa

LEARNING OUTCOMES

After reading this chapter, you should be able to:
- understand the different approaches to supervision
- develop skills in using critical reflection
- discuss different approaches to student supervision in fieldwork.

KEY TERMS

Administrative function
Adult learning principles
Apprenticeship approach
Articulated model
Competency-based approach
Critical incident analysis
Critical reflection
Educative function
Growth therapeutic approach
Learning by doing
Modernist perspective
Narrative record
Postmodernist perspective
Practice-reflection–theory-reflection process
Role systems approach
Student supervision in fieldwork placement
Supportive function
Think sheet
Work-integrated learning

INTRODUCTION

This chapter will begin with a definition of supervision and the different functions supervision has when you undertake fieldwork. Different models of supervision will be outlined, including the use of adult learning principles to guide the supervision process. The final section of the chapter will explore critical reflection and the tools for using critical reflection as an instructive and contemporary approach to supervision when you undertake fieldwork.

WHAT IS STUDENT SUPERVISION IN FIELDWORK?

Student supervision in fieldwork placement is the process within a professional relationship whereby fieldwork educators assist students to prepare for, reflect on and explore practice issues in order to develop competence in their professional practice. Specific examples of practice settings have been outlined in Part 1. The purpose of the supervisory process is to review and reflect on the work undertaken by you with the fieldwork educator.

The supervisory process is commonly described as having three principal functions:

- educative
- supportive
- administrative (Kadushin & Harkness 2002).

These three functions frequently overlap, and some functions are more dominant at different times throughout the fieldwork experience. For example, at the beginning of placement the fieldwork educator might focus more on the administrative function, providing you with access to organisational policies or protocols. The following section details the three functions.

The educative function

The supervisory process, for both you and your fieldwork educator, is primarily educative. The objectives of educative supervision are to promote professional competence, develop skills and understanding about practice, make the links between theory and practice and enable you to assess your abilities using a mutual process of giving and receiving feedback about performance within the organisation's learning opportunities. For example, the fieldwork educator might suggest to you to read about the particular approach to the work undertaken at the agency. The *educative function* is demonstrated in the discussion between you and your fieldwork educator about the link between your reading and practice within the organisation.

The supportive function

The *supportive function* of supervision assists you to develop, maintain and enhance a professional sense of self. The supportive process is one where the fieldwork educator acknowledges and responds to your emotional needs as these relate to the role of student.

The supportive function helps you to understand the processes of an event and the impact that event might have on you. It requires the fieldwork educator to empathise with your emotional reactions, validate feelings and integrate your experience into the context of your professional development. For example, the fieldwork educator might ask you to undertake a particular task. The supportive function is demonstrated in the opportunity provided by the fieldwork educator, after the task is undertaken, to discuss your feelings, outcomes and your process of understanding the task.

CLINICAL REASONING 12.1

Clinical reasoning is involved in the educative and supportive functions of supervision. Your fieldwork educator's clinical reasoning skills will be more advanced than yours. If you can't understand what is happening in a client-related situation, your fieldwork educator, using his or her clinical reasoning skills, will be able to give reasons why certain actions should be taken.

The administrative function

The administrative function assists you in gaining access to information and resources, and ensures your understanding and use of procedures within the agency. These will include both the formal and informal procedures in the agency. The *formal procedures* are generally documented and followed by all staff, and the *informal procedures* inform the culture of the organisation; for example, when and where lunch might be eaten, whether there's a roster for doing dishes in the agency staff room or how staff meetings are conducted.

The fieldwork educator is accountable to the agency through these procedures. It is the responsibility of your fieldwork educator to ensure that your learning process is consistent, through participation in learning opportunities within the organisation. Your fieldwork educator will also have a professional duty of care, according to his or her discipline. For example, to ensure that you are familiar with the administrative data collection requirements within the agency, the fieldwork educator might ask you to undertake some training in workplace information systems.

REFLECTION 12.1

The checklist

Cleake and Wilson (2007) provide a useful checklist for the student and fieldwork educator to work through during the beginning phase of fieldwork placement. The checklist, given in Table 12.1, provides an opportunity to ensure that both have the same expectations of the functions of supervision. Consider the tasks in the left-hand column. Are these tasks relevant, and should you act upon them in your situation? Note relevance and action in the right-hand columns.

Table 12.1: Function and task checklist for you and your fieldwork educator

Tasks	Before placement	During placement
To validate the student both as a developing professional and as a person		
To create a safe environment for the student to reflect on his or her practice and its impact on him or her as a person		
To clarify the boundaries between support and counselling and the issue of confidentiality in supervision		
To debrief the student and give him or her permission to talk about feelings raised by his or her work		
To help the student explore any emotional blocks to his or her work		
To explore issues of difference and discrimination that may be experienced by the student		
To monitor the overall health and emotional functioning of the student		
To clarify when the student should be advised to seek professional help		
Other (specify)		
To ensure that the student understands his or her role and responsibilities		
To ensure the student's work is reviewed regularly		
To ensure that the student has an appropriate workload		
To ensure that student activities are properly documented and carried out according to agency policies and procedures		
To ensure that the student knows when the supervisor needs to be consulted		
Other (specify)		

Source: Cleake & Wilson (2007: 57–8). Reprinted with kind permission of Cleake and Wilson © Thomson 2007

All three functions are incorporated into the supervisory process. In *work-integrated learning*, the supervisory process is also informed by *adult learning principles*. These principles are fourfold:

- the adult learner is an autonomous learner and able to direct her or his learning
- the adult learner brings life experience to learning. This life experience provides a valuable resource for new learning
- a higher level of learning is likely if the learner is able to use life experience in the generation of new knowledge
- new knowledge is directly applicable to real-life situations in the present rather than the future.

As a student and adult learner, a balance must be struck between the professional learning you need and the learning that may interest you, but may not be as immediately required or applicable to fieldwork placements.

REFLECTION 12.2

The experience of being supervised
The questions below provide the opportunity for you to reflect on your experiences of supervision. This provides the opportunity to use past experience to anticipate some of the fears and anxieties you might face when undertaking a fieldwork placement for the first time.

Reflective questions
What is your experience of being supervised? Consider, for example, an experience you have had in paid work experience or as a volunteer.
- What was the function of the supervision?
- What was useful about the supervisory experience?
- What was less useful about the supervisory experience?
- How might you have participated differently?

Approaches to work-integrated learning have changed over time. The following section provides an overview of the common approaches to fieldwork placement supervision, and explores in more detail the critical reflective approach to fieldwork. A key shift in approaches to supervision has been the move away from investing expertise in the fieldwork educator to a position where you are also an active contributor to fieldwork placement supervision (Beddoe 2000). However for the purpose of this chapter an overview of approaches to work-integrated learning will be provided, because you may encounter a variety of approaches used in the field.

APPROACHES TO SUPERVISORY PRACTICE

Approaches to supervisory practice provide ways of linking assumptions about practice, learning and teaching in different practice settings. They act as guides in developing styles of supervision, depending on the context, the nature of the relationship between fieldwork educator and student, and the parameters of the supervisory relationship. The supervision process is by its nature dynamic, and involves a constant evaluative aspect regardless of the model used. There is an overlap across the models presented, and an assumption that most fieldwork educators may use an eclectic combination of these, depending on the supervisory relationship and the individual's supervisory style. One typology for understanding different approaches to supervisory practice is the distinction between learning by doing and learning by integrating theory and practice. For example, the category of *learning by doing* has models that focus on learning through observation and doing the work. The category of *learning by integrating theory and practice* is concerned with the interrelationship between academic and work-integrated learning. Competent practice relies on prior cognitive understanding. This is sometimes referred to as the academic or *articulated model*.

The following section will use this typology to provide an overview of five different approaches to supervision in fieldwork, with particular emphasis on the critical reflection approach. Table 12.2 summarises these approaches to supervision.

Apprenticeship approach

The *apprenticeship approach* gives primary emphasis to learning by doing. Knowledge, skills, values and attitudes are transmitted to you by observing an experienced professional at work, and observing, emulating or modelling your own behaviour. It focuses on retrieval and formulation of professional responses (Knowles et al. 2005). In social work, for example, the apprenticeship approach was historically how social workers learnt their craft. In this approach, a range of tools monitor the student. They may include process recordings, audio or visual tapes, peer observation, one-way screens, team or casework meetings and co-leadership in groups. The apprenticeship

Table 12.2: Five approaches to supervision

Learning by doing	**Learning by integrating theory and practice**
Growth therapeutic approach	Critical reflection approach
(Siporin 1982)	(Bogo & Vayda 1986, Schon 1983, 1987, 1991)
Role systems approach	
(Kadushin & Harkness 2002)	
Apprenticeship approach	Competency-based approach
(Knowles et al. 2005)	(Bogo et al. 2002)

model generally omits reflective and conceptual activities. Table 12.3 details the strengths and limitations of the apprenticeship approach.

Growth therapeutic approach

The *growth therapeutic approach* assumes that, in order to facilitate growth and change for the client, you also need to undergo a personal growth experience. It is assumed that professional helpers will have a high degree of self-awareness (Siporin 1982). You may be encouraged to be reflective, and disclose personal dilemmas that may be elicited from the practice experience. For example, your fieldwork educator might expect you to reflect on your personal reaction to a particular fieldwork experience and focus on self-disclosure rather than discussing the work. There is a danger in this approach that, having explored and identified personal issues in supervision, professional instruction may be sacrificed. Table 12.4 details the strengths and limitations of the growth therapeutic approach.

Role systems approach

The *role systems approach* focuses on the interaction between you and your fieldwork educator. It is the fieldwork educator's responsibility to ensure that the most appropriate type of learning and teaching occurs. It requires negotiation of the structure, process and content of fieldwork, with the fieldwork educator disclosing to the student his or her explicit beliefs and approaches relating to fieldwork (Kadushin & Harkness 2002). Fieldwork educators will assume different roles with students, depending on their own developmental stage of being a fieldwork educator or their

Table 12.3: Strengths and limitations of the apprenticeship approach

	Strengths	**Limitations**
Apprenticeship approach	Focuses on retrieval and professional response as modelled by fieldwork educator	Traditionally limited to fieldwork educator's practice wisdom with task focus, and therefore omits reflective and conceptual activities

Table 12.4: Strengths and limitations of the growth therapeutic approach

	Strengths	**Limitations**
Growth therapeutic approach	Useful for marginal students	Process that focuses on personal reflection excluding the educational content
	Focuses on personal and professional growth	Exacerbates the power differential between fieldwork educator and student

Table 12.5: Strengths and limitations of the role systems approach

	Strengths	Limitations
Role systems approach	Recognises power imbalances between fieldwork educator and student	Negotiation of role expectations occurs in the context of unequal relationships

Table 12.6: Strengths and limitations of the competency-based approach

	Strengths	Limitations
Competency-based approach	Provides clear guidelines for assessment and evidence of student's performance	Reduces the unique practice opportunities offered by specific organisations There may be a shift from theory to acquisition of practice wisdom

theoretical orientation. Table 12.5 details the strengths and limitations of the role systems approach to supervision.

Competency-based approach

A *competency-based approach* defines learning objectives in specific, observable, behavioural terms. A variety of aspects of practice and associated competencies are identified and expressed as behavioural skills. Fieldwork educators are then able to rate student performance according to stages in skill acquisition, from understanding to behavioural integration. A fieldwork educator may focus on a range of tasks including, for example, values and ethics that are expressed as behavioural skills. The fieldwork educator might rate your performance for each competency, such as demonstrating congruency between one's activities and professional values (Bogo et al. 2002). Table 12.6 details the strengths and limitations of the competency-based approach to supervision.

CRITICAL REFLECTION AS AN APPROACH TO SUPERVISION

Critical reflection directs our practice towards the political and potentially emancipatory aspects of situations that may be changed. The use of critical reflection has evolved from the questioning and challenging of knowledge generation (Fook 2002).

From a *modernist perspective*, knowledge is understood in a linear, scientific and rational way, by which experts generate theory, and health professionals receive and apply this theory in practice (Fook 2002). A *postmodernist perspective* challenges this understanding of knowledge. Rather than understanding knowledge from only a theoretical perspective, postmodernists incorporate other types of knowledge generated by reflecting on personal experience and culture. In work-integrated learning, being able to make the links between theory, personal interpretation and experience and culture assists in developing your practice knowledge. On fieldwork placement, these links add depth to the meaning you ascribe to practice experiences.

Critical reflection is a tool used to make these links and to begin exploring the 'taken-for-granted' reasons for 'why we do what we do' in practice. The aim of critical reflection is to understand how our assumptions, values, beliefs and taken-for-granted reasons for *why we do what we do* have an impact on practice.

Critical reflection assists you in exposing how practice is affected by social structures and institutions, and how they may be reinforcing oppression and sustaining inequality. Critical reflection invites you to take responsibility for personal and professional identities, values, actions and feelings, and to understand their origins. By identifying the assumptions, ideas and values that you bring to a situation, you develop new ways of working and approaching the same situation.

Critical reflection also involves the application of the skills of challenge and confrontation. These skills are used to expose the dilemmas, ambiguities and paradoxes of practice, and to move practice towards anti-discriminatory practice (Fook & Gardner 2007). For example, critical reflection may involve you in naming the dominant and missing perspectives in the critical field practice incident.

By using critical questions, reflection on practice can lead to new ways of acting, by which means behaviours, contexts and values are challenged. Fieldwork placements offer you opportunities to grow and develop professionally, which is different from classroom-based learning.

REFLECTION 12.3

Critical reflections

Some critical reflection questions, listed below (based on Holland & Henriot 1995), can be used by you and your fieldwork educator to review practice, and add synthesis and evaluation to the consideration of fieldwork placement.

Critical reflection questions
- Which theoretical approach have I used to inform practice?
- Whose interests does this approach serve?
- Who is being disadvantaged or advantaged by this practice?
- Why do I think this is so? Are there inconsistencies in my thinking?
- How could I do things differently in my practice?
- What are the underlying assumptions of this theory?
- What knowledge is excluded?

THINK AND LINK 12.1

Chapter 20 discusses approaches to thinking through ethical issues that are related to vulnerable clients and patients. Some of these critical reflection questions are embedded in some of the approaches included in Chapter 20, although they are not presented as critical reflections.

Striving for critical reflection

As with any learning, our ability to engage in critical reflection is a work in progress. You may not always be successful or confident in your critical reflection, so it is important to have fieldwork educators who can help you revisit critical reflection processes and help hone your critical reflection skills. Critical reflection invites the health professional to recall life experiences that shape and influence how you see and experience the world. Using critical reflection takes time, commitment and a preparedness to reflect on and be aware of all that you communicate to people: your age, 'race', culture, sexuality and religious, political and social beliefs and background. Case Study 12.1 provides an opportunity for both you and your fieldwork educator to analyse, reconsider and re-question the issues that arise for you.

Case Study 12.1	Working with Mr Omar

Your fieldwork placement is at a community health centre. You have been working with Mr Omar for one month, and finding him difficult to engage. Mr Omar's interactions with you have been loud and aggressive. He consistently uses pointing and jabbing actions when interacting with you. Mr Omar has arrived at the reception desk again, asking to see you and claiming to be in crisis. This is the third time he has done this, so you have approached your fieldwork educator to see Mr Omar with you.

Questions for critical reflection

1   What might be happening for Mr Omar? (reflection on content)
2   What is happening for you?
3   What emotions or reactions are being stirred up for you?
4   Where might these have come from? (reflection on meaning)
5   How do you understand this?
6   Are there gender, age, socioeconomic or other considerations that might be having an impact on Mr Omar's or your own behaviour?
7   How could the interaction between Mr Omar and yourself be different? (critical reflection).

WORK-INTEGRATED LEARNING: TRANSLATING CRITICAL REFLECTION INTO CRITICAL ACTION

Learning critical reflective skills is only part of the challenge. Critical reflecting on practice situations needs to be followed by translation into action. Translating critical reflection into critical action can be challenging. Depending on one's personal life experiences, cultural background and social norms, critical reflection may be difficult for some individuals. However, these skills are central to work-integrated learning. Reflecting at the individual and community level can take many forms; for example, for a student on a fieldwork placement this may mean challenging stereotypes, gender roles or socioeconomic status. This may mean challenging the behaviour of the client, challenging the context in which you work and/or challenging the worker's own mindset.

Critical reflection on placement requires you to work systematically through the 'what', 'when', 'how' and 'why' of work experience. For example, using the structure of a *critical incident* exercise (see Reflection 12.4) can support the critical reflection process to arrive at a practical outcome.

REFLECTION 12.4

The critical incident
The following table provides an opportunity to critically reflect on a fieldwork placement incident.

Table 12.7: Critical incident technique

Situation	Describe briefly an incident that occurred during your placement
Name the facts	What led to the incident? What was the broader context of the incident? Who was there? What happened? Why did the incident occur?
List your actions	In as much detail as you can describe How you responded to the incident? What did you do?
List the outcomes of your actions	What was the consequence of your actions on: • you? • your client? • others in the agency?

Explain briefly any of these action outcomes	Negative outcomes Typical outcome for the agency Novel, challenging, demanding or unchanged outcome Made a difference to the incident The action had a significant personal outcome
Reflection	What previous knowledge or experience informed your action? List the skills used in this action. Write about the theory or theories that informed your actions. List the values that underpinned your actions. Do you think you acted ethically? Could you identify any ethical dilemmas for you? Describe them. What constraints (if any) had an impact on the actions you took?—for example, time, resources, agency policy, agency culture, your or your fieldwork educator's involvement. What did you feel during and after the incident? What did you find most demanding (if anything) about the incident? Did the outcome of the situation match your desired outcome? On reflection would you do the same again?
Learning	What did you learn from the incident about: • theory and knowledge? • values and ethics? • skills? • your own beliefs, attitudes, prejudices, values and ethics?

Source: adapted from Fook 2002

THINK AND LINK 12.2

Chapter 13 also uses tools for reflection. Try using these tools in conjunction with critical reflection.

TOOLS FOR CRITICAL REFLECTION

The phases of critical reflection use a *practice-reflection–theory-reflection process*. During this process, students can use a number of critical reflection tools. Fook and colleagues (2000) suggest a number of writing tools that can be used in critical reflection. These include critical incident analysis, journal keeping, think sheets and narrative records.

Critical incident analysis

A *critical incident analysis* includes a reflection on a specific incident using the following steps:

1 A description of the incident and those involved
2 The outcomes of the action for each involved in the incident, including positive and negative impacts of the actions
3 A reflection on the process, naming the types of knowledge or experience that informed the actions, the skills used and the theories underpinning the actions
4 Naming your learning from the incident: discipline-specific theory and knowledge; professional values and ethics; skills; personal beliefs and assumptions.

A journal

A journal is a record of significant events and personal responses to events, kept throughout the length of the placement and even beyond. The formatting and purpose of the journal can differ according to the expectations of you, your university and your fieldwork educator. However, before a journal is started you and your fieldwork educator need to clarify the purpose and content of the journal, and whether the content will be shared, and by whom. For example, the university may have an expectation that you keep a journal for the duration of the fieldwork placement; however, whether the fieldwork educator can read the journal needs to be clarified between your fieldwork educator and you at the beginning of placement.

Think sheet

A *think sheet* is a more structured, generalised writing exercise that encourages reflection on both behavioural and emotional responses to fieldwork placement experiences.

Narrative record

A *narrative record* is the retelling of events on fieldwork placement from a personal perspective. This can occur both in writing and/or conversation between you and your fieldwork educator. The retelling may include conversations with significant others and links with past or current experiences, and may also connect feelings with ideas and experiences. The narrative record tries to link the intellectual, spiritual, moral, social, physical and aesthetic dimensions of the narrative.

SUMMARY

This chapter has introduced different approaches to supervision in fieldwork placements. It provides an overview of four approaches to supervision in fieldwork, and explores in more depth a critically reflective approach to fieldwork placement.

DISCUSSION QUESTIONS

1   Name the different functions of supervision and provide an example of each.
2   What approaches to supervision resonate with you and why?
3   How might structured supervision include the three functions of supervision?

References

Beddoe, E. (2000). 'The Supervisory Relationship'. In L. Cooper & L. Briggs (eds). *Fieldwork in the Human Services: Theory and Practice for Field Education, Practice Teachers and Supervisors*. Allen & Unwin, Sydney: 41–54.

Bogo, M., Regehr, C. & Power, R. (2002). *Competency-Based Evaluation (CBE) Tool*. Faculty of Social Work, University of Toronto.

Bogo, M. & Vayda, E. (1986). *The Practice of Field Instruction*. University of Toronto Press, Toronto.

Cleake, H. & Wilson, J. (2007). *Making the Most of Field Placement* (2nd edn). Thomson, South Melbourne.

Fook, J. (2002). *Social Work: Critical Theory and Practice*. Sage, London.

Fook, J. & Gardner, F. (2007). *Practising Critical Reflection: A Resource Handbook*. Open University Press, Maidenhead.

Fook, J., Ryan, M. & Hawkins, L. (2000). *Professional Expertise: Practice, Theory and Education for Working in Uncertainty*. Whiting & Birch, London.

Holland, J. & Henriot, P. (1995). *Social Analysis: Linking Faith and Justice* (12th edn). Dove Communications, Melbourne.

Kadushin, A. & Harkness, D. (2002). *Supervision in Social Work* (4th edn). Columbia University Press, New York.

Knowles, M. S., Elwood, F., Holton R., III & Swanson, A. (2005). *The Adult Learner: The Definitive Classic in Adult Education and Human Resource Development* (6th edn). Elsevier, Amsterdam & Boston.

Siporin, M. (1982). 'The Process of Field Instruction in Quality Field Instruction in Social Work'. In B. W. Sheafor & L. E. Jenkins (eds). *Quality Field Instruction in Social Work: Program Development and Maintenance*. Longman, New York: 175–97.

Schon, D. (1983). *The Reflective Practitioner*. Temple Smith, London.

Schon, D. (1987). *Educating the Reflective Practitioner*. Jossey-Bass, San Francisco.

Schon, D. (1991). *The Reflective Practitioner: How Professionals Think in Action*. Basic Books, New York.

CHAPTER 13
MAKING THE MOST OF YOUR FIELDWORK LEARNING OPPORTUNITY

Helen Larkin and Anita Hamilton

LEARNING OUTCOMES

After reading this chapter, you should be able to:
- identify factors that influence your learning during fieldwork placement
- explain how your current skills, knowledge and attributes influence your personal learning opportunities and outcomes
- reflect on the actions you can take to facilitate your work integrated learning.

KEY TERMS

Discipline-specific knowledge
Evidence-based approach
Fieldwork learning framework
Goal-setting
Johari window
Personal attributes
Practice reflection
Work-integrated learning

INTRODUCTION

Health professions embed *work-integrated learning* or *fieldwork learning* into their programs as a required teaching activity. It is important that this learning be closely integrated with academic learning (Biggs & Tang 2007: 143), as it provides an opportunity for students to:
- apply knowledge and skills learned in university in real-life professional settings
- apply theories and skills to practice in all aspects of professional practice
- work collaboratively with all parties in multidisciplinary workplace settings
- practise with professional attitudes and social responsibilities in their respective professions.

This chapter explores the factors that influence fieldwork learning, and identifies how you can make the most of your fieldwork experience. The framework described will assist you to understand your central role in the learning process, and provides strategies for promoting critical reflection and professional growth and integrating theory with practice.

THE FIELDWORK LEARNING FRAMEWORK

The *fieldwork learning framework* (Figure 13.1) describes the personal and professional resources and attributes that contribute to developing your skills, knowledge and behaviours for professional practice. It emphasises the need to be continually *reflecting on practice*; *seeking advice*; *setting goals*; and *taking action* during fieldwork.

The framework emphasises a continuous cycle of learning over time. Different aspects of the framework become more or less important at various times during a fieldwork placement, or between placements, as you build on prior experience

Figure 13.1: The fieldwork learning framework

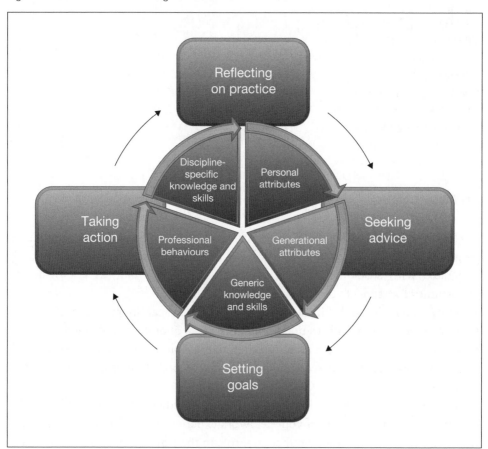

and learning and continue to develop professional and personal skills. Using the framework will help you to manage how you feel, think and act, and help you to make the most of your fieldwork learning opportunity. Throughout this chapter, specific tools are suggested that promote reflection throughout the cycle.

Personal and professional resources for learning

The inner circle of the framework consists of personal and professional resources and attributes upon which you can reflect. Each of these is described below, with suggestions on how to recognise and develop them during fieldwork learning. They include:

- personal attributes
- generational attributes
- generic knowledge and skills
- professional behaviours
- discipline-specific knowledge and skills.

Personal attributes

Before commencing fieldwork placements, you may express concern about your professional competence and the impact of this on your ability to perform satisfactorily. However, a common cause of difficulty is not your emerging professional skills and knowledge, but the personal attributes that you bring to the fieldwork placement. These include, but are not limited to, such things as: age and gender; learning style; cultural and family background; and the presence or not of a specific health condition or disability.

Aveling (2001) proposes that attributes such as those described above contribute to all of us being *marked* or *unmarked*, depending on the environment and context in which we are placed at any given time. For example, a male student amongst predominantly female students will feel marked by his gender. Alternatively, a female student will feel unmarked in this situation. Be aware of factors that might create a sense of being marked or unmarked. The unwritten norms of organisations, which define the context and environment, are often the ones that define who is marked or unmarked. A lack of awareness of these factors by you or your fieldwork educator can be a source of misunderstanding and confusion. Developing awareness through reflection and seeking advice are important steps in preventing negative or frustrating experiences.

Diversity is something to be affirmed and celebrated; however, it is important to recognise that sometimes our own and others' personal attributes (including fieldwork educators) may be misunderstood. Identifying this early in the placement ensures reducing opportunities for misunderstanding between you, your fieldwork educator and others in the workplace. Consider the following scenarios in Table 13.1.

Table 13.1: Personal attribute scenarios

I am a mature age student.	You may not be easily identified as a 'student' by other workers, or there may be higher expectations of you than may be made of younger students. Alternatively, you may relate more easily with others of a similar age.
I am a reflective learner and learn best through introspection.	Your fieldwork educator may expect you to be actively involved in fieldwork tasks, and expects you to discuss at length what you have done and why.
I am an international student and English is not my first language.	Apart from difficulties with language, your cultural and/or religious background may be different from that of others in the workplace. This may affect the way you go about fieldwork tasks.
I have a hearing impairment, but don't know whether to disclose this to my fieldwork educator.	By not disclosing, you remain 'unmarked' within the workplace. By disclosing, you enable your fieldwork educator and others to make accommodations for your learning needs. There is no right or wrong way, but requires some reflection and seeking advice.
My family has very high expectations of me, and I am worried that I am not going to do well.	If your primary focus is on not failing rather than on what you can learn, you will be more reluctant to immerse yourself in all of the available learning opportunities and to take risks with your learning.

Generational attributes

The generations born between 1982 and 2002, commonly known as Generation Y or Millennials (Prensky 2001), are thought to learn and communicate in a fundamentally different way from other generations (Arhin & Cormier 2007; Nimon 2007; Oblinger & Oblinger 2005, Pardue & Morgan 2008). If you are of this generation, it is likely that you: have learnt to multitask; favour graphics and multimedia over text; are able to communicate online; have minimal tolerance for delays; and, prefer Google to using the library (Oblinger & Hawkins 2005).

THINK AND LINK 13.1

If you are from Generation Y, then you might be more at ease with issues raised in Chapter 18. Chapter 18 outlines specific technology-enhanced learning strategies that can facilitate fieldwork learning.

Generational characteristics have implications for work-integrated learning beyond learning preferences. Your learning and communication style may be in direct contrast to those of your fieldwork educator or others in the workplace, and may result in your behaviour being viewed by others as uninterested or distracted, as shown in Table 13.2.

Table 13.2: Reframing generational attributes and behaviours

Generational attribute	Possible behaviour	May be interpreted by fieldwork educator as	Alternative action
Need to engage in multitasking and stay constantly connected	Checks messages on mobile phone in team meeting	The student is uninterested	Check phone messages during breaks. If you are waiting for an important message, discuss it with your fieldwork educator
Technologically savvy, and favours using multiple media to support learning	Feels disconnected if fieldwork setting does not have the same technology as university or home	Student is unable to work in the 'real world'	Explain some of the technology that you use at university and its application to the workplace
Expects instantaneous responses	Expects to be able to meet with fieldwork educator at minimal notice	Student is demanding and doesn't appreciate the supervisor's workload	Discuss the area of concern that you have, and ask when the fieldwork educator may be available to sit down and discuss this with you
Managing multiple priorities	Asks to leave early to be able to go to work. Falls asleep during a meeting	Fieldwork is not the students' priority, and they are not appreciative of the opportunities being provided	Determine your priorities. Plan your paid job well in advance so that you can manage the demands of fieldwork placement. Think about doing more work over the holidays so you can give greater priority to fieldwork

Generic knowledge and skills

Students frequently juggle fieldwork and academic workload with the demands of paid work, and perhaps voluntary or community work and caring responsibilities. These other experiences provide valuable skills in areas such as teamwork, time management, negotiating conflict, managing change, and leadership. Such generic work skills complement and add value to the discipline-specific knowledge and skills being learned at university. Utilising these generic skills is a key component of optimising learning in the fieldwork setting.

Professional behaviours

Some of the most critical behaviours for health professionals include demonstrating a positive regard for others, being able to maintain confidentiality and having excellent interpersonal skills. It can be challenging to remain positive and communicate effectively if the learning situation on your fieldwork placement is overwhelming and stressful.

Effective communication relies on being assertive, controlling anger and managing anxiety (Nelson & Low 2003). These factors can be difficult to manage when you are working in a hierarchical environment, working across disciplines in the junior role of student/learner. Communicating requires you to be an active listener, and speak clearly, objectively and honestly, while recognising that the other person has the right to disagree with you.

To communicate assertively, use first-person language to open your statement with 'I feel', 'I think' or 'I believe', and link it with the event that you wish to discuss. The case study below describes a typical fieldwork scenario, followed by alternative communication response examples.

Without reflection and advice Jenna may become stuck in a cycle of ineffective communication. Without an understanding of her own anxiety and anger she would be more likely to respond with ineffective or negative responses. By identifying her anxiety Jenna is taking steps to avoid being angry with herself and her fieldwork educator. By discussing it in an assertive manner (see Table 13.3) and considering how the situation could be improved, Jenna is taking steps to improve her communication skills in team meetings.

Case Study 13.1 | **Jenna, part 1**

Jenna was unexpectedly asked to speak at a team meeting about one of the clients she was working with. She was quite anxious about this, particularly in light of the fact that she was asked at the last minute. Jenna tried to collect her thoughts in order to clearly outline her role and progress with her client. However, as her anxiety increased, her presentation became rushed and disorganised. The fieldwork educator took over, and finished telling the team what Jenna had been doing. After the meeting Jenna felt angry with herself for not being able to think and speak clearly during her presentation. She was also angry with her fieldwork educator for putting her in that position, and then taking over.

Questions

1. Articulate the emotions that Jenna was feeling.
2. Have you felt like this at any of your fieldwork placements?
3. What might Jenna say to her fieldwork educator about the team meeting? (Hint: there are some alternative response types given in Table 13.3.)

Table 13.3: Alternative response types

Response type	Communication example
Aggressive	Jenna speaks loudly: *'It was completely unfair to expect me to suddenly present in the meeting today, and then take over when I wasn't able to do it properly'*
Passive aggressive	Jenna is quiet and smiles at her fieldwork educator after the meeting. While leaving she thinks to herself: *'I should never be put in that position. What kind of fieldwork educator is she anyway? I am not going to learn anything while I'm on fieldwork here!'*
Deferential	Jenna thinks to herself: *'Well, I messed that up, as usual! My fieldwork educator knows what she's doing by asking me to present without warning. I'll just have to see if I can improve … somehow'*
Assertive	Jenna asks to see her fieldwork educator later, and speaks privately with her: *'As you may know, I am quite anxious when presenting, so I felt awkward when you asked me to present at the team meeting. Is it possible to have time to prepare for meetings so I can manage my thoughts better and present clearly and concisely?'*

Discipline-specific knowledge and skills

Educational approaches in health care vary in the way work-integrated learning can be organised and delivered. According to discipline and year level, students develop a range of discipline-specific skills and knowledge through fieldwork placements, and a range of classroom, online, practical learning and assessment activities.

A key strategy for seeking advice regarding *discipline-specific knowledge* is obtaining evidence from the research literature. This *evidence-based approach* to fieldwork practice integrates a systematic search for, and critical appraisal of, the most relevant evidence, combined with clinical expertise and client preferences and values, to answer a fieldwork question (Fineout-Overholt et al. 2005). Through formal education, you will be learning how to implement the five steps of evidence-based practice (Fineout-Overholt et al. 2005: 338–40):

1 question framing
2 database searching
3 critical appraisal
4 implementation
5 evaluation.

Evidence-based practice is best undertaken in the practice context. However, your fieldwork educator may lack the support, time and resources to search for new evidence in day-to-day practice (Fineout-Overholt et al. 2005). Therefore, combining the experience of your fieldwork educator with your developing skills in evidence-based practice has learning outcomes for both parties, and positive healthcare outcomes for clients.

OPTIMISING YOUR FIELDWORK LEARNING OPPORTUNITIES

To make the most of fieldwork learning, you need to continually draw from your personal attributes; generational attributes; generic knowledge and skills; professional behaviours; and discipline-specific knowledge and skills. These are your personal resources for learning. This is best achieved by continually reflecting on practice, seeking appropriate advice, setting goals and taking action for learning.

Reflecting on practice

Reflecting on practice is one of the defining characteristics of a quality professional (Schön 1995). The reflective tool, presented in Table 13.4, is based on the *Johari window* (Luft 1969), which was designed to develop and enhance self-awareness. The window is divided into four panes or quadrants: *open, blind, hidden* and *unknown*.

In this reflection tool 'I' refers to you, and 'You' refers to the fieldwork educator. We all naturally communicate many things during our interactions with others, some we are aware of, some we are not. Using this tool promotes self-awareness, so that you and your fieldwork educator can explore your combined awareness of your current knowledge and skills, which will help you *set goals* and *take action* to improve practice (Smith 2007).

The *Open quadrant* includes those moments when you are aware of your skills and knowledge, and choose to share and demonstrate these with others. In this quadrant, students will not respond automatically to a question from a fieldwork educator with 'I don't know'. Instead, you can respond more positively with 'This is what I know': a more positive and productive way of communicating. You could use this tool with your fieldwork educator in a supervision session.

The *Hidden quadrant* includes those situations when you choose not to reveal your knowledge and skills. Students sometimes hide their abilities because they don't feel confident enough to use them in practice. Being able to discuss with your fieldwork educator what you can do, but are afraid to try, requires courage and trust, but it is worthwhile. Give your fieldwork educator a clear picture of how you see yourself, as this helps to develop your working relationship and opens the door to *seeking advice*.

Table 13.4: Reflecting on practice window

	Known to self	Unknown to self
Known to Others	**Open** I know it, can do it, can say it or show it	**Blind** You know I don't know it, do it or show it But I don't know what I don't know or do
Unknown to Others	**Hidden** I know it, can do it, but don't show or say it	**Unknown** We both can't see what I don't know or can't do

Source: Adapted from Johari window (Luft 1969)

The *Blind quadrant* includes issues of which you are unaware. Organisations often have unwritten rules of which novice health professionals are unaware. As a student it can be easy to break those unwritten rules, and it can be a shock when you are made aware of this. It can be as simple as using someone's coffee cup or as complex as acting inappropriately, without understanding the context of an issue. We all have blind spots, and we need to develop our awareness of them if we are to grow. When you find yourself feeling resentful or angry about any feedback, it is wise to seek advice from someone you trust. Ask that person if he or she thinks it is possible that you were blind to your behaviour.

The *Unknown quadrant* includes all those things of which both you and your fieldwork educator are unaware. You simply might not know what happened or why someone responded to a particular behaviour or comment. This can also include those areas of skills and knowledge that are difficult to practise; for example, responding to an emergency. This quadrant is the most difficult to predict.

Seeking advice

The ability to know when and how to appropriately seek timely advice is a core skill in any profession. It is a skill that requires practice. Some students are *deferential*, asking for advice too often and failing to trust their own judgment; while others are *overconfident*, failing to seek advice when they need to. The challenge is to find that middle ground, reflecting on what you honestly do and don't know is the best place to start.

THINK AND LINK 13.2

Chapter 17 is about learning from failure in fieldwork. If you have had difficulty in your fieldwork placement, read this chapter (Chapter 13) together with Chapter 17.

Case Study 13.2	Jenna, part 2

We continue to explore Jenna's experience of presenting unexpectedly at a team meeting. In order to support Jenna to better understand herself, the fieldwork educator suggested that they use the reflecting on practice tool. After carefully going through each window, both Jenna and the fieldwork educator were able to create a framework for a meaningful discussion about each other's thoughts, beliefs and behaviours, and consider how they might both contribute to improving Jenna's anxiety about presenting at team meetings.

Question

1   How does this solution differ from your suggestions in Part 1?

REFLECTION 13.1

Reflecting on practice window: Jenna's reflection on her own performance

	Known to self	Unknown to self
Known to others	**Open** I become anxious when speaking in team meetings	**Blind** You seem to have low confidence in speaking clearly at team meetings, but I have seen you speak clearly with clients
Unknown to others	**Hidden** I have done this before in case study presentations at university, but because this is a real team meeting I'm afraid of saying so in case I appear to be overconfident or I say the wrong thing	**Unknown** How would I manage at presenting to a large group such as a seminar? I haven't had an opportunity to do this before, but I feel very anxious about the idea

Outcome

Jenna and her fieldwork educator agreed that it would be helpful if Jenna had time to prepare for meetings. Jenna and the fieldwork educator discussed that her fears were common, and that many people had been in the same position when they were students. Jenna's fieldwork educator told her that she had observed Jenna working with clients and with other team members, and had observed evidence of specific knowledge, skills and behaviours valued by their profession. Jenna was pleased to hear that others thought she was performing well, but was unaware that she had been observed. Jenna's fieldwork educator asked to set a goal focusing on reducing her anxiety in team meetings. The unknown quadrant allowed Jenna and her fieldwork educator to explore opportunities for future practice, while at the same time reassuring Jenna that this would not be necessary for this particular placement

Warning! Don't wait for something to go wrong first. Use this tool as a guide when planning and preparing for fieldwork placement or on a regular basis to reflect on your practice and check your progress.

Setting goals

Goal-setting involves working out where you want to be and how you might get there. Based on what you know about yourself and your professional skills and knowledge, set goals that are achievable, but challenge and extend you further, allowing and helping you to grow. These should be developed in collaboration with your fieldwork educator. A simple goal-setting strategy is to write *SMART goals* (Specific, Measurable, Achievable, Related, Timely) to help you identify *how* you will achieve your goals, and *when* and *how* you will evaluate your progress. This may take the form of a formal learning contract. Be sure to review your progress, and continually re-evaluate your goals throughout your fieldwork placement.

A SMART goal for Jenna would be: 'To reduce anxiety about presenting at team meetings, I will clearly and concisely document my client summaries and give these to my fieldwork educator for review the day before the team meeting each week, so there is time to amend and rehearse before the meeting.'

Taking action

Lifelong learning as a professional starts at university, is demonstrated in fieldwork and is ongoing through your professional life. Acting on your agreed fieldwork learning goals is the most effective way to improve practice knowledge and skills, and help form good learning habits. Jenna identified that she is anxious about presenting in team meetings. In discussion with her fieldwork educator she was able to identify why she became anxious and create a plan to reduce her anxiety, and as a consequence improve her presentation skills. This example typifies the cycle of learning that continues throughout fieldwork, as you identify other personal and professional resources and attributes for learning.

Repeating the cycle

Depending on the duration of fieldwork placement, the fieldwork learning framework cycle will be repeated. Using the practice reflection tool (Table 13.4), review your learning goals, and consider with your fieldwork educator (and others) what your next learning goals could be. The focus of your goals may be any of the personal and professional attribute areas. Consider also, if any aspects have moved quadrants; for example, are you now aware of something to which you were previously *blind*?

SUMMARY

The model described in this chapter is designed to assist you to identify the factors that influence your learning within the context of fieldwork. Learning outcomes that arise out of fieldwork placements may be discipline specific in nature; more related to generic skills; or, an appreciation of how personal attributes facilitate or act as a barrier to successful learning during fieldwork. The best learning takes place when you are able to reflect on, seek advice, set goals and take action in relation to these factors.

DISCUSSION QUESTIONS

1 Which of the personal and professional attributes contained in the fieldwork learning framework do you feel are your strengths?
2 Which of these attributes do you feel you have had difficulty with in the past?

3   Identify examples in the past where you have communicated in the *Hidden* quadrant. Reflect on how you could have communicated in the *Open* quadrant in these situations.

4   What are the benefits of reflecting during fieldwork? What are the costs of choosing not to reflect?

References

Arhin, A. O. & Cormier, E. (2007). 'Using Deconstruction to Educate Generation Y Nursing Students'. *Journal of Nursing Education*, 46(12): 562–67.

Aveling, N. (2001). '"Where Do You Come From?" Critical Storytelling as a Teaching Strategy within the Context of Teacher Education'. *Discourse: Studies in the Cultural Politics of Education*, 22(1): 35–48.

Biggs, J. & Tang, C. (2007). *Teaching for Quality Learning at University* (3rd edn). McGraw-Hill Education, Berkshire.

Fineout-Overholt, E., Melnyk, B. M. & Schultz, A. (2005). 'Transforming Health Care from the Inside Out: Advancing Evidence-Based Practice in the 21st Century'. *Journal of Professional Nursing*, 21(6): 335–44.

Luft, J. (1969). *Of Human Interaction*. National Press Books, Palo Alto, CA.

Nelson, D. B. & Low, G. R. (2003). *Emotional Intelligence: Achieving Academic and Career Excellence*. Prentice Hall, Upper Saddle River, NJ.

Nimon, S. (2007). 'Generation Y and Higher Education: The Other Y2K'. *Journal of Institutional Research*, 13(1): 24–41.

Oblinger D. G. & Hawkins, B. L. (2005). 'The Myth about Students: "We Understand Our Students"'. *Educause*, 40(5): 12–13.

Oblinger, D. G. & Oblinger, J. L. (2005). *Educating the Net Generation*. Educause, Washington, DC.

Pardue, K. T. & Morgan, P. (2008). 'Millennials Considered: A New Generation, New Approaches, and Implications for Nursing Education'. *Nursing Education Perspectives*, 29(2): 74–9.

Prensky, M. (2001). 'Digital Natives, Digital Immigrants'. *On the Horizon*, 9(5): 1–6.

Schön, D. D. A. (1995). *Reflective Practitioner: How Professionals Think In Action* (new ed.). Arena, Aldershot.

Smith, J. K. (2007). 'Promoting Self-awareness in Nurses to Improve Nursing Practice'. *Nursing Standard*, 21(32): 47–52.

CHAPTER 14
ASSESSMENT OF CLINICAL LEARNING

Megan Smith

LEARNING OUTCOMES

After reading this chapter you should be able to:
- reflect upon the role and methods of assessment of clinical learning
- identify strategies to promote effective self-assessment.

KEY TERMS

Assessment
Assessment criteria
Midway assessment
Self-assessment

Case Study 14.1   Nicole's midway assessment

Nicole has been on fieldwork placement for three weeks. Today she is receiving her midway assessment and is feeling anxious. She thinks that she has been going OK, but is not sure what to expect during the assessment interview. She wonders how her fieldwork educator will rate her performance, and worries about the possibility of failing.

Questions

1. How would you describe your experiences of assessment on clinical placement?
2. Does this case study sound familiar to you?
3. Have you thought about how you prepare for and use assessment feedback in your clinical placements?

INTRODUCTION

Assessment is integral to your experience of your education, and is recognised as an important driver of the amount and type of your learning (Irons 2008). Although a common and familiar aspect of studying, assessment on fieldwork placement is a novel form of assessment for students who are more accustomed to exams and assignments. Strategies learnt to manage and succeed in traditional forms of assessment may not transfer successfully to the clinical environment. The aim of this chapter is to give you optimal help in preparing for assessment during your fieldwork placement. A key message promoted in this chapter is that you need to be an active partner in assessment, and develop sound skills in self-assessment.

It is important at the beginning of this chapter to highlight that clinical placements are primarily opportunities for learning, and assessment is just a measure of whether learning has taken place. You are expected to try new things and to make mistakes in the course of your learning. An important strategy for a successful assessment outcome is to show that you are learning and making adequate progress against the expected criteria.

This chapter begins by highlighting the differences between assessment in clinical settings and more traditional forms of student assessment. We will then look at the criteria used to assess clinical performance, and some examples from the range of health disciplines. Finally we will look at how to develop your skills in self-assessment as they apply to clinical placement.

WHAT IS SPECIAL ABOUT ASSESSMENT IN CLINICAL LEARNING?

By the time you commence your first fieldwork placement you are likely to be very experienced at assessment, having completed years of schooling and university study. However, not all assessment is the same, and the characteristics of assessment in the clinical settings are very different from those in exams and assignments (see Table 14.1 for a comparison).

You might notice important differences between these types of assessments. For example, fieldwork assessment is continuous over the duration of the placement. This ongoing nature of assessment means that you will continue to learn while you are being assessed. This is different from a final exam, which is a single task based on a defined body of material for which you are given a long time to prepare. However, during fieldwork placement you are likely to receive formal *midway feedback*, where you are given a mark or level of achievement using the same assessment forms that will be used at the end of the placement. You then have the opportunity to respond to this feedback to influence your subsequent results. Assessment in the clinical setting also assesses a greater amount and complexity of knowledge, skills and professional behaviours than can be contained in any single assessment that you might be used to.

Table 14.1: Differences between clinical assessment and assessment in formal academic settings

Assessment in formal academic settings (e.g. exams, assignments)	Assessment during fieldwork placement
• Single submission of an assignment or one-off examination • Extended period of time to prepare which can be controlled by the student (e.g. when you study) • Retrospective assessment of material previously studied • Single assessor • Limited or no chance to respond to feedback to influence marks • Limited frame of reference for criteria, e.g. may focus on narrow area of knowledge • More concrete criteria to address • Summation of understanding of material already learnt • Theory based rather than practice based	• Continuous assessment where aspects of your performance are repeatedly sampled and have an impact on the next assessment • Developmental process, allowing feedback to be integrated • Ongoing learning occurs while being assessed • May be multiple assessors • Multiple sources of data can be used to assess performance • Limited time for preparation and revision before assessment • Assessment under selected assessment conditions are used to predict your future practice as a health professional • Assessment is contextual and less controllable. Your performance may be influenced by the patient and others in the setting • Based on practice and performance rather than theory • Multiple criteria • More abstract complex concepts are being assessed • Assesses competency for entry-level practice as well as attributes that will develop over the course of your professional experience.

REFLECTION 14.1

Last-minute Ben

Ben is a third-year student who is used to completing his assessment tasks at the last minute. He has always reviewed the material covered during the semester in the week before the final exam. On his first day of fieldwork placement his fieldwork educator tests him on his knowledge of the anatomy of the upper limb while they are preparing to see a client presenting with a work injury. He has not studied this material before placement, and has had no time to prepare for her questions.

Questions

Think about your current approach to completing assessment tasks.

1 Will your current strategies be adaptable to the clinical setting?

2 What changes might you have to make?

3 What changes will Ben have to make if he is to be successful in placement?

WHAT IS THE ROLE OF ASSESSMENT IN CLINICAL LEARNING?

Successfully negotiating any assessment task is easier when you understand the purpose of the task. Assessment of fieldwork placement serves some very important purposes that can slip your notice when you become focused on meeting criteria required to pass a placement and the marks you will receive. You need to think about each placement assessment as a piece of the bigger picture that will lead to the awarding of your qualification and, more importantly, your right to practise as a health professional. This important role of being a practising health professional means that your assessment is in the interest of many other people beyond, you, your fieldwork educator and your university. For example:

- our clients and patients need to be confident that their health care is being managed by capable practitioners who will ensure they receive safe and effective care
- society requires and expects that health professionals provide a certain standard of care that all members of that profession have obtained
- our professional colleagues expect that those they work with can be trusted to do their job to a certain standard
- our colleagues in our specific disciplines expect that new members of that discipline maintain the minimum standard of care by which all members of the discipline are judged.

It is clear that being able to practise as a health professional requires you to achieve certain standards of practice. These standards form the basis of assessment on clinical placement. Many professions have defined these standards (for example, there are the Australian Physiotherapy Standards (Australian Physiotherapy Council 2006), the National Competency Standards for the Registered Nurse (Australian Nursing and Midwifery Council 2005) and the Australian Competency Standards for entry-level Occupational Therapists (OT Australia National 1994). Assessment of fieldwork placement, regardless of discipline, is usually based on these standards, and involves the collection of data to determine if these accepted standards or competencies are being met.

The assessment methods used to determine students' achievement of these standards vary according to your discipline. Typically, assessment during fieldwork placements will involve the completion of a form or grid by the fieldwork educator rating a student's performance. In some circumstances, disciplines have developed national forms against which students are assessed; for example, the Competency Assessment in Speech Pathology (COMPASS™) and the Student Practice Evaluation Form–Revised (SPEF-R), used in Occupational Therapy.

Although the use of a supervisor assessment grid is very common, other methods are used to determine achievement of standards. They can include submissions of clinical case studies, written reports of clinical situations, portfolios and logs, reflective diaries and clinical exams. In this chapter, the focus is on fieldwork educator assessments of competency, although the principles discussed will apply to these other forms of assessment.

CRITERIA AND MARKING SCALES

Although each discipline will have its discipline-specific standards of performance, there is a similarity in the behaviours and actions expected of entry-level practitioners regardless of discipline. Table 14.2 describes these typical criteria. These criteria have been linked to clinical activities that fieldwork educators might observe to reveal how you are meeting these criteria. During a single interaction with a client or patient, multiple aspects of your practice may be assessed.

Table 14.2: Assessment criteria used during clinical placements and activities used to reveal achievement of these criteria

Criteria	Activities that may reveal how well you are achieving these criteria
Discipline-specific skills and tasks These are often the aspects of our disciplines that we think are most important to learn, as they are visible to someone watching our performance. They can include communication skills, taking a client's history, hands-on skills and teaching skills	Observation of specific actions with a client/patient Exams and tests with and without clients present Practical sessions with other students
Combining and integrating knowledge, skills and attitudes in a series of actions typical of our discipline Clinical practice is not made up of isolated skills, but involves the effective integration of these skills	Giving you responsibility for all aspects of client's or patient's care, and observing how you sequence and progress this care Discussion of plans for future sessions
Knowledge When you start placement it is expected that you will have a certain level of knowledge that you have gained from the theory studied at university. An expectation of placement is that you are able to determine where this knowledge is relevant and apply this knowledge to the clinical setting, and that you will build on this knowledge over the course of the placement.	Direct questioning Tests and exams Observing the application of knowledge when explaining conditions and treatments to clients Referring to relevant knowledge when explaining clients' presentation to your fieldwork educator Inclusion of a broad range of knowledge in description of reasoning processes Written reports

(Continued)

Table 14.2 (*Continued*)

Criteria	Activities that may reveal how well you are achieving these criteria
Professional behaviour, communication and teamwork An important expectation of you on fieldwork placement is that you will learn acceptable professional behaviours. For some students, this can challenge the ways in which they act in many other facets of their life, and they need to learn to adapt their behaviour. Being a professional also means taking responsibility for your actions and wanting to improve the quality of the service you provide. This professional responsibility means that you will develop your capacity to assess and modify your own performance	Interactions with other health professionals Your ability to self-assess Interactions with clients Interactions with your fieldwork educator Behaviour when in group situations and locations How you spend your time when not engaged in client or patient activities Time you arrive at placement, take lunch and leave Your dress Discussions with your fieldwork educator that demonstrate your awareness of acceptable professional behaviours Examination of reflective journals and portfolios
Achieving positive outcomes for clients and not being harmful This means being safe and effective in your decisions and actions. It is important to note that as you develop, educators often provide you with more challenging situations to test your safety and effectiveness. You should be aware of the complexity of the circumstances you are being put into, and how you can adapt to these situations. You may initially be safe only to be assessed as unsafe if you don't respond to more challenging situations	Observation by educator and by others in the healthcare setting Comments by the client Your descriptions of actions and outcomes Your need for supervision; how well they trust you to be left alone
Reasoning and thinking processes An important element of being a professional is having the critical thinking skills and reasoning processes that underpin decision-making. Educators will ask you questions to encourage you to talk about and explain your thinking. Being able to describe your reasoning processes is an essential element of being assessed. Students might show all the technical skills, but be judged not to have achieved the expected level because they cannot demonstrate an understanding of the reasoning needed to monitor and guide the application of technical skills	Direct questioning about your reasoning Written intervention plans Written case reports Patient or clinical notes Presentations to your fieldwork educator, fellow students or other health professionals about a client or patient Letters to other health professionals Discussions about clients in team meetings

(Continued)

Table 14.2 (*Continued*)

Criteria	Activities that may reveal how well you are achieving these criteria
Work-readiness	Providing you with more independence
Educators can also look at the extent to which they feel a student is ready for practice in the workplace as a new graduate. This criterion would apply more so to placements occurring at the end of the course	Increasing time pressures
	Providing more complex clients or patients who are typical of a new graduate workload

THINK AND LINK 14.1

Consider the assessment criteria and activities of Table 14.2 together with the practice window (Table 13.4) in Chapter 13. What have you learnt about yourself?

REFLECTION 14.2

Your assessment

Locate the assessment criteria and forms that will be used to assess your performance on fieldwork placement.

1   How do the criteria in these forms compare to those listed in Table 14.2?
2   Are there any additional criteria you need to think about?
3   What are the ways that these criteria may be assessed in your discipline?

RATINGS OF PERFORMANCE

An essential part of passing a placement is being aware of the criteria that are being used to judge your performance. Often assessment criteria have a scale against which a student's performance is rated. These may be limited to 'Satisfactory' or 'Unsatisfactory', or there may be a more extensive scoring system. Typically, your performance is rated according to the extent to which you have met the criteria or performed expected behaviours. Depending on the assessment criteria, you will often be judged against how you are expected to be performing at a particular point in a placement. You may be performing at a satisfactory level mid placement, but if there is no change over the course of the placement then your results at the end may be rated as lower than they were previously.

Consider this example. Anne, a final year student, received good grades during her midway assessment. She was confident she was doing well, and didn't make a conscious effort to increase her knowledge or skills further. She continued to practise in the same way, even though her fieldwork educator gave her increasing challenges in the placement. At the end of her placement her results were lower than they had been mid placement, because she had been expected to reach a higher level by the end of the placement. When being assessed, it is important to establish what is expected as the minimal level of performance, and how this is expected to change over the duration of the placement.

What if you fail?

It is worth clarifying the notion of failure as it refers to an assessment of fieldwork placement. Failure doesn't mean that you have failed as a health professional, although it may feel like this. Failure usually means that you haven't reached the expected criteria within the timeframe expected. Fieldwork educators experience a considerable dilemma if a 'Fail' grade is awarded. This decision is never taken lightly, and would only be made after careful consideration of the assessment criteria, and often in consultation with academic staff from the university.

THINK AND LINK 14.2

Chapter 17 discusses failure on fieldwork placement. Consider the different student responses to failure in Chapter 17 against the practice window in Table 13.4 and the assessment criteria discussed in this chapter.

Students are often concerned that single instances of poor performance will adversely affect their assessment. Fieldwork educators seldom look at a single performance in isolation. Yaphe and Street (2003) identified that assessors of medical students formed an initial impression of students, and then engaged in a process of testing to ensure that this initial impression was accurate or needed revising. Fieldwork educators observing a student might ask themselves questions such as: Is this performance consistent with other behaviours I have seen? Has the student recognised the problem and resolved to amend it? Is this a behaviour that the student was given feedback on before and it hasn't changed?

Failing is less likely to occur if you are aware of the criteria and have understood the level of performance that is expected. It is important that you have developed your own ability to assess your performance against the criteria, and modify your performance as needed rather than being solely dependent on feedback from others.

REFLECTION 14.3

Your acceptable standards

1 What sorts of behaviours and performance standards do you think are the minimum acceptable standard?
2 How are you going to establish this level of expected performance?
3 What would inadequate performance look like to you, and is your perception accurate?

DEVELOPING SKILLS IN SELF-ASSESSMENT

Self-assessment requires students to learn skills in assessing their own performance and a decreasing dependence upon external forms of assessment. An important argument for this approach is that practising health professionals are continually required to learn new information, apply this to their practice and assess how well they are performing and using this new knowledge. Boud (2000: 152) argues for the importance of self-assessment to future practice.

> In order for students to become effective lifelong learners, they need also to be prepared to undertake assessment of the learning tasks they face throughout their lives. They should be able to do this in ways which identify whether they have met whatever standards are appropriate for the task in hand and seek forms of feedback from their environment (from peers, other practitioners, from written and other sources) to enable them to undertake related learning more effectively.

Learning to self-assess requires you to seek out ways to determine the quality of your own performance and how well you are learning the skills of practice. Self-assessment skills require a sound internal understanding of the required performance, and the ability to compare your own performance accurately against the observable and published standards.

In Table 14.3, findings from research conducted with nursing students (Crawford & Kiger 1998) has been used to provide you with a framework to help you develop skills in self-assessment. Included in Table 14.3 are some case examples to guide the application of the strategies. This table is also designed to help you use the assessment of others effectively while also developing your own skills in self-assessment. You will notice that the suggested strategies change over the course of the placement as your self-assessment skills mature.

Table 14.3: Developing self-assessment skills throughout a clinical placement

Stage of the placement	Characteristics of stage (adapted from findings of Crawford & Kiger 1998)	Suggested self-assessment strategies	Case example
Beginning of the placement: adapting to the new environment	• Reading objectives, protocols • Observing and practising procedures	• Become familiar with the assessment criteria	Toby has just started his new placement. This afternoon he will be completing his first task of conducting an assessment of a new client.

(Continued)

Table 14.3 (*Continued*)

Stage of the placement	Characteristics of stage (adapted from findings of Crawford & Kiger 1998)	Suggested self-assessment strategies	Case example
	• Seeking role models to identify expected standards • Questioning and seeking reassurance • Building relationships • Acting 'like a student'	• Clarify interpretations of the criteria and how and when they may be assessed. • Identify examples of how qualified staff self-assess their performance	Toby decides to spend the morning carefully watching his educator conducting an initial assessment, reading assessments completed by other staff in the centre and checking with his educator about whether there are any particular practices used in the centre. Toby has previously read the assessment criteria his educator will use to evaluate his performance and recognises that during his initial assessment aspects of his performance such as his communication, clinical reasoning and professional behaviour could be assessed
During the placement: getting comfortable and seeing the opportunities for learning	• Discriminating between other staff as role models • Finding good role models • Asking more specific and probing questions to guide learning • Needing less direct supervision • Developing own standards	• Start confirming that your judgment of the expected standards is accurate • Start making self-appraisals and testing that these are accurate • Compare your performance against the assessment criteria	Toby has been on placement now for two weeks, and his educator has scheduled a meeting to discuss his midway assessment. Toby has prepared for the meeting by completing his own version of the assessment. During the placement Toby has been checking how his sense of performance compares with the qualified professionals and his peers.

(*Continued*)

Table 14.3 (*Continued*)

Stage of the placement	Characteristics of stage (adapted from findings of Crawford & Kiger 1998)	Suggested self-assessment strategies	Case example
		• Listen and critically appraise feedback • Compare your educators' feedback with own judgment • Discuss differences or mismatches	He is prepared for some differences between his own perception and that of his educators, and plans to understand any discrepancies that exist and to focus on the feedback, in particular how it affects his developing self-judgment skills
Towards the end of the placement: mastery of the placement	• Feeling comfortable about ability in the area • Acting more like a health professional than a student • Greater mastery of own performance and needing less supervision • Comparing own performance against own standards	• Continually apply self-assessment, rechecking the accuracy under new conditions • Don't expect perfection; learn to be realistic about the standard expected at your stage • Focus on future learning and development of practice	Toby is feeling more confident about his ability to assess his performance, and feels he is realistic about what is expected of him. He has also implemented a number of strategies to improve his performance and learn from the outcomes of his experience. He has started to broaden the sources of data upon which to base his assessment, and is focusing on the outcomes he is achieving with his clients and their feedback. He knows there are things he still needs to improve, but doesn't think that his final assessment will hold any surprises

WAYS OF COLLECTING DATA ABOUT YOUR PERFORMANCE

In Table 14.3, ideas were introduced that can support your developing sense of self-assessment. Below is a summary of these ideas related to sources of information about the quality of your performance on fieldwork placement. Consider how the integration of these sources of information can provide you with an overall understanding of your performance.

- *Client appraisal*: Have you ever asked your clients to give you feedback on your performance? They could provide you with valuable information on aspects such as your communication. This feedback could be direct, but you can also look for indirect markers of your clients' satisfaction, such as the comments they make to your supervisor and other staff, their keenness to come back and see you or their attendance at appointments.

- *Client outcome*: How well have you helped the client achieve positive health outcomes or the goals you have set for the time you are with the client? How long has it taken to achieve these outcomes? What changes to the client's health have occurred as a direct result of your actions, and how much have you depended on the ideas of your supervisor? It is worth noting that this source of data can be difficult when you are a member of a team where everyone is contributing to the client's outcome.

- *Fieldwork educator input*: How does your assessment of your performance compare to their expectations? How do they collect information to form their assessment? Why do they use these methods? The emphasis here is on actively using the input of the supervisor rather than being a passive recipient.

- *Peer assessment/comparison*: How does your performance compare with that of your peers and qualified health professionals? What does this comparison tell you about your own performance?

Challenges to the use of self-assessment

Emphasising and practising self-assessment is desirable, but can also be challenging. A potential risk in not balancing self-assessment with external input is that you may miss out on input to guide you in determining acceptable standards. As a result, you may over- or underestimate the level of performance that is expected. There is the potential that poor self-assessment skills will reinforce misconceptions and perpetuate inappropriate behaviours. A further advantage of having input from others is that it provides a means for you to develop strategies to meet desired criteria. Without this input you may be unsure of what to do.

On the other hand, when you are being assessed by someone else, it is easy to become dependent upon this assessment. You may try to act in a way you think will lead to a positive assessment. It is easy to value external feedback highly and value self-assessment less. The risk of relying on external feedback is that you learn to please others rather than respond to the task in front of you. In future practice, where direct supervision and feedback will not be as readily available, you may be unable to determine how well you are performing and how to respond if problems arise with your performance.

THINK AND LINK 14.3

Chapters 15 and 16 discuss placements where self-assessment may be an important part of the fieldwork placement assessment. Consider the issues raised here in this section of Chapter 14 in relation to issues raised in Chapter 15 and 16.

Molloy & Clarke (2005) identified that students tended to view their educators as experts who diagnosed and helped to fix problems, and adopted a passive or received approach to assessment. This was in spite of the student's previous experience and skills in being able to self-appraise. Molloy and Clarke also identified that fieldwork educators also saw themselves in this diagnosis role. The particular challenge is to recognise where the opportunities to engage in a dialogue with clinical educators exist, and to introduce your own self-appraisal. Although early in practice a more guided approach may best support you, it is less desirable as you mature. A further challenge in self-assessment can be the impact of cultural and language differences, particularly if you don't feel comfortable critiquing or confronting the opinion of a teacher or person in charge.

There are times when there is going to be a mismatch between your self-appraisal and a clinical educator's appraisal. Rather than viewing this as a failure of self-assessment, it is important to reflect upon and explore with your fieldwork educator why your individual expectations may have been mismatched. Without this approach it is tempting to undervalue self-assessment. If you do not discuss the different expectations between you and your fieldwork educator, it may also result in overvaluing of your own opinion, and you may mistakenly attribute any mismatch to feelings that you have not been adequately assessed or received adequate or useful feedback or that personality clashes exist between you and the educator.

In spite of the challenges, learning to self-assess is important. Assessment is an integral component of clinical placements. An understanding of the purpose of the assessment, the criteria used for the assessment and an active engagement in the assessment process will all contribute to an enhanced and positive learning experience.

SUMMARY

- Models of clinical assessment are usually based on standards expected of qualified health professionals.
- Assessment on fieldwork placement involves the collection of data on your performance from multiple sources and integrating these to give a complete understanding of your readiness for professional practice.
- The ability to accurately self-assess is as critical to learning on clinical placements as preparation for clinical practice.
- Learning to self-assess is a skill to be learnt in the same way as learning to practise in your discipline.
- Self-assessment on fieldwork placements is challenging, and requires active effort from students and their supervisors.

DISCUSSION QUESTIONS

Having read this chapter, consider these questions to reflect upon the key messages.

1   Are you aware of the assessment criteria that will be used to assess your performance on fieldwork placement?
2   How might your current views and approaches to assessment have to change to prepare you for assessment in the clinical setting?
3   How are you going to develop your skills in accurate and critical self-assessment?

References

Australian Nursing and Midwifery Council (2006). *RN Competency Standards* <http://www.anmc.org.au/professional_standards/index.php> accessed 27 January 2009.

Australian Physiotherapy Council (2006). *Australian Standards for Physiotherapy* <http://www.physiocouncil.com.au/file_folder/AustralianStandardsforPhysiotherapy Summary> accessed 27 January 2009.

Boud, D. (2000). 'Sustainable Assessment: Rethinking Assessment for the Learning Society'. *Studies in Continuing Education*, 22(2): 151–67.

Crawford, M. W. & Kiger, A. M. (1998). 'Development through Self-assessment: Strategies Used during Clinical Nursing Placements'. *Journal of Advanced Nursing*, 27: 157–64.

Irons, A. (2008). *Enhancing Learning through Formative Assessment and Feedback*. Routledge, London & New York.

Molloy, E. & Clarke, D. (2005). 'The Positioning of Physiotherapy Students and Clinical Supervisors in Feedback Sessions'. *Focus on Health Professional Education: A Multi-Disciplinary Journal*, 7(1): 79–90.

OT Australia (1994). *The Australian Competency Standards for Entry-Level Occupational Therapists* <http://www.ausot.com.au/inner.asp?relid=11&pageid=22> Accessed 27 January 2009.

Yaphe, J. & Street, S. (2003). 'How Do Examiners Decide?: A Qualitative Study of the Process of Decision Making in the Oral Examination Component of the MRCGP Examination'. *Medical Education*, 37: 764–71.

CHAPTER 15
A MODEL FOR ALTERNATIVE FIELDWORK

Rachael Schmidt

LEARNING OUTCOMES

After reading this chapter, you should be able to:
- discuss how alternative fieldwork can augment your professional skill acquisition and broaden professional knowledge
- describe the elements of support essential for enhancing student supervision in an alternative fieldwork model.

KEY TERMS

Alternative fieldwork
Community-building project work
Community neighbourhood house
Conventional fieldwork placements
Fieldwork education
Host centre
Information pack
Occupation Wellness Life Satisfaction (OWLS) program
Peer skill performance evaluation
Role-emerging fieldwork
Self-evaluation
Tutorial programs

INTRODUCTION

Over the last decade, increased health student numbers have placed pressure on conventional fieldwork placements, especially in urban clinical centres (Barney et al. 1998). *Conventional fieldwork placements* are defined as those placements where the student has a fieldwork educator from the same profession, and placement occurs in a setting where the profession of the fieldwork educator has had a presence for many years. In response to increased student numbers, innovative models of fieldwork have evolved to creatively meet service gaps and to provide challenging and relevant fieldwork placements for your skill development. These innovative fieldwork models have a number of names, including alternative or role-emerging fieldwork, nontraditional or nonclinical or *alternative placements* and *community projects* (Overton et al. 2009). This form of fieldwork is often located in less traditional locations, without direct profession-specific services, thus requiring an innovative approach to student supervision. Alternative fieldwork has an impact on your role as a student and the practice skills you acquire. Part of your student role, then, is to familiarise the staff at your fieldwork placement with your role and the potential skills you can offer within their service. You must take responsibility for identifying your specific learning objectives as dictated by the fieldwork service and location.

Background

Alternative fieldwork provides you with a wider variety of learning activities. Unlike clinical fieldwork, alternative fieldwork often occurs in the community, where identified gaps in services are addressed by student-directed projects to enhance and build on an existing service (Overton et al. 2009). Known as *host centres*, typically these services offering fieldwork placements rarely employ staff from your specific health professional group, and so you may have limited access to staff from your specific health profession. It is therefore likely that employees of your host service may not have a clear understanding of the professional role or the breadth of services your profession has to offer. This means that your student role involves educating the staff about your profession. As the name implies, *role-emerging fieldwork* suggests that the student-driven activities demonstrate and communicate the potential of the your professional role within the host centre, to raise the community's understanding of your profession's service possibilities, and in doing so encourage employment for future graduates (Adamson 2005; Overton et al. 2009).

Alternative fieldwork placements are often located in non-urban settings, which may be initially confronting for you, because of the distance between you and your *discipline-specific fieldwork educator* or *remote supervisor*. Distance communication demands active input for you and your remote supervisor (Barney et al. 1998). In the absence of an onsite discipline-specific fieldwork educator, onsite student support is provided by *generic staff* acting as fieldwork educators or host facilitators, to facilitate student projects with appropriate resources and local knowledge.

Access to discipline-specific supervision that is undertaken remotely is typically provided by a combination of periodic site visits, regular electronic and phone contact, and is optimised if student and educator actively collaborate. Ensuring that you feel well supported by your educational facility and the hosting centre relies on adequate fieldwork preparation and an early fieldwork placement orientation to ensure all stakeholders are familiar with the combination of roles and responsibilities. In rural or remote environments where you are required to leave your home base, assigning small groups of students to one placement has the added benefit of providing peer and social support to ease the issues of separation from family and potential social isolation that can have an impact on the success of the fieldwork experience.

THINK AND LINK 15.1

Chapter 10 gives some practical advice on how to prepare for rural and remote placements.

You are more likely to be successful in fieldwork if you are a competent self-directed learner. Additionally, alternative models of fieldwork are best suited to students who are nearing graduation, as you are more likely to have developed a better understanding of your professional identity.

COMMON ATTRIBUTES THAT YOU ACQUIRE FROM ALTERNATIVE FIELDWORK PARTICIPATION

Self-directed learning and managing stress

Your success in community building projects and role-emergent fieldwork hinges on your ability to cope and manage your own learning, especially as your daily activities may not be supervised as closely as in clinical settings. You need to be confident and independent in managing your time, decision-making and setting goals, and problem-solving. Confident communication skills are required, as you may need to advocate for yourself in seeking effective supervision from offsite discipline-specific educators, in seeking resources from your host centre and in educating and advocating for yourself with host staff.

REFLECTION 15.1

Gaps in learning
- What strategies do you currently use to identify your gaps in learning?
- How do you ensure that the information you have gathered to address fieldwork issues is relevant, current or trustworthy?
- Could you explain your profession to another person?

An independent learner

In fieldwork, ongoing supervision should assist your development as an independent learner, with a graded educational information flow and exchange as required, and provide ongoing support both professionally and socially (Barney et al. 1998).

Those students with well developed self-directed learning skills, who are confident and competent adult learners, tend to engage in the challenge of community-building projects. If successful, challenging fieldwork fosters your lifelong learning in practice, and in developing competence and confidence in clinical decision-making (Doherty et al. 2009). Take every opportunity to develop your communication skills through actively discussing the successes and challenges of your daily sessions with host workers, as well as with the discipline-specific fieldwork educator, to enrich your fieldwork experience. Also, if you have a clear sense of your intended professional identity and role, you will thrive within the role-emerging model of fieldwork, and you may find you are more willing to seek employment within this environment or similar location in the future (Barney et al. 1998).

THINK AND LINK 15.2

If you have access to the Internet during your alternative fieldwork placement, you might prefer to keep in touch with others via online technologies. Chapter 18 discusses several online technologies that can be used to keep in touch with others, as well as sites that provide information on evidence for your professional knowledge and skills.

Communicating about your profession and establishing your professional identity

If placed in student pairs, you have the added benefits that peer support affords, such as in shared learning and reflection on practice in collaboration, which assists in developing clarity within your professional role. *Community-building project work* in particular provides an opportunity for you to talk about your role and work with aligned professionals to illustrate how your profession can contribute, through your professional skills as a productive team member. For instance, in a setting that does not receive occupational therapy services, you (if you are an occupational therapy student) learn to articulate confidently, to those who are not familiar with occupational therapy, what the profession can offer within your specific fieldwork environment. Such professional exchanges enhance your professional thinking and language, as discussion with host staff can highlight role differences and demonstrate the overlap of professional skills and thinking.

Learning to communicate with clients and their families about your professional role assists in developing your confidence in explaining the role of your profession, and thus strengthens the sense of your professional identity.

ENHANCING THE LEARNING EXPERIENCE WITHIN AN ALTERNATIVE FIELDWORK PLACEMENT

The most challenging aspect of any alternative fieldwork exercise is how best to support the student in developing their professional identity. Thomas and colleagues (2005) have cautioned that role-emerging placements can be challenging for students with poor knowledge of their professional role. The following section provides practical ideas for support that can be given to you as you work in an alternative fieldwork placement.

Clear goals and understanding of aims of fieldwork

To facilitate early orientation before any student placement, an exchange of *information packs* will help all stakeholders understand the specific fieldwork-related roles, goals and expectations. Establishing clear learning goals suitable to each setting is important for successful fieldwork placement. However, unlike conventional placements where student roles are clear, in an environment where workers may have poor specific professional service knowledge, it is essential to establish your student role clearly with all stakeholders before placement.

For the university, fieldwork planning should commence well before the placement starts, when clear learning outcomes are identified to match the service gaps or projects identified by the host centre. Information given to host staff should include the intended length of the fieldwork, the assigned students' names and contact details, the fieldwork goals, the student role descriptions, a brief discipline-specific profile and the expectations of the services to be driven by the student cohort. In preparation for fieldwork, you should make contact with your assigned host fieldwork facilitator to ensure you are expected on the days assigned, that you have all items required to arrive safely and you are prepared for work. Keeping everyone informed facilitates timely exchange of information and can extend the learning possibilities for all concerned.

Be active in your learning

Clarifying your fieldwork objectives and your student role early in the placement reduces anxiety and enhances a feeling of engagement from day one. Although not ideal, where an orientation activity is omitted, you should initiate and request assistance in orientating to your fieldwork environment, and ensure you are introduced to the relevant personnel within your first week of placement.

As alternative fieldwork rarely provides discipline-specific fieldwork supervision, it is your responsibility to be an active participant in the fieldwork activities. You are responsible for developing your portfolio of practical skills, actively engaging in self-reflection and group reflection, evaluating your own performance and actively sharing, searching and evaluating relevant literature to support your learning. If available, utilise student peers to practise assessment activities, seek performance feedback, discuss intervention session outcomes, practise your interview questions and discuss case studies to develop your clinical reasoning and to link theory to practice through reflection (Courtney & Wilcock 2005).

Support through tutorials

For alternative fieldwork placements, specifically designed *tutorial programs*, delivered face to face or online, are important to support the student as well as challenge students in skill development, practice reflection and professional thinking. These tutorial activities are often delivered by discipline-specific tutors or fieldwork educators. Tutorial activities should allow time for students to reflect on practice roles, engage in theory-in-practice reasoning, discuss case studies and share fieldwork experiences between students in order to understand their professional purpose.

A responsive tutorial program aims to enhance your independent learning and inspire your critical thinking, which is aligned with applied practical and professional performance. Also, regular tutorial sessions allow an opportunity for your discipline-specific fieldwork educator to monitor your progress in defining learning goals and developing your clinical reasoning, coping strategies and practice techniques.

Supervision and facilitation

Feeling supported as a student is paramount, especially where physical access to discipline-specific supervision is restricted. All fieldwork students feel most supported when they perceive they have access to their onsite facilitators and offsite discipline-specific fieldwork educators, either in person or electronically. Communicating indirectly, via email or telephone, requires a higher level of skill for all stakeholders to ensure the message is truly conveyed and supervision is supportive. Therefore building rapport between you and your discipline-specific fieldwork educator may take longer and require more effort to ensure both are being heard. Scheduling regular, formal phone supervision enables your discipline-specific fieldwork educator and you time to prepare, thus facilitating a reflective approach to your learning. Email communication offers informal support, especially for random questions requiring quick answers for unresolved difficulties, issues or specific discussion.

In preparation for professional practice, initiate your own research in relation to your questions before meeting with your host fieldwork educator or your discipline-specific educator. Critical analysis of the literature adds depth to the discussion with your peers and educators and develops your critical reflection, while addressing your gaps in knowledge. Independent critical thinking in combination with your clinical reasoning are essential professional skills for managing complex professional practice.

REFLECTION 15.2

My professional role
How would you describe to those who don't know (concisely in plain language) what your profession does and what your professional role is?

Discipline-specific fieldwork educator visits

Where practical, periodic site visits by a discipline-specific fieldwork educator is ideal. This may be undertaken by a clinician working in an aligned area or location, or by an academic professional. To optimise these periodic supervisory sessions, planning before the site visit should include a clear agenda, including problem-solving and specified learning outcomes. Onsite supervision provides you and your discipline-specific fieldwork educator with an active exchange of professional information, practice skill evaluation and clinical thinking, through observation, demonstration and discussion. Periodic discipline-specific fieldwork educator site visits also provide an informal opportunity to network with host staff, thus building stronger alliances between fieldwork and educating facility and to establish clearer professional roles for present and future students.

Peer mentors

Providing adequate discipline-specific supervision to you from a distance is always a challenge. The informal support offered by student peers or mentors can assist in reducing any anxiety you may feel. A student peer, with recent fieldwork experience and local knowledge, acting as a mentor can assist with your orientation and provide insider knowledge to enable you to seek appropriate resources and deal with placement issues early to avoid further difficulties (Hurley et al. 2003). Peer support eases the pressure on the host (generic) fieldwork educator, and if you feel well supported you will require less orientation and emotional support, especially early in the placement.

THINK AND LINK 15.3

Chapter 16 discusses interprofessional learning fieldwork. In this type of fieldwork, the student does not always have a discipline-specific fieldwork educator. Read about interprofessional learning, and compare this type of fieldwork to alternative fieldwork placement.

Your evaluation

Finally, the evaluation of your performance as a student by your discipline-specific fieldwork educator, who is not physically present onsite, presents a challenge. In addressing this challenge, undertaking fieldwork in pairs or small groups of students provides an opportunity to formalise peer appraisal through *peer skill performance evaluation*. Providing constructive student-driven feedback, aligned with specific learning goals of one's peer, takes practice and support to develop effective peer evaluation. LoCicero and Hancock (2000) recommend both a structured halfway and end-of-placement evaluation for peer performance evaluation. Providing halfway feedback allows considered time to highlight issues and set achievable goals for the final half of the placement. Participating in a peer evaluation process provides you with an additional experience, both as the evaluator and the evaluated, which broadens the skill set of any student.

THINK AND LINK 15.4

For more information on assessment, Chapter 14 discusses assessment, including self-assessment.

OWLS program

To exemplify the strengths and challenges of an alternative fieldwork model, the *Occupation Wellness Life Satisfaction (OWLS) program*, presented in Case Study 15.1, is one working model focused on developing participating students as competent independent learners (Courtney & Wilcock 2005; Diener 2006). Designed by Deakin University's Occupational Science and Therapy program, the OWLS program originated to address the challenge of providing sufficient, relevant and valuable fieldwork opportunities for occupational therapy students within regional Victoria (Diener 2006).

OWLS is a community-based fieldwork placement that involves students working in diverse environments without onsite occupational therapy fieldwork educators. The program aims to provide student-driven services in nonclinical settings. The OWLS experience challenges all students to refine their skills, identify their learning needs, selectively seek knowledge through independent research, collaborate in remote supervision and initiate and build professional networks.

Case Study 15.1	The OWLS program

The OWLS program was designed initially along a role-emerging fieldwork model within a regional community to encourage the participating students to consider rural practice in the future (Barney et al. 1998; Paterson et al. 2004). In providing student-driven occupational therapy services in 'areas of unmet needs and to expand services to keep pace with the community needs' (Diener 2006: 3), the fieldwork extends the range of professional, generic skill base and competencies of the student and encourages critical thinking desirable for proactive community-based occupational therapy practice.

Students are allocated to the OWLS program as one of their fulltime fieldwork placements, either in third or fourth year. Within any OWLS week, all students attend

(continued)

---

one tutorial day, then in pairs they attend two consequent days each in two host services. These two host services are in a mainstream school and within a community service. In host centres, OWLS students receive daily onsite support from non-occupational therapy facilitators and remote supervision from Deakin-employed occupational therapists (Courtney & Wilcock 2005).

In the mainstream school sites, the student projects are directed towards skill development of school-age children, either individually or in groups. Within the community sites, mostly students work with adult clients within service teams in health, disability, work-related programs or leisure-related services.

In participating in the two settings, the students gain a breadth of experience in learning to think creatively, juggle work roles in two diverse genres, manage their time and be well prepared. These are all valuable skills for future practice.

The weekly OWLS tutorial addresses specific fieldwork education, such as establishing students' roles, responsive and trend-setting practices, service enhancement, health promotion and program development. Constructive peer evaluation and reflective practice are used to monitor skill development and clinical thinking.

Remote discipline-specific supervision is essentially undertaken electronically, with the occasional onsite supervisory visits, depending on the student service provision and the autonomy of the students participating. Student peer mentors provide additional informal support to alleviate student anxiety and assist in addressing fieldwork issues early to avoid accelerating difficulties and ease pressure on the host centres and the supervising educators.

Fieldwork performance is peer evaluated. Each student evaluates his or her own fieldwork performance for one placement, and the student partner's performance in the second placement. Specific student coaching is addressed within the tutorial program to ensure peer evaluation provides constructive feedback for enhancing professional practice development. Additional assessment includes fieldwork reflective exercises, literature reviews and class presentations.

A significant proportion of Deakin graduates surveyed stated that their participation in the OWLS program was the most significant fieldwork experience in preparing them for practice (Doherty et al. 2009).

Questions

1   Have you experienced an alternative fieldwork placement?
2   What did you learn?

CLINICAL REASONING 15.1

The following are tips for alternative fieldwork placements such as OWLS:

- *Be aware of nonverbal behaviours of your clients*, as these provide essential information about how a person is managing in his or her physical and social environment.
- *Keep your clients engaged*: Wherever possible, practise collaborative decision-making, by inviting your client or clients to assist in making choices, to ensure that everyone is aware of the chosen activity's goals before commencing.
- *Be prepared*: Even the best-laid plans may be thwarted by unscheduled changes, especially with children, so plan for the unexpected and think creatively. Ensure your playbox is well stocked, and have three simple games that can be adapted (according to age) ready at any time, so when caught on the hop, you have a choice of activities ready for some appropriate playful fun.

Case Study 15.2	Eliot

Eliot is halfway through her alternative fieldwork program. She describes her first full-time placement as being challenging but exhilarating. *Already halfway through and there is so much to know!* She is learning so much, and looks forward to every Monday when she can meet up with the other students participating in the same fieldwork program. She loves the exchange of their fieldwork stories, especially the highs and lows associated with fieldwork practice.

Monday starts with a tutorial program. Eliot is excited by this morning's tutorial, as they have been learning to administer a new paediatric assessment and an innovative approach to engage challenging children. This content comes just at the right time, as she has recently received four new referrals for handwriting difficulties for children aged seven years. Each Tuesday and Wednesday Eliot attends a nearby primary school, followed by a placement in a neighbourhood house on Thursdays and Fridays. The majority of her planning occurs on Mondays, when she has access to discipline-specific educators, student peer support and university resources.

At the primary school, Eliot and her fellow student Jo have been invited by the physical education teacher to design and facilitate two graded *perceptual motor programs (PMPs)* for the early years primary children. The students discuss their ideas with the PE teacher, who is very keen to learn more of their role in the school and to ensure that all his pupils are challenged appropriately by the PMP activities. Eliot enjoys this weekly challenge of designing appropriate fun activities, and targets the games to engage children, as she has observed a range of developmental levels. As each school day is busy, Eliot and Jo like to plan ahead to ensure that their sessions with pupils are task focused, in order to optimise the goals set for the children.

Eliot has also organised an assessment with a new pupil during a supervisory visit. In anticipation of performing in front of their remote supervisor, the students practise assessment procedures on each other early in the morning. Eliot booked the multipurpose room with the school administrator earlier, and now needs to send a reminder email to the teacher about appointment time and the purpose of the pupil's assessment. Eliot intends to work on the assessment report after school, when access to the school's computers is more likely.

Through the week, Eliot also attends a *community neighbourhood house* that caters for programs directed to building parenting skills for local families. She attends this part of her alternative fieldwork placement with student Michael. They have met with the neighbourhood house director, and she has requested that they design a number of parents' group activities as part of a year's program to be held in the local park. To help them prepare, Michael and Eliot watch a DVD on positive parenting skills, while drinking their morning coffee. Coincidentally, a recent tutorial was directed to the fundamentals of program development and evaluation, so they feel they have some good ideas to discuss with the planning group scheduled for the afternoon.

The students are feeling really positive about their involvement in this community setting, as they have begun to connect with some of the parents during their Healthy Cooking class each Friday morning. A lively discussion during the cooking class is directed to possible poster designs and captivating messages for an anticipated neighbourhood event in the local shopping precinct. The parents are keen to collaborate with the computer-savvy students in designing a number of posters addressing Healthy Shopping Choices. As the week winds down, Michael and Eliot meet with Jill, who is their peer mentor. Jill will assist them to work on the content of their information package for the neighbourhood house staff. They share stories about their experiences and performances with their mentor, who notices their developing confidence in speaking about their role with the parent groups. In confiding with their mentor, they admit, however, to still having difficulty articulating the role potential of their profession within this particular environment. Their plan is to research the topic during breaks next Monday when at university. Their mentor suggested discussing this topic with their peers and so they decide to research in preparation for the next tutorial session.

Questions

1   What generic skills are being developed by Eliot?
2   Are there any discipline-specific skills that Eliot is learning? What are they?

SUMMARY

Alternative fieldwork models expose students to a breadth of fieldwork environments and related work cultures that expands their own professional thinking and knowledge. Students gain a broad range of generic professional skills, as well as specialist skills that assist in developing confident and resilient professionals. Working in less traditional settings provides real-time opportunities for students to develop an insight into how other professional groups think and act within a specific setting, and helps to clarify their own role as distinctive from but also often complementary to other disciplines. Alternative fieldwork programs require considered preparation, empathetic supervision and collaborative teamwork to provide supportive and challenging fieldwork for students. Positive experience in alternative fieldwork programs equips the future graduate with a much-needed diverse range of professional skills required to cope and thrive as a health professional when delivering competent and confident professional services for complex practice environments.

DISCUSSION QUESTIONS

1   How would you best prepare for an onsite supervisory session, provided by a remote discipline-specific fieldwork educator, to ensure that the limited time was used wisely? Prioritise your list.
2   If you were assigned the role of student peer mentor, what approach would you take in providing support to your assigned students in fieldwork?
3   In an alternative fieldwork setting, how would you describe your professional role to a non-discipline-specific worker? Be as clear and succinct as possible.
4   What are the steps you would take, if you were placed in an alternative fieldwork environment, to find out about a profession-specific approach to an assessment procedure or process?

References
Adamson, L. (2005). 'Inspiring Future Generations of Occupational Therapists'. *Australian Occupational Therapy Journal*, 52: 269–70.
Barney, T., Russell, M. & Clark, M. (1998). 'Evaluation of the Provision of Fieldwork Training through a Rural Student Unit'. *Australian Journal of Rural Health*, 6: 202–7.
Courtney, M. & Wilcock, A. (2005). 'The Deakin Experience: Using National Competency Standards to Drive Undergraduate Education'. *Australian Occupational Therapy Journal*, 52: 360–2.

Diener, M. (2006). Deakin University's Occupation, Wellness and Life Satisfaction Centre: working locally to achieve diverse competencies. 14th Congress of the World Federation of Occupational Therapists, 23–28 July 2006. WFOT Congress Abstracts.

Doherty, G., Stagnitti, K. & School, A. (2009). 'From Student to Therapist: Follow up of a First Cohort of Bachelor of Occupational Therapy Students'. *Australian Occupational Therapy Journal*, 56: 341–9.

Hurley, K. F., McKay, D. W., Scott, T. M. & James, B. M. (2003). 'The Supplementary Instruction Project: Peer Devised and Delivered Tutorials'. *Medical Teacher*, 25: 404–7.

LoCicero, A. & Hancock, J. (2000). 'Preparing Students for Success in Fieldwork'. *Teaching of Psychology*, 27: 117–20.

Overton, A., Clark, M. & Thomas, Y. (2009). 'A Review of Non-Traditional Occupational Therapy Practice Placement Education: A Focus on Role-Emerging and Project Placements'. *British Journal of Occupational Therapy*, 72: 294–301.

Thomas, Y., Penman, M., & Williamson, P. (2005). 'Australian and New Zealand Fieldwork: Charting the Territory for Future Practice'. *Australian Occupational Therapy Journal*, 52: 78–81.

CHAPTER 16
INTERPROFESSIONAL LEARNING: WORKING IN TEAMS

Nick Stone

LEARNING OUTCOMES

After reading this chapter, you should be able to:
- discuss the key interprofessional learning concepts and principles
- explain why interprofessional learning has become essential for all health professionals
- identify important factors that can help and hinder interprofessional learning
- raise self-awareness about your own interprofessional beliefs, assumptions and preferred and non-preferred interaction styles
- identify strategies to use your own IP strengths and to continually improve your capacity to enhance multidisciplinary teamwork.

KEY TERMS

Constructive controversy
In-placement review
Interprofessional education (IPE)
Interprofessional fieldwork placement
Interprofessional learning (IPL)
Interprofessional practice (IPP)
Post-placement
Teamwork

INTRODUCTION

This chapter will cover the following topics:
- What is interprofessional learning (and what is not)?
- *Why* interprofessional learning?
- Does interprofessional learning 'work'?
- What makes good teamwork?
- Professional stereotypes
- Assessing IPL fieldwork
- Ensuring a good start to IPL fieldwork

- In-placement review
- Post-placement debrief and reflection.

| Case Study 16.1 | Nice to meet you, too? |

You've just driven three hours to arrive in the small coastal town where you have chosen to go on a rural interprofessional fieldwork placement. There you are joined by a student from another health discipline whom you've never met. You're sharing accommodation together, and will need to work closely throughout the two weeks to complete all the tasks successfully. You're quite excited, but also a little nervous, because the main assessment task—a community-based project—will rely heavily on you being able to work well with a total stranger.

On arrival you meet the other student, but get the impression that she is not very interested in interacting with you. This is a bit puzzling, as this is supposed to be a voluntary interprofessional placement, and you expected other students to be just as motivated as yourself. Over the first day you try to engage her, asking her about her course, her interests and how her discipline would typically approach the different health care situations you encounter. She seems reluctant to discuss anything, and only seems interested in talking with her same-discipline preceptor by herself.

On the second day she reveals that:

a   she didn't really want to do this placement, but had to make up her required 'rural time'

b   she doesn't believe she can learn anything useful from a student in your discipline

c   she is planning to go home on the first bus tomorrow.

Questions

1   How would you probably react? What are the possible consequences of this reaction?

2   What might be the best way to respond? Discuss this in pairs, and try to reach agreement.

3   What assumptions does this student seem to be making about interprofessional learning? How valid are these assumptions?

4   Which health disciplines do you think might (or might not) have been involved, and why?

5   What could have been done to avoid such a situation in the first place?

6   Which, if any, health disciplines would not be able to learn anything valuable from which other health disciplines? Justify your response in discussion with others.

7 What beliefs about professional hierarchies are you aware of (real or imagined)?—for example, that certain disciplines are better, deserve more power or authority, or know more than others.

WHAT IS INTERPROFESSIONAL LEARNING?

Understanding the language we use, and clarifying with our colleagues what particular terms mean, are particularly important for successful interdisciplinary teamwork. Going the extra yard to ensure you understand each other helps to avoid unnecessary misunderstandings that can cause team conflict and dysfunction. A good example is the variety of interpretations of terms such as *interprofessional learning (IPL)* and *interprofessional education (IPE)*. The following short case reveals an interesting interpretation:

Case Study 16.2	The Dean's savings scheme

The Dean of a large university health faculty stood up energetically to speak during a seminar to explore ways to implement interprofessional education: 'It's a great idea; I can see some real benefits coming out of this,' he exclaimed.

I sat up quickly in surprise. I had been working for years in the area, but so far had seen little real support for IPE from the top.

The Dean went on: 'For one thing, we can put at least three or four different first year disciplines in the same lectures. We've got big enough lecture theatres and they need to know the same anatomy, physiology, pharmacology ... We could really get some economies of scale!'

Questions
1 What's your reaction to the Dean's idea? What would you (like to) say to him?
2 What did the Dean apparently understand by the term IPE?
3 What is your understanding of the term IPE?
4 How might strengthening IPL, in pre- and post-registration settings, affect the costs (financial and otherwise) of providing health care?
5 What experiences have you had so far (or seen or heard of) that relate to IPE or IPL?

Case Study 16.2 may also relate to the confusing range of terms used to describe IPL (see Table 16.1).

Table 16.1: Terms associated with IPL

Prefixes	Adjectives	Nouns
common cross- inter- joint multi- pan- shared trans-	professional disciplinary	education development learning practice training

REFLECTION 16.1

Write down what you understand to be the similarities and differences between the adjectives and nouns in Table 16.1. Feel free to do the same for the prefixes, although these are harder.

A recent snapshot across health agencies and universities in the state of Victoria revealed a wide range of interpretations about what IPE means (Stone & Curtis 2007). Like the Dean above, the most common definition (by about 40 per cent of respondents) stated that students are simply being co-located; for example, sitting in the same lecture theatres, potentially with no interaction at all. Only a handful, less than 5 per cent, mentioned that IPE should explicitly include collaboration, interprofessional practice (IPP) and teamwork as central goals.

IPL tends to be used as an umbrella term (see Figure 16.1) by most researchers working in the area. It is an important choice, because it places top priority on people *learning* in teams *with*, *from* and *about* each other, regardless of disciplinary background.

IPL can be seen to include IPE, as in pre- and post-registration courses, continuing professional development or training, as well as all the informal opportunities that arise to learn *with*, *from* and *about* other health professionals across the career lifespan. IPL is also often considered to include interprofessional practice (IPP), in recognition that effective health practice necessarily involves ongoing learning. A useful IPL definition that has been widely adopted is:

> Occasions when two or more professions learn with, from and about each other to improve collaboration and the quality of care (Barr et al. 2006: 2).

Some definitions also include the patient, client or carer as a part of the IP team. This reflects advances in technology, pharmaceuticals and professional knowledge, which mean that some simpler treatments can take place in the home, often using patient self-management.

Figure 16.1: IPL umbrella terms

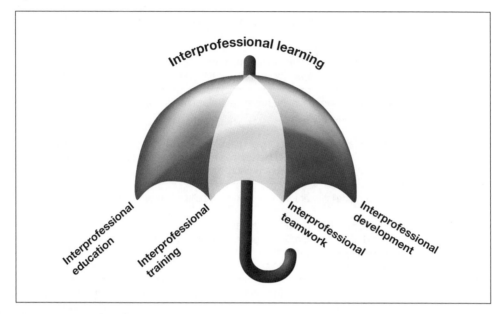

AND WHAT IS IPL NOT? MYTHS AND REALITIES

Just as there are many different interpretations about what IPL means, there are also some common myths and misunderstandings about IPL that deserve attention (see Table 16.2).

WHY INTERPROFESSIONAL LEARNING?

Over recent years there has been growing recognition that most health and social care now requires the collaboration of a range of health professionals. Multidisciplinary teams are now recognised as the most appropriate way to manage the chronic and

Table 16.2: IPL myths and realities

Myth	IPL means all healthcare situations can be addressed by a multidisciplinary team
Reality	There will always be certain health conditions and issues that can be appropriately managed by individual health professionals and single disciplines
Myth	IPL means everyone in the healthcare team has the same power to make important decisions
Reality	Differing professional scopes of practice and expertise, legal responsibilities, disciplinary and traditional hierarchies mean that some people in healthcare teams will always have more authority than others in particular decisions
Myth	IPL is an idealistic fantasy that is too difficult to achieve in the real world
Reality	IPL already exists: there have always been examples of excellent IPP in the field and occasionally in education programs. However, there is now a worldwide recognition that IPL is not only desirable, but essential for the emerging models of health care
Myth	IPL will blur professional identities and will cause confusion about roles and responsibilities
Reality	Learning more about the roles of other health professions actually helps to clarify and strengthen one's own professional identity and place within the healthcare system, much the same as travel abroad and experiencing other cultures can help to better understand your own culture
Myth	IPL will lead to a lowering of professional standards, which will compromise the quality and safety of health care
Reality	There is no solid evidence to support this claim. IPL leads to better communication and workplace relations, which can only improve the quality and safety of health care.

complex health conditions that constitute the major burden of disease. For example, Australia's National Health Priority Areas are:

- Cardiovascular health and stroke
- Cancer control
- Mental health (with a focus on depression)
- Injury prevention and control
- Diabetes mellitus
- Asthma
- Arthritis and musculoskeletal conditions

<www.aihw.gov.au/nhpa> Accessed 9 May 2009

Efforts towards the prevention of these diseases demand effective multidisciplinary health teams.

REFLECTION 16.4

Who is involved?

1   Which health professions would typically be involved in the treatment of each of these National Health Priority areas?
2   How can they be involved in their prevention?
3   Are there any National Health Priority areas that would not require effective interprofessional collaboration?

THINK AND LINK 16.1

Working in teams with people with chronic diseases often brings up ethical issues. Chapter 20 discusses ethical decision-making with vulnerable clients or patients.

So far, however, most courses include little deliberate interprofessional preparation. If students graduate with good teamwork skills, it is likely to be the result of personality and chance factors rather than by strategic intent. The costs of absent or *ineffective* interprofessional practices can range from mild to catastrophic. A mild example might be an unsatisfying workplace, in which there is little sharing of knowledge or trust among the different professionals involved. This can lead to unnecessary duplication of services, communication breakdown and other inefficiencies.

A more serious case was the Bristol Royal Infirmary Inquiry (<www.bristol-inquiry.org.uk>) in the United Kingdom, which found that in the early 1990s, poor interprofessional communication and teamwork were major factors leading to an infant death rate that was about double what would have been expected. Since this inquiry and subsequent health system and service improvements, the infant death rate at the infirmary dropped from 29 per cent to 3 per cent. Results were published in the *Guardian* newspaper (<www.guardian.co.uk/society/2004/oct/08/hospitals.uknews>).

Closer to home, in response to a perceived crisis in patient safety and quality of care, the ACT and federal governments are undertaking the first major Australian intervention to improve interprofessional practice.

IPL and IPP are increasingly seen as building blocks to progress in health care.

(Braithwaite et al. 2007)

This initiative involves not only interprofessional collaboration, but also collaboration across sectors: state and federal governments, universities and healthcare agencies.

Recent Australian research by Haller and colleagues (2009) appears to confirm what has been called the 'killing season' in the UK. In Australia this 'season' occurs around February when new medical trainees arrive at hospitals. Rates of serious complications were found to be up to twice as high compared with later in the year. Haller and colleagues found these preventable errors were happening regardless of trainees' levels of clinical experience. They believed that their unfamiliarity with the new environment—for example, hospital rules and procedures, location of patient information and roles of other health professionals—were leading to 'breakdown in communication and poor interprofessional interactions, two well-identified causes of errors and undesirable events' (5). Their recommended improvement strategies included interprofessional meetings and training, similar to those adopted by 'high reliability' industries such as aviation, nuclear power and offshore oil production, in which training in teamwork and free communication are regarded as essential to reduce the risks of preventable errors (McCulloch and Mishra et al. 2009: 109).

These examples may appear reactionary; that is, acting after the horses have bolted. However, there are a number of inexorable long-term trends that also demand much more and better IPL. The ageing population means there is already a shift from episodic, one-on-one treatment in acute settings towards community-based and ambulatory care in non-acute settings, such as in the home. As mentioned above, multiple disciplines are now often needed to work together with clients to manage chronic complex diseases. These include preventable, so-called 'lifestyle' diseases, such as cardiovascular and pulmonary conditions and metabolic diseases such as diabetes. It is now also widely agreed that management of these diseases needs increased attention to preventative approaches, such as health promotion, education and community capacity building.

REFLECTION 16.5

Upstream and downstream
1   What is meant by 'upstream' factors in health care?
2   Please identify examples of upstream and downstream factors for a specific disease.
3   To what degree is it a health professional's responsibility to help prevent disease?
4   Are some professions exempt from this responsibility? Discuss.

DOES IPL 'WORK'?

We first need to clarify what we mean by 'work'. In promoting IPL, we assume causal links between IPL, IPP and improved health outcomes. That is, by implementing and improving IPL, we expect a consequent improvement in the capacity of health professionals and, in turn, an improvement in health indicators among individuals and communities. These links are illustrated in Figure 16.2.

Figure 16.2: Links between IPL and outcomes

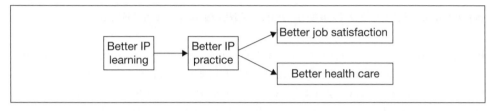

To prove such links exist, especially using traditional biomedical research models such as randomised controlled trials, has proven challenging to say the least. It is questionable whether these models are appropriate when trying to evaluate complex social systems (Stone 2006a). There is, however, a diverse, solid and growing research evidence base to support the assumption that successful interprofessional practice (IPP) can lead to significantly improved outcomes, as outlined below.

Effects of successful IPL
- Interprofessional team and health service effectiveness and efficiency
- Job satisfaction among interprofessional team members
- Respect for and understanding of the roles of health professional colleagues
- Patient health outcomes.

Obviously, these links rely on IPL being implemented *successfully*. The evidence suggests that IPL is likely to be successful when specific conditions are being met, as outlined below (Stone 2006b).

Conditions that support successful IPL
- Focus on clear learning objectives that are understood, valued by and shared by all participants
- Explicit aiming to improve patient and client health outcomes
- Conditions that are flexible enough to allow the targeting of general content relevant to all professions involved, but also including discipline-specific components
- Explicit attention to learning about teamwork, and assessing the dynamics of interprofessional collaboration (especially self-assessment)
- Project planning jointly negotiated by students, clinical supervisors and local community stakeholders
- The involvement of participants who have chosen to participate and who have been actively involved in making arrangements

- Provision of multiple opportunities for students to engage in IPL throughout their education and professional life
- Being situated in applied settings, such as fieldwork, rather than academic classes.

WHAT MAKES GOOD TEAMS WORK AND GOOD TEAMWORK?

In a situation such as interprofessional fieldwork, attention to factors that enhance team functioning are especially important. There is often nowhere to hide out in the field. Team members typically rely on each other in order to get the job done. David and Roger Johnson (1999, 2009) have been actively researching collaborative learning and teamwork for nearly half a century, and are regarded as world leaders in this area. The brothers have identified five key conditions for successful teamwork that are very relevant and useful for guiding IPL in the field:

- *Positive interdependence*: 'swim together or sink together': team members understand that they must learn together to accomplish the goal; they need each other for support, explanations and guidance. Rewards and incentives relate to the group, not individuals.
- *Individual accountability*: the performance of each group member is assessed against a standard, and members are held responsible for their contribution to achieving goals. This means there is no room for 'social loafing', or people not pulling their weight.
- *Promotive interaction*: the tasks require that students interact closely, rather than, for example, each person going off to complete a fragment of the task individually.
- *Group processing*: the group uses language that shows they understand important group processes so they can discuss and reflect on their collaborative efforts and develop ways to improve.
- *Development of small-group interpersonal skills*: Most people do not automatically develop the skills required for successful teamwork. These skills include giving constructive feedback, reaching consensus, decision making, negotiation, conflict resolution and involving every member.

Adapted from Johnson & Johnson 1999

REFLECTION 16.6

Teamwork conditions
1   Is it realistic to expect all of the conditions listed above to be evident in teamwork?
2   Which ones seem easiest and hardest to put into effect (and why)?
3   What sorts of behaviour help and hinder these conditions?
4   What issues and obstacles might arise, and how could you address them?

Simply trying to avoid conflict, or expressing disagreement impolitely, are rarely helpful in team situations, even though they can be tempting options amid the stresses typical of health and social care delivery. In fact, a hallmark of excellent teamwork is accepting the fact that tension and disagreement will inevitably occur, then working out ways to resolve the conflict while preserving respectful working relationships. Interprofessional fieldwork is especially prone to interdisciplinary differences of approach and opinion: it is therefore essential to develop effective strategies for dealing with these differences.

Recognising these realities of human nature and group dynamics, the Johnsons have recently focused on areas such as *constructive controversy*, and using team conflict to help teams effectively and creatively achieve their goals. This idea, which encourages people to develop the skills to disagree respectfully, seems much more realistic than assuming everyone needs to agree on everything all the time. Johnson and Johnson (2009) offer eight practical guidelines for controversy in teamwork.

Guidelines for constructive controversy in teamwork

1 Be critical of ideas, but not people. You can challenge the ideas of the other participants while still affirming their competence and value as individuals.
2 Understand that if someone questions your ideas, it is not a criticism of you as a person.
3 Focus on coming to the best decision possible (in the client's interest), not on 'winning' or 'saving face'.
4 Positively encourage everyone to participate and to share relevant information.
5 Listen to everyone's ideas, even if you do not agree.
6 If unsure, restate what you think someone means (paraphrase).
7 Try to understand both sides of the issue. Show you can see the issue from the opposing perspective.
8 Be prepared to change your mind if the evidence clearly indicates so.

Case Study 16.3	An illustration of structured post-fieldwork IPL reflection

Following are some excerpts from an IPL *post-fieldwork placement* tutorial discussion. It was a structured session designed to guide reflection and self-assessment on the students' IPL experiences during their two-week program. The students belonged to four different health disciplines, and had been placed together at an alcohol and drug service in a regional town.

(continued)

As you read, identify which of the Johnsons' conditions and guidelines for effective teamwork (above) are suggested. Also try to guess which disciplines are represented (S1–4 denotes students from each discipline, PM refers to the project manager and author):

The discussion

S1: It was actually easy for me to work with the others because they were just blatantly honest with each other [laughter] no matter what you said. I think a sense of humour helped in making sure we were all comfortable.

S2: We definitely learned a lot from each other.

S3: I really enjoyed getting to look at three [other] disciplines. I tried to imagine what it would be like to be only working with one other discipline but I couldn't. I wrote in the online thing [discussion] that we all saw a patient from [the service] and then we all sat around and did a case conference kind of thing. We all put in our two cents which was really good. It felt like we were being interprofessional.

S2: We all had common goals with the project, but because we all come from different perspectives we all had different ideas on what it would be about. We went through a flat stage where it was going to end up being a 50-page document, and we had to cut it and cut it. Things that S4 thought was important, say about joints or something, I would go 'Joints? Who cares?' and just delete it. And then S4 would come back and put it back in. It was really hard deleting stuff, because we'd only known each other for five or six days and we didn't know how each other would react. So we had to just swallow our pride and say, 'Go for it, delete what you want.' It was a really interesting procedure.

S4: And learning about your own strengths and weaknesses and learning about how best to use other people's strengths and weaknesses—to get the project done ... S1 was really busy doing typing and getting information together.

PM: So [discipline 1] students are good for typing? [laughter]

S4: That's generalising, but it is my weakness.

NS: [Discipline 4] students are good at inviting themselves around to other people's places to eat.

S2: [Discipline 3] students are pedantic ... It's a very interesting experience.

S3: [Discipline 2] students do all their work in the first few days then just lie on the bed ...

PM: You guys are the first group of four, so what advice would you give other students [going into that situation].

S4: It's a really good dynamic; it allowed a fair bit of flexibility.

S3: We didn't always work together.

S4: Sometimes we worked in twos, threes or fours. Whatever was easiest.

S3: We had a timetable and we just said, 'Well, you just go and organise yourselves.'

S2: I think an advantage we had was that our preceptors were so easy going, like we would turn up ten minutes late, it's a country way of life. One day I went with S4, who introduced me to the [same discipline preceptor] and he said, 'Oh, I thought I was having a [discipline 3] student but it doesn't matter.' It made it really nice to have a really flexible timetable.

S2: I think we made the most of having all the different disciplines. We had lots of really lengthy discussions about each other's professions and what we all do. We made the most of it.

Questions (for pairs or small groups)

1   What factors appear to have made this placement so satisfying for all concerned?
2   Both Case Study 16.1, at the start of the chapter, and Case Study 16.3 above allude to health professional stereotypes (both lighthearted and otherwise). Please identify other health profession stereotypes in Case Study 16.3, as well as any others that you or others may hold. Discuss the usefulness, accuracy and limitations associated with these stereotypes.

PROFESSIONAL STEREOTYPES

Stereotyping is a result of the way our minds naturally make sense of the world by forming mental categories from our experiences. They may be based on little or no valid evidence (uninformed stereotypes), or may have some accurate aspects based in reality. Not all stereotyping is negative; indeed, positive stereotyping of students by teachers, for example, can lead to superior achievement and educational success. Stereotypes can become problematic, because they often involve particular mental associations, including value judgments. Adler (2007) has drawn together decades of social psychology research about stereotypes to point out that they can be helpful to working relationships and productivity.

When are stereotypes helpful?

- *Consciously held*: rather than pretending you don't have any stereotypes, be aware of impressions or biases that may be lurking at the edge of your conscious thinking. You may not be aware of stereotypes' influence on your reactions until you bring them to the surface; for example, by discussing their possible origins with trusted colleagues.
- *Descriptive vs evaluative*: focus on describing what you have seen, heard or read rather than making value judgments. For example, instead of claiming that another discipline's approach to health care is better or worse than your own, identify some points of similarity and difference, and discuss their relative merit.
- *Accurate*: does it match the weight of available evidence? Ask yourself what else you need to know or find out to form a balanced and defensible impression.
- A *'first best guess' if there is no other information*: Sometimes what little we know is all we have to go on. This 'guess' can be modified later when and if further evidence comes to light.

ASSESSING IPL FIELDWORK

Assessment is a powerful driver of learning, so it is important to make assessment closely matched, or even integrated with key learning objectives. Self-assessment is a particularly powerful method to maximise and consolidate the learning gains involved in IPL. The list below offers a range of IPL sample objectives that form the basis for a number of subsequent activities further below, including self-assessment methods.

THINK AND LINK 16.2

Chapter 14 discusses assessment and has a section on self-assessment. Refer to Chapter 14 for more information on assessment criteria, as well as issues related to self-assessment.

IPL fieldwork objective and examples

'Umbrella' objective: to enhance the attitudes, knowledge and skills associated with successful interprofessional practice.

Examples of interprofessional attitudes

- Interest and commitment to ongoing IPL
- Resilience to persist with IPL, even when it may present new challenges

- Willingness to share skills and knowledge with other health professionals
- Valuing collaboration as a preferred option, when possible
- Inclination to value and respect others' contributions, as well as challenging them
- Interest in learning about, with and from other health professionals
- Humility, such as being open to suggestions from others who might challenge your existing habits, recognising that multiple scopes of practice are often better than one.

Examples of interprofessional knowledge
- Knowing the roles, responsibilities and capabilities of other health professionals
- Understanding appropriate referral protocols and procedures
- Knowledge of factors that enhance and inhibit interprofessional collaboration
- Knowledge of processes of group formation, teamwork and collaboration
- Understanding issues and sensitivities specific to other health professions
- Understanding the complexity of many health issues, and that there may be a number of different valid perspectives, models and approaches to health care
- Awareness of the ways in which effective IPP can benefit patient health outcomes, as well as health professionals' job satisfaction
- Knowledge of common barriers to IPL, and strategies for addressing them
- Recognising the sorts of health issues that are best addressed through IPP
- Awareness of one's own preferred and non-preferred ways of approaching tasks.

Examples of interprofessional skills
- Demonstrating trust in and respect for colleagues
- Negotiating roles and responsibilities to establish clear shared expectations
- Communicating problems and possible solutions in constructive ways
- Expressing your own needs and concerns in appropriate ways and contexts and at appropriate times
- Accurately self-assessing your own IP skills (identify strength and improvement areas)
- With a range of colleagues, engaging in reflective discussion focused on IPP
- Making an active contribution to collaborative tasks (such as case conferencing, planning projects and conducting evaluations or research)
- Encouraging others to participate in collaborative activities
- Facilitating conflict or tension resolution
- Empathic listening (for example, attentive body posture and facial expression), showing an understanding and respect for another's point of view
- Maintaining harmonious working relationships while under stress
- Checking for meaning; for example, paraphrasing or summarising what someone else has said
- Maximising your ability to establish a positive, client-focused working relationship quickly.

ENSURING A GOOD START TO IPL FIELDWORK

The following advice has proven valuable to many other students. You will need to adjust or ignore some points, depending on the context and nature of your IPL fieldwork experience. Similarly the timing will vary; it may suit to do this the week before the placement or on the first day. Ideally, there will be an academic or administrative facilitator who has some IPL insight and experience:

- Start establishing a positive rapport with your fellow students by holding a face-to-face meeting, a teleconference or an online chat or asynchronous discussion forum.
- Exchange contact details and a little about your personal and academic backgrounds, including what you think is most important in IPL and any particular interest areas.
- Discuss logistical arrangements, such as travel and accommodation (if relevant), timetables, negotiation of shared learning tasks and any other concerns, issues or information that are still needed.
- Establish a positive working relationship by clarifying your respective expectations and hopes for the placement.
- Identify where your respective expectations and learning objectives are similar and different, such as discipline-general and discipline-specific areas.
- Discuss how you might manage to accommodate everyone's core goals and where you are prepared to make compromises.
- Anticipate possible placement problems, and generate problem-solving strategies. Make sure you know what to do if things go wrong, such as personal health or safety issues, or if the placement is not meeting your expectations.
- Familiarise yourself with the above principles of effective IPL and teamwork and sample learning objectives, and identify any terms, language or meanings that are unclear.

IN-PLACEMENT REVIEW

Abundant research and experience emphasise how essential it is to allocate preset times during placements dedicated to evaluating progress, reflecting on student IPL and identifying any problems and ways to manage them. Typically, there are few opportunities for preceptors to meet and discuss interprofessional practice during the placement. If these things are left to chance, they tend not to happen in the context of busy healthcare provision. It is usually a false economy to hold meetings only when something goes wrong; by then it may be too late to fix a problem that a preemptive consultation might have addressed. As in health care itself, prevention is often far more effective and efficient than waiting for disease to emerge.

At the very least, there should be one in-placement review during a typical field-work placement, preferably at least one a week. This is one of the few opportunities fieldwork educators will usually have to reflect on IPL in situ, and they typically find the experience very rewarding. They can also use the information shared to contribute towards their formal assessment requirements of their students.

The purpose of the *in-placement review* is to:
- provide some structured mental space and time to review the placement
- ensure both fieldwork educators and students touch base with each other, clear up any questions, and raise and address issues
- share and discuss experiences and impressions so far, and relate them to learning objectives
- assess the extent to which students have had the opportunity to address interprofessional learning objectives
- identify any gaps in student learning or interest areas, and make plans to plug them.

REFLECTION 16.7

Frequently asked questions (FAQs) and answers (As) on the in-placement review

FAQ: Who should be involved?

A: Both fieldwork educators and students.

FAQ: Should IPL be directed by fieldwork educators?

A: No. Students should take as much initiative in raising topics or issues as fieldwork educators. Only students can represent their own experiences, needs and interests.

FAQ: How long should the review go for?

A: About an hour should be sufficient for the formal review process. However, there should be continual discussion and informal review processes throughout the fieldwork placement.

FAQ: What preparation is required?

A: Students should address the items below before participating in the review:

1 Make some notes on your overall reactions and impressions of the placement so far

2 What have been the most interesting things you have learned so far?

3 What have been the most difficult aspects of the placement so far?

4 Which IPL objectives have you been able to address most?

5 Which IPL objectives would you like to address but have not had the opportunity to do so far?

6 How could your fieldwork educators help make the placement more satisfying?

7 How could you help to make the placement more satisfying?

8 Other Issues, needs or comments.

POST-PLACEMENT DEBRIEF, REFLECTION AND DISCUSSION

Ideally this will take place at the very end of the fieldwork placement while everything is fresh in mind. Some suggested objectives and associated activities follow.

Table 16.3: Post-placement objectives and activities

Objective	To share and reflect on the placement experience
Activity	Write down two or three highs, and two or three challenges of the placement. Then in turns, share one or two of these experiences*
Objective	To review the placement in terms of the given student learning objectives
Activity	Look at the list of example IPL objectives, and identify which you addressed more, and which less than others. Do you have any related additional objectives you have addressed or feel would be relevant?
Objective	To identify issues or problems that arose, as well as possible or actual solutions applied
Activity	Identify problems and issues that arose, how you tackled them and what you have learned that might help in future similar situations. Identify scenarios that could be used for PBL to help prepare future students
Objective	To review the fieldwork placement with reference to the principles of collaboration and the literature on interprofessional education and practice
Activity	Review the Johnsons' conditions and guidelines, as well as the factors that facilitate successful IPL
	For each activity, identify what you witnessed, or saw a lack of, during your placement that related to the various points. Most important of all, what have you learned about your own IP skills, knowledge and attitudes?
Objective	For students to co-present, in pairs, any formal assessment tasks (for example, a community-based project)
Objective	Identify ways in which you might continue your interprofessional education
Activity	How might you be able to continue your interprofessional education even in the absence of structured programs focusing solely on IPL?
	Is it likely that one placement is likely to have long-term effects on the development of your IPP-related knowledge, skills and attitudes?
	What sort of opportunities could you find or create to consolidate and extend your IPL?

* All information needs to be treated confidentially. You should feel safe being open, even if it is not all positive news.

SUMMARY

This chapter has covered the issues involved in IPL. Students who undertake IPL are often confronted with their own stereotypes of how students from other disciplines behave. For a successful IPL placement, students learn how to work effectively in teams. IPL is best carried out in fieldwork placements because it is here that true interprofessional work is seen in action. IPL is not sitting in a lecture with other students from other disciplines.

DISCUSSION QUESTIONS

1   What are my assumptions about IPL?
2   If I were to work with students from three other professions, which professions would I choose first? Why?
3   How is health care enhanced by effective teamwork between professions?

References

Adler, N. J. (2007). *International Dimensions of Organizational Behavior* (5th edn). South-Western, Cincinnati, OH.

Barr, H., Freeth, D. Hammick, M., Koppel, I. & Reeves, S. (2006). 'The Evidence Base and Recommendations for Interprofessional Education in Health And Social Care'. *Journal of Interprofessional Care*, 20, 75–8.

Braithwaite, J., Westbrook, J. I., Foxwell, A. R., Boyce, R., Devinney, T., Budge, M., Murphy, K., Ryall, M., Beutel, J., Vanderheide, R., Renton, E., Travaglia, J., Stone, J., Barnard, A., Greenfield, D., Corbett, A., Nugus, P. & Clay-Williams, R. (2007). *An Action Research Protocol to Strengthen System-wide Interprofessional Learning and Practice.* BMC Health Service Research, 7: 144. <www.pubmedcentral.nih.gov/articlerender.fcgi?artid=2212639> published online 13 September; accessed 8 February 2009.

Johnson, D. & Johnson, R. (1999). *Learning Together and Alone: Cooperative, Competitive, and Individualistic Learning.* Allyn & Bacon, Boston.

Johnson, D. W. & Johnson R. T. (2009). 'Energizing Learning: The Instructional Power of Conflict'. *Educational Researcher*, 38(1): 37–51.

Stone, N. (2006a). 'Evaluating Interprofessional Education: The Tautological Need for Interdisciplinary Approaches'. *Journal of Interprofessional Care*, 20(3): 260–75.

Stone, N. (2006b). 'The Rural Interprofessional Education Project'. *Journal of Interprofessional Care*, 20(1): 79–81.

Stone, N. & Curtis, C. (2007). *Interprofessional Education in Victorian Universities.* Report for the Department of Human Services: Victoria. Available from the author.

CHAPTER 17
LEARNING FROM FAILURE

Eva Nemeth and Lindy McAllister

LEARNING OUTCOMES

After reading this chapter, you should be able to:
- discuss student difficulties in the fieldwork placement
- understand what it is like to experience failure in fieldwork placements
- be prepared to learn from failure.

KEY TERMS

Learning in fieldwork
Narrative inquiry
Perspective transformation
Readiness to learn
Transformative learning

INTRODUCTION

Learning in fieldwork placements occurs within workplace settings 'with complex interlocking arrays of people and activity' (Boud & Edwards 1999: 174). Your learning as a student on fieldwork placement can be influenced by the interplay of this complex array of variables, which include your knowledge, skills, attributes and dispositions; your capacity to manage time, tasks, yourself and others; your reflective and clinical reasoning skills; your capacity to transform theoretical knowledge into practice; and the nature of fieldwork educator–student relationships. Given the potential for interplay between the array of variables, it is not surprising that students at times experience difficulties with or even fail their fieldwork placements. Such students have been variously described in the literature as being marginal borderline, strugglers, poor, inadequate, incompetent performers, at-risk or failing students (see Hicks et al. 2005; Shapiro et al. 2002).

STUDENTS EXPERIENCING DIFFICULTIES IN THEIR FIELDWORK PLACEMENTS

Key characteristics of students who experience difficulties with fieldwork placements (see, for example, Hicks et al. 2005) are summarised in Table 17.1. Although these characteristics can serve as warning signals, they do not portray the complex interactions between student characteristics and the many demands required when learning in fieldwork environments.

Table 17.1: Characteristics of students experiencing difficulties in fieldwork

Characteristic	Example
Behavioural difficulties	Negative personal characteristics, such as dishonesty, defensiveness, a lack of awareness or ownership of the problem and a lack of commitment or motivation
Interpersonal problems	Poor communication skills, lack of assertiveness, overassertive or demanding behaviour, lack of integrity or lack of compassion
Cognitive problems	Learning difficulties (such as poor writing skills and poor memory), poor critical thinking or clinical reasoning skills, an inability to integrate knowledge, poor conceptual knowledge and understanding, poor planning and rigid thinking
Clinical skills deficits	Poor application of knowledge to fieldwork; poor diagnostic, planning or therapeutic skills
Mental health or emotional problems	Mental health problems, inability to manage anxiety and stress or depression
Difficulties adapting to the dominant culture	Difficulties such as poor communication skills, inability to interpret body language, poor understanding of rules and beliefs operating within the dominant culture—all of which can affect student interactions with others and student adaptation to fieldwork settings

THINK AND LINK 17.1

Chapter 13 has some practical exercises on self-reflection. Refer to Chapter 13 for the practice window, which may be helpful to you if you suspect you may have some characteristics listed in Table 17.1.

It is surprising that there is little literature available describing students' experiences of difficulty and failure in their fieldwork placements, given that those students who experience difficulties in fieldwork have an impact upon all stakeholders involved in fieldwork education: other students, fieldwork educators, clients and university programs. Understanding students' experiences of difficulties or failure may assist in better preparing and managing such students by identifying factors that have an impact on their learning and strategies that might optimise their learning.

This chapter draws on research that investigated the experiences and perspectives of students who encountered difficulties or failure in fieldwork placements (Nemeth 2008). The methodology of this study utilised a qualitative research methodology called *narrative inquiry* (van Manen 1990) which was integrated with a *hermeneutic phenomenological approach* (Connelly & Clandinin 1990). Through narrative analysis of indepth interviews with seven students, abstractions that were common to students' experiences and those that were different among students who participated in this study were identified. It became clear that each student was talking about aspects of being 'ready to learn' from the experience of failure in the fieldwork placement (Nemeth 2008). *Readiness to learn* refers to students' readiness to use the experience of failure in a fieldwork placement as a catalyst to alter perceptions of themselves or their worldview. When such altered perceptions occur, the experience of failure in a fieldwork placement can become a transformative learning experience.

Although the research discussed in this chapter focused on speech pathology students, presentations of the research at numerous health professional development events suggest that the implications of the research have broad applicability in the preparation and support of students across the human service professions. This chapter presents data drawn from two speech pathology students' experiences, accounts and understandings of failure in their fieldwork placements. The stories reveal how one student was ready to learn from this experience of failure whilst the other was not. The concepts of *readiness to learn* and *transformative learning* are discussed, and suggestions are provided to support learning for students experiencing difficulties or failure and their fieldwork educators.

Case Study 17.1   Chris's story of failing fieldwork

Chris was a final year speech pathology student when she experienced failure in her final paediatric fieldwork placement. Throughout the first three years of the undergraduate program, Chris experienced difficulties with academic exams and had sought assistance from the university to improve her skills in answering exam questions. Thus, at the start of her final placement, Chris had perceived herself as being less academically capable than her peers and as having strong clinical skills.

Chris felt fatigued at the start of her final fieldwork placement because it occurred immediately following completion of her academic exams. Chris also found it difficult to cope with the daily two-hour travel to attend that fieldwork placement, and by mid-placement she felt that her skills were inadequate for her stage of learning.

> I was finding things really hard ... I knew I was having problems. You're sort of at that stage in the course you know what's expected of you ... By the way I was crying every night because I was just so upset. I was feeling so incompetent. ... That was the thing: this is really my last child placement. If I can't cope here, how am I going to cope by myself?

She attempted to improve her skills by searching for solutions, such as referring to lectures to help access her theoretical knowledge, as much as time permitted. Previously Chris's fieldwork 'had always gone well, so that's what I hung onto' as a source of strength, yet she was aware that her clinical skills and knowledge were suddenly inadequate.

> It was just awful … I've always hung onto clinic as my strong point and academically I haven't gone so well and suddenly I wasn't going well at clinic and I thought, 'Oh, I've got nothing now.'

Chris was aware that her skills were inadequate. However, she was 'devastated' by her mid-placement assessment, which showed failure. Despite her hopes that her skills might not have been as poor as she had feared, upon seeing her results, she realised, 'Oh, this is reality; this is the truth.' Failure was not only personally confronting and challenging but resulted in her losing confidence in her abilities. Chris relinquished control for her sessions with her client 'to [my fieldwork educator] because I just felt so incompetent and I just couldn't go on'.

However, towards the end of her placement Chris became more confident to make mistakes.

> I didn't want to make a fool of myself. At the beginning of the placement I probably wasn't willing to answer any questions. I'd just say, 'I don't know.' At the end of the placement … it felt better to have a go at things than to leave it unanswered.

Failure gave Chris permission to 'not know', and thus she could risk saying the wrong thing because her lack of knowledge was now exposed. Chris was also receptive to her fieldwork educator's appraisal and assessment of her clinical skills as inadequate. She did not solely deflect reasons for her difficulties to external sources, although she could acknowledge both external factors (such as her limited time availability to read relevant clinical theory) and her clinical deficiencies, which influenced her fieldwork educator's decision to fail her. Her inherent strength, insight and self-awareness meant that she was 'robust' enough to acknowledge her deficiencies, which contributed to her less than adequate performance.

Due in part to Chris' awareness of her difficulties and her receptiveness to confirmation of failure at her mid-placement evaluation, Chris became more open and honest with her fieldwork educator. This allowed her fieldwork educator to assist her in learning effectively. In fact, Chris maintained a good relationship with her fieldwork educator.

> It was weird because usually if you have a bad experience you usually sort of blame it on your clinical educator, but she was really good and … sort of perceptive that … I was worried about things. She was so supportive.

Chris and her fieldwork educator worked collaboratively so that Chris could improve her skills. Chris expressed anger about past fieldwork experiences and the failure of her previous fieldwork educators to prepare her for the demands on a final year student. Yet she was not angry about the circumstances in her placement, where failure actually occurred. She acknowledged that her skills were inadequate, and allowed herself to accept the unpleasant reality of this acknowledgement.

Chris's openness and receptiveness to her fieldwork educator's appraisal of her inadequate clinical performance, in conjunction with her accurate self-appraisal of her deficient clinical skills and willingness to accept that those skills were deficient, meant that she could account for failure in a fair and balanced way. Chris felt that her skills improved considerably as a result of her experience of failure.

> Like I said, you don't like to have those sorts of life experiences, but in a way it helped me realise what I needed to know, and how I needed to do it, sort of thing. I can look back now and say that it was really great but at the time it was very traumatic.

Questions

1   Have you had an experience like Chris's? If so, did you have similar feelings? Why?
2   Do you think that you can learn from failure?

Interpreting Chris's story

Chris's story suggests she possessed considerable awareness of her clinical deficits, and that her insight into issues affecting her poor performance, plus her receptiveness to her fieldwork educator's feedback, meant that she was ready to learn. Her perception of having had strong clinical skills before this placement may have helped her ward off feelings of inadequacy about her poor academic results and her intelligence. However, through the experience of failure, Chris altered this perception to incorporate new information that her clinical skills were weak. This altered perception was reintegrated, and became part of how she then perceived herself. Thus she experienced a *perspective transformation* (in her case, realising that she could no longer view herself as having strong clinical skills), which suggests that she was ready to learn from failure in a clinical placement. Once she experienced the perspective transformation, she could focus on improving her clinical skills so that she could achieve entry-level clinical competence, accepting that this required a further fieldwork placement. Failure became a catalyst for her to experience a perspective transformation.

By way of contrast to Chris' readiness to learn from her experience of failure, Rita's story provides an example of a student who was not ready to learn from her experience of failing her clinical placement.

| Case Study 17.2 | Rita's story of failing fieldwork |

Upon matriculation from school, and before enrolling in the speech pathology undergraduate program, Rita had enrolled in another degree and boarded at one of the colleges at a university campus. In comparison to previous life experiences from a country town, her newfound freedom was unprecedented. She frequently drank alcohol to excess and failed her academic subjects.

Rita decided that a career in speech pathology might suit her more. However, upon moving in with some relatives Rita felt isolated, bored and lonely. During this same period, Rita broke up with her boyfriend and began to experience more significant feelings of low mood:

> I went insane. I was very depressed. I had never been so depressed in my whole
> entire life, you know. It lasted about 3 months … People talked to me and I just start
> crying. It was horrendous. I was just so depressed really just wanted to die I felt so
> bad … It was awful. I was like suicidal, not suicidal because you're too apathetic to
> do it. Like I couldn't be bothered. You know when you're so depressed you sleep so
> much … I just wanted to die.

Despite these feelings and even suicidal thoughts, Rita did not seek professional assistance to overcome her problems. Toward the latter part of the second year of her course, Rita flatted with her sister and secured a part-time job to help support herself financially. Her priorities at the time were paid work so that she did not have to rely on her parents' financial support. Consequently, she was working up to three shifts per week.

> I think when I moved out [from my relatives' place] that's when I really lost it. I started
> drinking and drugs and stuff.

In her final year, Rita's difficulties with her fieldwork placement came to the fore. Rita reported that her fieldwork educator felt that she had poor organisational skills and failed to prepare adequately for her sessions.

> My clinical educator initially said … I am a disorganised person, which unfortunately
> is probably not good in speech pathology … So I worked quite hard. Well I didn't
> work hard but like I made sure I was organised for her.

Rita's lack of taking responsibility for adequate client management came to the fore toward the end of her placement.

> 'I was going to do [a particular assessment] …' And she said, 'Have you looked at the
> assessment?', and I said 'No', and she said, 'What! You should have [prepared the
> assessment].' Like, I was really [casual] about it but she said, 'You know, you can't
> just go look at it and then do it.'

Rita felt that her fieldwork educator overreacted to her inadequate preparation for the assessment and 'picked on' her.

She said … 'I thought you'd changed … You can't go on, if you're going to be like this.' And I was sitting there saying 'yeah yeah', and inside, saying, 'I hate you, I hate you!'

Although Rita was aware that she should have been better prepared for her assessment of a client, she felt angered by what she saw as an overreaction by her fieldwork educator. Rita did not acknowledge that her inadequate clinical preparation and inability to take responsibility for her work were the reasons she was failed at her end-placement evaluation.

Questions

If you had a placement with Rita, would it have been an easy placement for you? Consider whether Rita's attitude would have affected you, and whether you would have had to do Rita's work as well.

Interpreting Rita's story

Rita's story suggests that she had been receptive to hearing and attempted to placate her fieldwork educator's concern that she was disorganised early on in her placement. But when she was later failed for the same issue, Rita showed scant regard for the seriousness of her inadequate preparation for client care. Rita displayed many of the characteristics of failing students listed in Table 17.1. Her compromised clinical skills and failure were of little consequence to Rita, despite feeling anger toward her fieldwork educator for failing her. It is possible that her limited self-awareness and lack of insight into the need to take her clinical work seriously were also byproducts of her lifestyle choices and deteriorating mental health, all of which may have had an impact upon her ability to appraise her situation in a fair and balanced manner.

Although Rita remained angered by the experience, failure was not a catalyst for experiencing a perspective transformation. Instead, Rita returned to her habitual way of being, unchanged by the experience. She was not ready to learn, because she showed limited self-awareness and little insight into her behaviours and their consequences, and she lacked receptiveness to hearing that her skills were insufficient to warrant passing. Fortunately for Rita, some time after the conclusion of her failed fieldwork placement, Rita sought professional help for her problems.

READINESS TO LEARN

Figure 17.1 depicts students' readiness to learn. We return to Chris's and Rita's stories to explain the diagram in terms of how a student may or may not be ready to learn from a fieldwork placement where he or she experiences difficulty or failure. Figure 17.1 depicts how failing a fieldwork placement causes disturbance to students' habitual ways of perceiving themselves.

Both stories illustrate the next stage in the diagram: how students try to make sense of their experience of failure by determining why failure has occurred. The way in which students account for failure, together with their insight and self-awareness, influence whether students are ready (or not) to learn from their experience of failure. Chris accounted for failure in a fair and balanced way, and was robust enough to consider that her skills were poor. Thus she could experience failure as a catalyst for a transformative learning experience. She was ready to learn from the experience of failure in a transformative way, as is denoted on the left hand side of Figure 17.1.

Figure 17.1: Readiness to learn from failure in a fieldwork placement

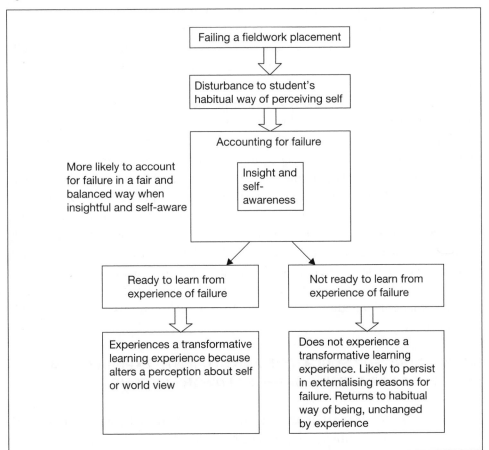

Rita, however, although angered by her fieldwork educator's reaction to her inadequate performance, felt that her fieldwork educator overreacted to her lack of preparation. Rita externalised blame for her problems, and was less able than Chris to account for failure in a fair and balanced way. Furthermore, Rita's poor insight and self-awareness also influenced her lack of readiness to learn from her experience of failure.

TRANSFORMATIVE LEARNING

Wade (1998: 717) defined *transformative learning* as a 'dynamic, uniquely individualised process of expanding consciousness whereby an individual becomes critically aware of old and new self-views and chooses to integrate these views into a new self definition'. This is compatible with Mezirow's (2000) description of a *perspective transformation* as requiring an individual to question what is being done incorrectly and correct distortions in reasoning and attitudes. According to Mezirow (1991: 14), a perspective transformation is the 'process of becoming critically aware of how and why our presuppositions have come to constrain the way we perceive, understand, and feel about our world; of reformulating these assumptions to permit a more inclusive, discriminating, permeable and integrative perspective'.

Chris experienced a perspective transformation because she reintegrated a new perception of herself that arose because of her experience of failure, which ultimately added to her self-knowledge, the importance of which has been acknowledged in clinical education (Higgs & Titchen 2000). In contrast, Rita attributed her failing largely to external factors, and returned to her habitual way of being, unchanged by her experience. Rita's mental health status and lifestyle choices appeared to have influenced her habitual way of being, her self-awareness and her insight, which seemingly compromised her readiness to learn from failure. Her experience of failure in her fieldwork placement therefore was not a catalyst for a perspective transformation. Nonetheless, when the experience of failure is transformative, as for Chris, students are more likely to be able to improve their skills by addressing their deficiencies in an authentic manner. Perhaps such individuals are more likely to function as self-directed learners because they are able to acknowledge and learn from their deficiencies. It is possible, therefore, that individuals who can experience a perspective transformation may be the types of adult learners and professionals who are proposed by authors as important for the health professions (McAllister & Lincoln 2004).

SUGGESTIONS FOR EDUCATORS AND STUDENTS EXPERIENCING DIFFICULTIES OR FAILURE IN THE FIELDWORK SETTING

The following reflections assist students and their fieldwork educators working with students experiencing difficulties or failure in fieldwork.

We have found that, even though it may seem that students have a myriad of difficulties that contribute to their failing grade, there are often one or two key issues that underpin their difficulties. For example, if it appears to be a time management difficulty, it may be that students do not know how to treat their patients because they do not have a constructive framework from which to work. With students who 'talk too much', we would explore reasons for this behaviour, such as whether students felt uncomfortable with silences, whether students felt compelled to tell patients everything they know to assert themselves as professionals, or whether

---

REFLECTION 17.1

Suggestions for students: questions to ask yourself when told you are failing
- Might there be some truth in what my fieldwork educator is saying about my performance in my fieldwork placement?
- How aware am I of my own behaviour and skills generally?
- How would my peers, friends and family perceive me and my self-awareness?
- How self-aware and insightful am I about my performance in the fieldwork setting?
- How do I perceive my performance in my fieldwork placement compared with my fieldwork educator's assessment of my performance?
- How can I try to account for my difficulties in a fair and balanced way? (Speak with your fieldwork educator or others who can be frank with you about this.)
- What other resources can I utilise to assist my learning?
- Are there any other career choices that might suit me better?

REFLECTION 17.2

Reflection by students with difficulties in fieldwork
- Reflect upon what aspects of your own knowledge, behaviours, attitudes, learning abilities, emotional and stress issues, mental health or adaptation to the dominant culture may be contributing towards difficulties.
- Acknowledge that having difficulties in a fieldwork placement can be a highly charged and emotional event, and that it is a normal reaction to try to determine or even agonise over why difficulties have occurred.
- Discuss with your fieldwork educator your perceptions of why you are having difficulties, while considering the possible accuracy of your fieldwork educator's perceptions.
- Use other students, fieldwork educators or university staff to gain alternative perspectives if your relationship with your educator is problematic.
- View the experience as an opportunity for self-growth.
- Consider how you can use the experience as a catalyst for a transformative learning experience.

REFLECTION 17.3

Suggestions for educators: prompting educators' reflections on their students' readiness to learn

- Was the student ready to learn from his or her experience?
- If so, what did the student learn? If not, reflect upon the reasons that person might not have been able to.
- Did the student experience a change in perception?
- If so, did you assist in facilitating that changing perception? How?

they felt fearful of hearing and having to deal with their patients' feelings of loss or grief. Below we provide suggestions for fieldwork educators dealing with students who experience difficulties in fieldwork placements.

Diagnosing the problem
- Demystify the problem.
- Look beyond just the student's presentation: try to get to the heart of the issue.
- Diagnose the key areas that need to be targeted to assist student competence most efficiently.
- Consider students' awareness and ability to account for their difficulties and failure in a fair and balanced way.
- Ensure that your expectations are reasonable, realistic and explicitly stated.
- Reflect on whether the difficulty is the student's problem or your problem.

Managing the problem
- Alert students to their difficulties, indicating whether they may not pass their placement as soon as possible.
- Air your concerns sensitively.
- Try to promote students' awareness and ability to account for their difficulties by being open and honest, yet empathic, to ensure that an effective educator–student relationship is maintained.
- Work with them to implement structured strategies to help ameliorate their difficulties.
- Be ready to listen to students' perspectives as well as gain their perspectives of why they feel they are experiencing failure.
- Ask students to reflect upon your perspectives, and consider possible alternative perceptions.
- Be prepared to alter perceptions about yourself from what students tell you.
- Be aware of the power differential between you and students. Ultimately you are responsible for failing students, and therefore it can be difficult for students to address their concerns with you.

- Be alert to possible mental health and emotional issues.
- Discuss with students how lack of competence relative to their stage of learning can have an impact on their future placements, and future clients and colleagues, if their skills continue to be problematic.

THINK AND LINK 17.2

Chapter 14 discusses assessment from the student's perspective. Refer to Chapter 14 for more information on how you can be more aware of assessment criteria and how to address the assessment process.

SUMMARY

This chapter suggests that an important consideration for students who experience failure is to consider their readiness to learn from the experience. Failure could be seen as a detour that provides opportunities for transformative learning experiences that ultimately increase student self-knowledge and readiness to learn. Gaining students' perspectives about their experiences of struggling or failing in placements could well assist students in becoming ready to learn from their difficult placements. In addition, do not underestimate the importance of fieldwork educators considering their own behaviours, expectations and interaction styles that may be contributing to a difficult placement with a student.

DISCUSSION QUESTIONS

1 What might I ask my fieldwork educators in earlier placements to ensure that I am learning adequately?
2 What does my health profession demand of me for my final fieldwork placement?
3 Would I be ready to learn if faced with failure on a fieldwork placement?

References

Boud, D. & Edwards, H. (1999). 'Learning for Practice: Promoting Learning in Clinical and Community Settings'. In J. Higgs & H. Edwards (eds), *Educating Beginning Practitioners.* Butterworth Heinemann, Oxford: 173–9.

Connelly, F. M. & Clandinin, D. J. (1990). 'Stories of Experience And Narrative Inquiry'. *Educational Researcher*, June–July: 2–14.

Hicks, P. J., Cox, S. M., Espey, E. L., Goepfert, A. R., Bienstock, J. L., Erickson, S., Hammoud, M. M., Katz, N. T., Krueger, P. M., Neutens, J. J., Peskin, E. & Puscheck, E. E. (2005). 'To the Point: Medical Education Reviews Dealing with Student Difficulties in the Clinical Setting'. *American Journal of Obstetrics and Gynecology*, 193(6): 1915–22.

Higgs, J. & Titchen, A. (2000). 'Knowledge and Reasoning'. In J. Higgs & M. Jones (eds), *Clinical Reasoning in the Health Professions* (2nd edn). Butterworth-Heinemann, Oxford: 22–32.

McAllister, L. & Lincoln, M. (2004). *Clinical Education in Speech-Language Pathology*. Whurr, London.

Mezirow, J. (1991). *Transformative Dimensions in Adult Learning*. Jossey-Bass, San Francisco.

Mezirow, J. (2000). *Learning as Transformation: Critical Perspectives on a Theory in Progress*. Jossey-Bass, San Francisco.

Nemeth, E. (2008). Learning from failure: Speech pathology students experiences of failure in a clinical placement. Unpublished Master of Health Science (Honours) thesis, Charles Sturt University.

Shapiro, D. A., Ogletree, B. T. & Brotherton, W. D. (2002). 'Graduate Students with Marginal Abilities in Communication Sciences and Disorders: Prevalence, Profiles and Solutions'. *Journal of Communication Disorders*, 35: 421–51.

van Manen, M. (1990). *Researching Lived Experience: Human Science for an Action Sensitive Pedagogy*. University of Western Ontario, London, Ontario.

Wade, G. H. (1998). 'A Concept Analysis of Personal Transformation'. *Journal of Advanced Nursing*, 28(4): 713–19.

CHAPTER 18
USING ONLINE TECHNOLOGY

Anita Hamilton and Merrolee Penman

LEARNING OUTCOMES

After reading this chapter, you should be able to:
- describe key Web 2.0 tools that support learning
- understand how to search, store and share information using Web 2.0 tools
- know how to verify online information.

KEY TERMS

Avatar
Blog (weblog)
Blogger
Collaborative writing tools
Healthcare Blogger Code of Ethics
Impression management
Net Code of Conduct (HONCode)
Online social networks
Open blog
Podcast
Post
RSS
Social software
Virtual worlds
Web 2.0
Wiki

INTRODUCTION

We begin this chapter with online technology, particularly Web 2.0, because Web 2.0 represents an evolution in how the Internet is used. O'Reilly (2005), who is considered to be the father of Web 2.0, states that the success of Web 2.0 lies in the fact that it has provided tools that have embraced the power of the Internet to harness collective intelligence. The Web 1.0 Internet changed from being a unidirectional repository to search and download information to becoming a multidirectional virtual environment, where people can interact with each other, build networks, collaborate and share ideas, form questions, give information and create communities around topics of shared interest. Until recently, healthcare practitioners have been slow to adopt online technology as a means of seeking and sharing knowledge for practice

(Kamel Boulos & Wheeler 2007; McLean et al. 2007; Seeman 2008), but this is slowly changing.

The rapid adoption of Web 2.0 tools by sectors such as business, education and politics has not been shared by health care. There are several reasons to explain the slow uptake of online social software tools by healthcare practitioners, including:

- the healthcare workplace culture values 'clinical contact and occasions of service' (McCluskey & Cusick 2002: 66) in preference to time spent on professional development
- ongoing professional development is seen as a personal responsibility (Jantzen 2008)
- health professionals have limited access to the Internet at work (Schaper & Pervan 2007)
- confidentiality, professionalism and self-protection concern healthcare practitioners, which may prevent them from utilising Web 2.0 tools in practice (Baerlocher & Detsky 2008).

Web 2.0, with its capacity to connect students, practitioners, researchers and the public, has enormous potential to carve a niche between workplace-based questions and research to develop knowledge from multiple perspectives. Although health care is behind other sectors in adopting Web 2.0 tools for practice, best practice models are emerging (Kamel Boulos & Wheeler 2007; Seeman 2008), with early adopters of online technology across health professions identifying the importance of online technology in the future of healthcare education and practice. These innovators are advocating the utilisation of Web 2.0 tools such as wikis, blogs and podcasts created *for* and *by* healthcare practitioners (Kamel Boulos & Wheeler 2007; McLean et al. 2007). The Internet is now a virtual space for information sharing and knowledge transfer beyond traditional methods.

RELIABILITY OF ONLINE INFORMATION

During fieldwork you may find that it is difficult to access your usual sources of information, such as your educational institution's library resources or teaching staff or your peers. You may decide to access online resources using the Internet and bring these to the practice setting. Concerns exist around tools that enable anyone to be the author, therefore guidelines for ethical development of online healthcare resources have been created (Letendre 2008). These guidelines include *Healthcare Blogger Code of Ethics* (Figure 18.1) and the *HONcode* (Figure 18.2). Scepticism is healthy, and all consumers of online healthcare information and evidence need to consider the reliability of the information they plan to use.

Figure 18.1: Healthcare Blogger Code of Ethics symbol

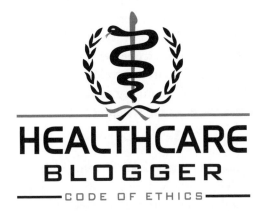

Figure 18.2: HONcode symbol

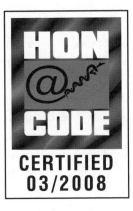

In order to check if a blog, podcast or wiki is reliable and trustworthy, it is important to identify who created the blog and what their credentials or experiences are. Do they cite peer-reviewed sources of information, and do they display the *Health on the Net Code of Conduct (HONCode)* logo. If using information from one of these sources, ensure that they have cited their sources, and if you can, source these for use in your own learning. If there are no references, use information from blogs, podcasts or wikis judiciously, understanding that it is one person's or group's opinion, and not peer-reviewed in the formal sense. However, rigorous debate is occurring among supporters of Web 2.0, who state that blogs and wikis that encourage comments or are open to user input are in fact using a peer-review process.

KEY ONLINE TOOLS TO SUPPORT AND ENHANCE LEARNING

Healthcare professionals are discovering, exploring and using the freely available Web 2.0 tools to find, store, share, create and promote healthcare information

(Seeman 2008). In this section we will define and give examples of a range of online *social software* tools you could use to support your fieldwork learning. We will also discuss how you can evaluate the reliability of information. The tools covered in depth are weblogs (blogs), collaborative writing tools, online social networks, podcasts, syndication feeds (RSS), virtual worlds and wikis. Additional tools have been outlined in the Web 2.0 tools summary table (Table 18.1), and all key websites are listed alphabetically at the end of the chapter.

Blogs

Blogs (weblogs) are websites that individuals known as *bloggers* create and maintain (Junco & Cole-Avent 2008). Usually a blog is about a single topic or theme, and items are posted on a regular basis, with the most recent entries appearing at the top. Each entry is called a *post*, with most bloggers allowing others to respond by *posting* comments. Blogs can be developed and maintained by individuals or groups, even with little technical ability, and can be either private (with the blogger deciding who can view his or her blog) or public (open for viewing by anyone with Internet access). A blog can include text, pictures, video, audio, Internet links and RSS feeds, and the list grows as technology advances.

A growing number of health professionals maintain a professional blog. Many report that through their blogs they are discovering other people with similar interests, and have formed international online communities of practice (Kamel Boulos & Wheeler 2007). This trend has also occurred among blogs created by people living with an illness or disability, where people share stories and offer support to others experiencing a similar life event. Blogs offer us an opportunity to gain insight into others' experiences and to ask questions.

As a reflective student, you may find that a blog can provide you with a forum to record thoughts, experiences, impressions and struggles. While blogs can be valuable tools, students and health professionals should be careful about the content of their reflections. If confidential information is recorded, then blog settings must be set to private, or shared only with your fieldwork educator. If the blogger chooses an *open blog*, then confidential or identifying information cannot be used. Open blogs are best if they focus on the individual's learning rather than experiences of the clients or the fieldwork agency.

Two blogging sites are recommended here: Blogger for its simplicity, and WordPress for its sophistication.

- Blogger, owned by Google, can be set up in about 10 minutes. It has a range of basic templates, from which you can add text, pictures, video, audio, Internet links and RSS feeds (see below for explanation of RSS feeds). You can set your blog to be public or private.

- In WordPress you can also add text, pictures, video, audio, Internet links and RSS feeds, but it offers a wider range of templates, and the capacity for you to upload documents such as PowerPoint or portable document format (pdf) files. A key feature is that each post in a WordPress blog can be set at a different level of privacy. These can be private posts, accessed only by the blogger, posts accessible to selected people using a password, or posts that are fully open to the public. Some bloggers have used WordPress as an e-portfolio, including text, presentations, audio, video and images. For a small yearly subscription, users can upgrade from 4GB of storage upwards to 25GB.

Case Study 18.1 | Meg the blogger

Meg became a blogger to record her experiences during her gap year before starting university. After starting at university, Meg was surprised that few students had blogs, and was concerned when one of the academic staff told students not to cite blogs, Wikipedia or any other non-peer-reviewed information in their academic work. Meg could see that blogging did not have a place in University life.

Some time later, Meg was undertaking fieldwork away from home and was finding it challenging. Meg thought to discuss her feelings with her supervisor, but was anxious that she would be perceived as being ill equipped for her future profession. Meg felt isolated.

Remembering the value of her earlier blog, Meg decided to start blogging again. She wanted to record her thoughts and feelings, so she set up a private blog in WordPress. Meg followed the guidelines for reflective journals, using pseudonyms for clients, supervisors and her location. Meg made sure that her blog was closed down each time she left the computer.

Meg used a range of applications, such as text and graphics, and even recording audio using a digital recorder and uploading as audio files to her blog. She found a mindmapping tool online, and used this to reflect on her practice dilemmas. The mindmaps were uploaded to her blog as pdf files, and she used them for ongoing reflection and to track her learning.

One day Meg's fieldwork educator showed her a professional portfolio that she had developed over her career. It was a collection of documents, photos and certificates detailing her professional development and career highlights. She explained that she also *journaled* when she was working in new areas of practice. Meg could see the parallel, and realised that she was creating a multimedia electronic portfolio. Meg mentioned it to her fieldwork educator, and offered to show her the blog. The next day Meg adjusted her settings in her WordPress blog, and allowed her fieldwork educator to access a specific post that illustrated her learning during the fieldwork placement.

The fieldwork educator said that the blog had provided her with new insight into how a student might feel during fieldwork, and asked Meg if she felt comfortable sharing this with the other members of the team, which Meg did. Meg left fieldwork strengthened in her resolve to continue to add to her blog and redirect it towards being an e-portfolio tool for the next phase of her learning, lifelong professional development.

Questions

1   Do you keep a blog?
2   Do you think that keeping a blog throughout fieldwork would work for you?
3   What other technology(ies) do you use to learn?

Collaborative writing

Collaborative writing tools can be used by one or more people in real time or asynchronously. A number of collaborative writing tools exist, such as Zoho Writer and Google Documents. As each document is web based, and has its unique URL, groups of people can work on a document, spreadsheet or presentation, overcoming the need to keep track of different versions. Once completed, the final version can be uploaded back to the relevant program. These tools are appealing to healthcare workers, as they can be used to organise meetings, take notes or create joint documents, enabling us to work smarter and more efficiently.

This chapter is an example of collaborative writing, as it was developed using Google Documents, with authors in the northern and southern hemispheres completing the writing process asynchronously. In fieldwork, collaborative writing tools could be used as part of a student's reflective learning cycle, with the student completing an online reflective journal and the supervisor adding comments to aid reflection. Similarly, groups of students could collaborate to complete fieldwork assignments or to create documents, such as information pamphlets, for their fieldwork facility.

Credibility of information in a collaborative document lies with the authors, who are known to each other. Reliability of the collaborative writing tools can be a concern if the company running the program decides to remove it from the Internet. Users of collaborative writing tools are recommended to back up their work to a reliable place, such as their own hard drive, a pen drive or an external hard drive. Students should also be aware that computer hackers may access their documents, just as they do hard drives of computers. Therefore, while the companies developing the software confidently assure the user of privacy, students need to consider the type of information they store in collaborative programs, and always pay careful attention to privacy.

Online social networks

Online social network sites support the maintenance of existing social networks, or help people connect with strangers who may share interests or activities. Sites vary in the types of applications and communication tools they offer users, such as mobile connectivity, blogging and photo- or videosharing (Kamel Boulos et al. 2007), but the most important feature they offer is to make a user's network visible to others, thus opening up the possibility of making new connections and new networks. There are over 40 major social network sites on the Internet today, with the two most popular in the English-speaking world being Facebook and MySpace (Junco & Cole-Avent 2008). A different type of social networking site is Ning, where users set up their own social networks based on special interests.

As more students from the millennial or Y Generation (Junco & Cole-Avent 2008) enter university, most have well-developed online social networks and profiles. Social network sites display social connections and give information about identity. When students commence studies to become health professionals, they are learning about the appropriate identity signals of their chosen profession, but may not understand how the healthcare sector expects them to portray themselves.

While you are studying to become a health professional it is important to consider management of your online profile (DiMicco & Millen 2007), as boundaries between personal and professional lives have become permeable since the advent of Web 2.0. DiMicco and Millen's (2007) research looked at people who had developed a Facebook profile while at university, and had continued using it as they transitioned to the workforce. By analysing the online profile and photos, they concluded that three groups existed:

- the 'Reliving the college days' group, who were not managing their online identity for the work environment
- The 'Dressed to impress' and 'Living in the business world' groups were managing their self-presentation better, indicating they are aware that both professional colleagues and old friends would view their profiles.

With an increasing number of employers now using the Internet to research job applicants, we recommend that you take some time with 'impression management' of your online profile and privacy settings. *Impression management* entails developing a professional online profile that is potentially visible to future employers, clients and colleagues.

REFLECTION 18.1

My online life
- Do you have an online presence?
- Have you thought that one day a potential employer may search the Web looking for information about you?
- This may not occur, but what was your reaction to such a suggestion?

Podcasts

Podcasts grew in popularity, largely after the advent of portable MP3 players, because of their capacity to capture and share class lectures in higher education settings (Hendron 2008). The name *podcast* evolved from the use of Apple iPods; they are downloadable audio or video files.

Keeping up to date with healthcare information has become easier since podcasting began, as you can download audio and video podcasts on topics of interest. To subscribe to podcasts, there is free software through iTunes. To locate podcasts, CNET Podcast Central and Podcast.com are currently two popular Web-based podcast listing services. Sites like MedReader specifically focus on healthcare information, and also include podcasts. YouTube, which is the largest resource for video podcasts, includes healthcare information by both qualified practitioners and the general public.

Podcasting is becoming an increasingly popular way to share information with people who have difficulty with text. To start creating your own podcast visit How to Podcast, which offers step-by-step instructions on how to create your own podcast and upload it to the Internet. An example of a healthcare podcast is Jonathan Singer's podcast site All Things Social Work.

Syndication feeds (RSS)

RSS stands for Really Simple Syndication, Rich Site Summary or RDF Site Summary (McLean et al. 2007). RSS allows you to subscribe to alerts from Internet news services, blog or podcast updates, journal table of contents alerts and even Pubmed searches. Subscribing to RSS feeds means that you no longer have to visit your favourite websites or blogs for updates; rather you are informed of updates. It is simple to subscribe to any site that has the RSS symbol (Figure 18.3) but rather than explain it here, it is simpler to go online to Commoncraft, the URL located in our list of resources at the end of this chapter.

To start receiving RSS feeds, you will need to set up a reader or an aggregator to receive subscribed updates. We suggest using either Google Reader or Bloglines. Bloglines offers you the opportunity to search other feeds or blogs using keywords,

Figure 18.3: RSS symbol

and Google Reader offers you the option to share your RSS feeds with others, thus enhancing everyone's access to online information.

Virtual worlds

Multi-user *virtual worlds* are computer-based, simulated multimedia environments that are designed to enable users to interact with each other using digital objects. Each user has a customisable graphical self-representation known as an *avatar*, which has its own name and can be adapted to have unique features (Kamel Boulos et al. 2007). Currently the most popular virtual world is Second Life, with 8.9 million *residents* in 2008 (Seeman 2008). Second Life is an example of the emerging world of Web 3.0, a 3-D social network, where people collaboratively create and edit objects and interact in a virtual world.

Second Life is evolving rapidly, and Kamel Boulos and colleagues (2007) identify the following capabilities that are applicable to healthcare education and practice:

- multimedia content, such as audio, video or TV collections
- information spaces: document collections in 3-D virtual libraries
- new places and cultures
- multiplayer games, including educational, health-related games
- virtual and real-life goods and services
- healthcare information and skill development
- interaction and networking with other people and communities
- attendance at and participation in lectures, conferences, festivals and concerts.

Healthcare education initiatives are emerging in Second Life, with Healthinfo Island being the biggest healthcare initiative so far. An example of a new and innovative project is a Second Life Education New Zealand (SLENZ)-funded project to design, build and evaluate a virtual birthing unit by midwife Sarah Stewart and her colleagues (Stewart, personal communication, 22 February 2009).

Wikis

Wiki, which means 'hurry' in the Hawaiian language (McLean et al. 2007), is another example of software that facilitates collaborative writing. A wiki is a collection of linked webpages that are able to be contributed to, edited or updated by its users (Kamel Boulos & Wheeler 2007). Like blogs, wikis can have different levels of access, such as reader, writer, editor or administrator. However, a wiki does not show contributions in reverse chronological order; they are incorporated into the whole site and the changes are only evident when you view the 'history' of the wiki. The history can also be used to 'roll back' to previous versions of the wiki, which is useful if an unwelcome contribution has been made.

A wiki can include text, pictures, video, audio, links to its own wiki pages, Internet links and RSS feeds; the list grows as technology advances. Two wiki programs are recommended here:

- PBWorks is a hosted program that is free to register to use. It is one of the simplest wiki programs to use, and can be quickly set up and easily personalised. To learn how to set up your own wiki, visit its website and click on the link to the user manual

Table 18.1: Web 2.0 tools summary table

Web 2.0 tool	Description	Tools to get started
Blog	A blog (or weblog) is a website where items are posted on a regular basis with the most recent posts at the top. Usually a blog is about a single topic or theme	Blogger Wordpress
Collaborative writing	Collaborative writing tools facilitate editing and reviewing of a text document by multiple individuals, either in real time or asynchronously	Google Documents Zoho Writer <http://writer.zoho.com/>
Online scholarly databases	A freely accessible Web search engine that indexes the full text of scholarly literature across an array of publishing formats and disciplines	Pubmed BMJ Google Scholar
Multi-user Virtual World	Virtual world where the user is represented by an avatar and can interact with other avatars in a 3-D virtual environment	Second Life (SL) Croquet Project
Personalised home pages	A personalised home page lets you assemble all your favourite widgets, such as note pages, feeds, social networks, email, videos and blogs on one fully customisable page	iGoogle myYahoo

Web 2.0 tool	Description	Tools to get started
Podcast	A podcast is a series of audio or video digital-media files that is distributed over the Internet by syndicated download (RSS), through Web feeds, to portable media players and personal computers	CNET Podcast Central <Podcast.com> YouTube
Photosharing	Photosharing is the publishing or transfer of a user's digital photos online, thus enabling the user to share them with others (whether publicly or privately)	flickr Picasa
Social bookmarking	Users save links to Web pages that they want to remember and/or share. These bookmarks are usually public, but can be saved privately or shared with specified people or groups	Delicious CiteULike
Syndication (RSS) feeds	You can subscribe to syndicated Web feeds so that the Internet updates you—you don't have to remember to check for updates for your favourite blogs or websites	Google Reader MedReader Bloglines
Social network sites	Online communities of people who share interests and activities, or who are interested in exploring the interests and activities of others	Facebook MySpace Bebo Ning
Voice over Internet Protocol (VoIP) and Synchronous Communications	VoIP services convert voice into a digital signal that travels over the Internet to a computer or a phone or another computer	Google talk AOL Instant messaging Gizmo5
Wiki	A wiki is an interactive Web page designed to enable anyone who accesses it to contribute or modify content	MediaWiki PBWiki Wikispaces

- MediaWiki is the wiki program used by Wikipedia. It is free to download but it needs to be hosted. This program requires some computer technical knowledge to set up and manage. If you are in a setting that has its own IT department, you can ask members of the department to download and manage MediaWiki for your project.

The best-known wiki is Wikipedia, the online encyclopedia. It is an open wiki, which means it can be modified by anyone. Wikipedia is sometimes criticised as being unreliable; however, a comparison made with the online Encyclopaedia Britannica showed the accuracy to be very similar (Giles 2005, as cited in McLean et al. 2007: 175).

Wikis are useful for tasks that require collaboration by a group of people; for example, a group project or development of a community resource. A community resource wiki called Health Evidence Search was developed by health professionals and a University librarian to share information about reliable online databases to search for healthcare evidence. This is an example of Web 2.0 technology facilitating dissemination of Web 1.0 information. Get a Note From your Doctor is an example of a peer-reviewed wiki that is expert moderated, with only approved physicians able to post (Seeman 2008).

SUMMARY

It is estimated that the speed at which knowledge becomes obsolete is currently between two and five years (Ryan 2003), and with the explosion of health-related knowledge new ways to manage information are needed. Web 2.0 has changed the way people manage information, as it has provided a virtual environment where health professionals can reflect on their experiences and ask questions with others, and develop online communities of practice.

Health professionals, not just students, are continually reminded that there is new information for practice that they need to access and critically appraise. This situation is magnified by the fact that health professionals need to cope with everchanging health service demands. With the speed of change, information in texts and journals can quickly become outdated; therefore use of the online resources to stay up to date has become vital. Although guidelines for sharing healthcare information online through blogs and wikis exist, we all need to source review and evaluate the evidence carefully, regardless of the source of the material online or in print.

Web 2.0 is not a fad (Seeman 2008), and it is simply a matter of time before we start hearing about Web 3.0. Knowing how to effectively use Web 2.0 tools to optimise learning is crucial to building capacity by healthcare professionals in knowledge generation and knowledge translation for the future.

DISCUSSION QUESTIONS

1   What steps can you take to ensure that online healthcare information you access is credible and trustworthy?

2   What issues need to be considered if you were to blog about your experiences with a challenging client or fieldwork setting?

3   Why is 'impression management' in social network sites such as MySpace or Facebook so important?

4   What might you do to ensure that information you provide on your blog or wiki is perceived as credible and trustworthy by readers or visitors?

References

Baerlocher, M. O. & Detsky, A. S. (2008). 'Online Medical Blogging: Don't Do It!' *Canadian Medical Association Journal*, 179(3): 292.

DiMicco, J. M. & Millen, D. R. (2007). Identity Management: Multiple Presentations of Self in Facebook. Proceedings of the 2007 International ACM Conference on Supporting Group Work. <http://portal.acm.org/citation.cfm?id=1316624.1316682> accessed 20 February 2009.

Hendron, J. G. (2008). *RSS for Educators: Blogs, Newsfeeds, Podcasts, and Wikis in the Classroom* (1st edn). International Society for Technology in Education, Washington, DC.

Jantzen, D. (2008). 'Reframing Professional Development for First-line Nurses'. *Nursing Inquiry*, 15(1): 21–9.

Junco, R. & Cole-Avent, G. A. (2008). 'An Introduction to Technologies Commonly Used by College Students'. *New Directions for Student Services*, 124: 3–17.

Kamel Boulos, M. N., Hetherington, L. & Wheeler, S. (2007). 'Second Life: An Overview of the Potential of 3-D Virtual Worlds in Medical and Health Education'. *Health Information and Libraries Journal*, 24: 233–45.

Kamel Boulous, M. N. & Wheeler, S. (2007). 'The Emerging Web 2.0 Social Software: An Enabling Suite of Sociable Technologies in Health and Health Care Education'. *Health Information and Libraries Journal*, 24: 2–23.

Letendre, P. (2008). Perils and joys of blogging: Electronic letter to the editor. *Canadian Medical Association Journal*. <http://www.cmaj.ca/cgi/eletters/179/3/292#19949> Accessed 18 February 2009.

McCluskey, A. & Cusick, A. (2002). 'Strategies for Introducing Evidence-based Practice and Changing Clinician Behaviour: A Manager's Toolbox'. *Australian Occupational Therapy Journal*, 49: 63–70.

McLean, R., Richards, B. H. & Wardman, J. (2007). 'The Effect of Web 2.0 on the Future of Medical Practice and Education: Darwikian Evolution or Folksonomic Revolution?' *IT and Health*, 187(3): 174–7.

O'Reilly, T. (2005). *What Is Web 2.0? Design Patterns and Business Models for the Next Generation of Software*. <http://oreillynet.com/pub/a/oreilly/tim/news/2005/09/30/what-is-web-20.html> Accessed 1 May 2008.

Ryan, J. (2003). 'Continuous Professional Development along the Continuum of Lifelong Learning'. *Nurse Education Today*, 23(7): 498–508.

Schaper, L. & Pervan, G. (2007). 'ICT and OTs: A Model of Information and Communication Technology Acceptance and Utilisation by Occupational Therapists (Part 2). *International Journal of Medical Informatics*, 76: 212–21.

Seeman, N. (2008). 'Web 2.0 and Chronic Illness: New Horizons, New Opportunities' (electronic version). *Healthcare Quarterly*, 6: 104–10. <http://www.electronichealthcare.net> Accessed 1 May 2008.

Further Reading

Arrington, M. (2008). *Facebook No Longer The Second Largest Social Network*. <http://www.techcrunch.com/2008/06/12/facebook-no-longer-the-second-largest-social-network/> Accessed 18 February 2009.

Boyd, D. M. & Ellison, N. B. (2007). 'Social Network Sites: Definition, History, and Scholarship'. *Journal of Computer-Mediated Communication*, 13(1): 210–30.

Donen, N. (1999). 'Mandatory Practice Self-Appraisal: Moving towards Outcomes Based Continuing Education'. *Journal of Evaluation in Clinical Practice*, 7: 297–303.

Gwozdek, A. E., Klausner, C. P. & Kerschbaum, W. E. (2008). 'The Utilization of Computer Mediated Communication for Case Study Collaboration'. *Journal of Dental Hygiene*, 82(1): 1–10.

Lowry, P. B., Curtis, A. & Lowry, M. R. (2004). 'Building a Taxonomy and Nomenclature of Collaborative Writing to Improve Interdisciplinary Research and Practice'. *Journal of Business Communication*, 41: 66–99.

Potts, H. W. W. (2006). 'Is E-health Progressing Faster than E-health Researchers?' (electronic version). *Journal of Medical Internet Research*, 8. <http://www.jmir.org/2006/3/e24/> Accessed 1 May 2008.

Prensky, M. (2001). 'Digital Natives, Digital Immigrants'. *On the Horizon*, 9(5): 1–6.

Schembri, A. M. (2008). 'Why Social Workers Need to Embrace Web 2.0'. *Australian Social Work*, 61(2): 119–23.

Tassone, M. R. & Heck, C. S. (1997). 'Motivational Orientations of Allied Health Care Professionals Participating in Continuing Education'. *Journal of Continuing Education in the Health Professions*, 17(2): 97–105.

Townsend, E., Sheffield, S., Stadnyk, R. & Beagan, B. (2006). 'Effects of Workplace Policy on Continuing Professional Development: The Case of Occupational Therapy in Nova Scotia, Canada'. *Canadian Journal of Occupational Therapy*, 73(2): 98–108.

Useful Websites

All Things Socialwork: http://socialworkpodcast.com

Blogger: www.blogger.com/start

Bloglines: www.bloglines.com

CNET Podcast Central: www.cnet.com/podcasts

Commoncraft: www.commoncraft.com

Facebook: http://facebook.com

Get a Note From your Doctor: www.ganfyd.org

Google Documents: http://docs.google.com

Google Reader: www.google.com/reader

Healthcare Blogger Code of Ethics: http://medbloggercode.com/the-code

Health Evidence Search Wiki: http://healthevidencesearch.pbworks.com

HONCode: www.hon.ch/index.html

How to Create a Podcast: www.how-to-podcast-tutorial.com

MedReader: www.medreader.com/

MediaWiki: www.mediawiki.org/wiki/MediaWiki

Midwives and Second Life SLENZ project: http://sarah-stewart.blogspot.com/search/label/second%20life

MySpace: www.myspace.com

Ning: www.ning.com

PB Wiki user manual: http://pbwikimanual.pbwiki.com

Podcast.com: http://podcast.com

RSS in Plain English: www.commoncraft.com/rss_plain_english

Second Life: http://secondlife.com

Top educational locations in Second Life: http://healthcybermap.org/sl.htm

WebCite: www.webcitation.org/5aDEkONrK

Wordpress: http://wordpress.org

YouTube: http://Youtube.com

Zoho Writer: http://writer.zoho.com

PART 2 CHECKLIST
MAKING THE MOST OF YOUR FIELDWORK PLACEMENT

MODELS OF SUPERVISION

- [ ] Reflect on the type of supervision that suits you best.
- [ ] How do you like to learn?

MAKING THE MOST OF YOUR FIELDWORK LEARNING OPPORTUNITY

I have reflected on the following in relation to myself:
- [ ] my personal attributes
- [ ] my generational attributes
- [ ] my generic knowledge and skills
- [ ] my professional behaviours
- [ ] my discipline-specific knowledge and skills.
- [ ] To make the most of my fieldwork placement I will: reflect on my practice; seek appropriate advice; set goals and take action
- [ ] I will use the practice window when I need to.

ASSESSMENT OF CLINICAL LEARNING

- [ ] Have I read the assessment criteria and assessment form before taking up my placement?
- [ ] Have I reflected critically upon the means by which I will be able to demonstrate my achievement of the criteria?
- [ ] Am I able to link the criteria to activities I will carry out on placement, and sources of feedback?
- [ ] Have I planned to rate myself on the assessment form before meeting with my clinical educator?
- [ ] Have I established what the minimal standard of performance looks like?

☐ Do I have a plan for managing any mismatch between my self-assessment and that of my fieldwork educator?

☐ Have I spoken with my fieldwork educator about how I should progress throughout my placement?

A MODEL FOR ALTERNATIVE FIELDWORK

☐ I am clear on the aims for my fieldwork.

☐ I realise that my host fieldwork educator is not from my profession.

☐ I will aim to learn how to articulate to others what my profession does and what my role is.

☐ I will actively seek out support from peers, mentors, discipline specific staff and host staff

INTERPROFESSIONAL LEARNING: WORKING IN TEAMS

If I want to have a successful placement I will:

☐ start establishing a positive rapport with my fellow students by holding a face-to-face meeting, a teleconference or an online chat or asynchronous discussion forum

☐ exchange contact details and a little about my personal and academic backgrounds, including what I think is most important in IPL and any particular interest areas

☐ discuss logistical arrangements, such as travel and accommodation (if relevant), timetables, negotiation of shared learning tasks and any other concerns, issues or information that are still needed

☐ establish a positive working relationship by clarifying my expectations and hopes for the placement

☐ identify where my respective expectations and learning objectives are similar to and different from those of the other students

☐ discuss how I might manage to accommodate everyone's core goals, and where I am prepared to make compromises

☐ make sure I know what to do if things go wrong, such as personal health or safety issues, or if the placement is not meeting my expectations.

LEARNING FROM FAILURE

▢ Do I think I am failing?
▢ Am I having difficulties?
▢ I will discuss my concerns with my fieldwork educator before my midway assessment.

USING ONLINE TECHNOLOGY

▢ When using online technology, I know to be aware of sites that are evidence based.

PART 3
ETHICS, LAW AND RESPONSIBILITIES

Chapter 19:   Fostering Partnerships with Action   251

Chapter 20:   Ethical and Supported Decision-making   263

Chapter 21:   The Three Rs: Roles, Rights and
              Responsibilities   281

Chapter 22:   Legal Issues   299

This section takes a step back and considers the wider issues surrounding fieldwork placements, such as the role of the stakeholders involved and who has responsibility for what. Fieldwork placements are governed by professional standards, university academic standards, government legislation and policies of the individual agencies and institutions that accept students on placement. Your role as a student within these structures is vitally important. As part of your role, this section also discusses your responsibilities and legal obligations, as well as legal implications of your behaviour while on placement. This section extends the discussion about working with vulnerable clients and how to make ethical decisions when working with such clients.

CHAPTER 19
FOSTERING PARTNERSHIPS WITH ACTION

Michelle Courtney and Jane Maidment

LEARNING OUTCOMES

After reading this chapter you should be able to:
- understand students' engagement with partnerships in fieldwork education from a critical perspective
- understand the role of key stakeholders in fieldwork education
- understand the importance of fieldwork partnerships
- discuss students' roles in fieldwork partnerships.

KEY TERMS

Core business
Forcefield analysis
Government
Horizontal partnerships
Individual professional
Integrated fieldwork practice
Profession
Stakeholders
Triple helix partnering model
University
Vertical partnering model

INTRODUCTION

There is a growing body of literature acknowledging the significant professional and pedagogical drivers for *integrated fieldwork practice* (Beddoe & Maidment 2009; Courtney 2008). You were aware of the requirement for fieldwork placement when you signed up for your studies as a health and human services professional. You will now have a clear understanding of the specific requirements for fieldwork placement as they are listed in your course handbook. You will fulfil these specific requirements within the day-to-day real world of health and human services. The real-world dynamics of fieldwork placement are complex. It's important for you to have some understanding of these dynamics to function positively during your fieldwork placement.

The aim of this chapter is to provide a practical introduction to the day-to-day dynamics of fieldwork placement in the health and human services. We will be taking a big-picture view of fieldwork placement. We'll discuss who's who in fieldwork, and why it's important that we all work together positively, including you in your role as a consumer of fieldwork education.

We begin this chapter discussing the key stakeholders in fieldwork placement: the profession; the university; the government; the individual professional; and you the student. Using a broad-brush approach, we will introduce some important aspects of the perspective of each of the stakeholders. We will discuss why partnerships matter in placements and conclude with the important role that you play in fieldwork placement partnerships.

KEY STAKEHOLDERS

Although there are differences between each health and human service profession, they have in common fieldwork placement as a requirement of qualifying studies. The key stakeholders involved in fieldwork placement consistently support the advantages of work-integrated learning. Stakeholders creatively, positively and consistently explore ways to optimise the provision of fieldwork placement in the day-to-day real world of health and human services. Nevertheless, given that placement is not the core business of any of the key stakeholders, these groups do not see fieldwork placement from a common perspective. It's important to begin to understand the differing perspectives of other stakeholders, so you can work effectively right from the start of your engagement.

Fieldwork placement involves different specific requirements for each profession; for example, differing hours, definition of roles, delineation of suitable facilities and guidelines for adequate supervision. There are also varying relational models between the professions and the universities. For example, placement may be undertaken during a qualifying degree, or during a graduate (post-professional) period. Further examples of relational models include universities who make direct payments to facilities for fieldwork placement as opposed to models involving no direct payment.

Despite these differences, each health and human services profession has key stakeholders in common, including the profession, the university, the government, the individual professional and you the student. The need to balance the needs and expectations of stakeholders is constant, as well as imperative for the effective delivery of fieldwork placement.

The following is a broad-brush view from the perspective of each of the key stakeholders. Not all the issues will be discussed, and the level of detail is not exhaustive. The purpose of the discussion below is not to provide an in-depth synopsis of the discourse surrounding fieldwork education, but to shed light, for you, on the day-to-day dynamics of fieldwork placement.

The profession

A *profession* is the collective organisation of each specific work role undertaken by individual members of the health and human services workforce. Professional associations are the peak bodies representing the collective of the individual members of each profession. Examples include OT Australia (Australian Association of Occupational Therapists) and AASW (Australian Association of Social Workers). In the context of this chapter, the core business of the profession is to define and assure standards of practice (including qualifying education) in the interests of the community; while concurrently advancing the standing of the profession within the community in the interests of the members of the profession.

The profession wants well-educated health and human services professionals. The profession needs to set standards for entry into the profession as well as standards for qualifying education. It will have a belief about the minimum number of fieldwork placement hours required to qualify, therefore sets the specific requirements for fieldwork placement.

The profession is an influential key stakeholder in fieldwork education. Nevertheless, it is not the core business of the profession to provide fieldwork education.

The university

A *university* is an institution that delivers higher education and advanced specialist knowledge through the integration of teaching, research and practice in the health and human services. In the context of this chapter, the core business of the university is to provide courses leading to suitably qualified members of the health and human services workforce.

The university is an influential key stakeholder in fieldwork placement. Nevertheless, it is not the core business of the university to provide fieldwork placement.

The government

The *government*, whether federal or state, is the organisation that provides funding sources for higher education as well as large areas of the Australian community's health and human services. In the context of this chapter, the core business of the government is to provide support for the needs, objectives and vision of the whole Australian community, both now and into the future.

The government wants people to work in the health and human services. The volume and complexity of that work is dramatically increasing and, now and into the future, workforce shortages are serious. Both federal and state governments are aware that this issue is critical. They are dedicating considerable resources to addressing the problems of getting the work done in the health and human services, including the development and securing of an adequate health and human services workforce.

Standards of services remain important to the government, but are not directly and solely linked to the standards set down by the professions.

The government is an influential key stakeholder in fieldwork placement. Nevertheless, it is not the core business of the government to provide fieldwork placement.

The individual professional

The *individual professional* is the individual person doing specialist work within health and human services. Examples include occupational therapists, social workers, nurses, speech pathologists and physiotherapists.

In the context of this chapter, the core business of the individual professional is to provide the knowledge, skills and expertise required to deliver services that optimise outcomes in the interests of clients in health and human services.

Individual professionals want to meet the needs of clients through working in the health and human services. They also want to advance the visibility and influence of their profession. Individual professionals want to see an expanding workforce of well-educated and articulate colleagues in the field, primarily to meet the needs of a growing client base. At the same time, they take on a very demanding role, and the available resources are stretched. Their attention and energy must be devoted to giving the best services to their clients.

Individual professionals are influential key stakeholders in fieldwork education. Nevertheless, it is not the core business of the individual professional to provide fieldwork education.

The student

The final key stakeholder for discussion in this chapter is *you*! The student is the person who is the consumer of higher education, including fieldwork placement. You may be consuming fieldwork placement during your qualifying studies, after you have completed your coursework or as paid employment during your early working life. In the context of this chapter, your core business is to undertake fieldwork placement to fulfil the requirements for entry into the profession and therefore eligibility to join the health and human services workforce.

Students are keen to earn eligibility into the health and human services profession while balancing this aim with other life demands. As a consumer of higher education, the student is demanding more flexibility in the delivery of coursework, including using online and other digital technologies. Comparatively, there remains limited flexibility in fieldwork placement. Students understand that the relationship with the individual professional (fieldwork educator) is paramount.

At the same time, students can be in the position of creating additional work as well as placing stress on other resources (such as computer access and desk space). Importantly, you the student are at the point of convergence between all the other key stakeholders. *You* are linked to and influenced by all the other key stakeholders in fieldwork placement.

Students are influential key stakeholders in fieldwork education. Nevertheless, it is not the *core business* of students to provide fieldwork placement.

IMPORTANCE OF FIELDWORK PARTNERSHIPS

The landscape for field education in Australia and other western nations is subject to constant flux, where rapidly changing economic and political imperatives have a constant impact upon workforce demand, employment opportunities, and health educational priorities and policies. In order to respond quickly to change and promote sustainability within health service delivery, the government, tertiary and industry sectors must now operate interdependently.

The last two decades in higher education have been characterised by increasing emphasis on partnering between education providers, industry and government. The potential gains for each of these stakeholders in finding common synergies have been widely documented (Hirsch & Weber 1999; Etzkowitz 2008; Patrick et al. 2008), with a growing realisation that more can be achieved for all parties through cross-sector collaboration than by operating separately. As such, there has been increasing recognition of the mutual benefits associated with cross-sector partnering in education and research. Specific drivers for partnering include: pooling resources and expertise; addressing identified areas of skills shortage; promoting professional development opportunities for industry staff through engagement with learning and research opportunities; improving retention among staff and student groups; fostering research and development opportunities between industry and higher education to address identified concerns; making indirect cost savings; information sharing; accessing different types of knowledge and skill; and drawing upon alliance networks and expertise to respond quickly to competitive pressures and funding opportunities.

While there are significant economic, commercial and pedagogical drivers for partnering, there are also qualitative advantages to be derived from collaboration between the government, industry and higher education sectors. These factors include the generation of goodwill and credibility in the community; using coalitions to promote diverse participation and social justice objectives; and the demonstration of relevance and responsiveness to identified need; while fostering a creative milieu for the hatching of new ideas, development and research. These factors provide potent individual and organisational intrinsic motivation for initiating, supporting and maintaining cross-sector alliances.

REFLECTION 19.1

Understanding stakeholder imperatives
This is an exercise to do in pairs.

As discussed earlier in this chapter, there is a range of different stakeholders in fieldwork, including the professional associations, learning institutions, government and service delivery organisations.

- *Step 1*: Think about each of the different government, industry and professional stakeholder interests in fieldwork education, and identify which factors might be considered 'not negotiable' for these parties in negotiating educational fieldwork. Make a list of these. (Consider legislation, values and ethics, accountability, management principles such as communication and minimisation of risk, and organisational requirements).
- *Step 2*: Ask yourself: what sorts of information and processes can I identify that might have been used in negotiating the terms of my discipline's fieldwork arrangements?
- *Step 3*: Ask yourself: what factors within the economic and political context do I think might have influenced the terms of my fieldwork placement arrangements?

THINK AND LINK 19.1

Reflection 19.1 also alludes to your role, rights and responsibilities. Chapter 21 discusses in depth the three Rs. This chapter may add thoughts to your reflections in Reflection 19.1.

Partnering models

Partnering models have commonly been classified as either *vertical* or *horizontal* (van Ginkel 1999). *Vertical partnerships* refer to partnerships between organisations where one partner or group of partners acts as consultants (commissioned experts) to others wishing to make changes in their structure, functioning or methods of service delivery. *Horizontal partnerships* occur within a flat structure of governance, with expertise being shared between the partners, and the relationship is acknowledged as symbiotic. In these types of arrangements it is not uncommon for relational interactions between stakeholders to occur at strategic executive, operational and technical levels of the partnering organisations.

Most recently, the complex interchange of collaboration and innovation derived from industry, government and higher education cross-sector partnerships has been conceptualised as a *triple helix* (Etzkowitz 2008): the interconnected spiral relationship between these three stakeholders, where spirals are rarely equal, with one party acting as the core around which the others rotate. The institution that acts as the core spiral changes over time, depending upon the changing lifecycle, drivers and motivations of stakeholder interests in the collaboration. The helix formation manages to capture the more complex contemporary nature of relationships inherent in bringing together trilateral interactions between the three sectors, whereas traditional partnership arrangements were more likely to include only two sectors, such as university–industry or government–university.

Professional fieldwork in higher education is one significant area where the interests of each of these stakeholders intersect, creating a milieu for significant innovation, collaboration and potential conflict. We now turn our attention to the way fieldwork placements act as a microcosm for reflecting the broader debates in government education and employment policy, higher education pedagogical and marketing concerns, and industry capacity building.

Why do fieldwork partnerships matter?

The Work Integrated Learning (WIL) Report (2008) documents a recent scoping investigation into work-integrated learning in Australia. While the authors of this report were careful to note that fieldwork placements were just one type of work-integrated learning activity, they did highlight the centrality of cross-sector partnerships between university, government and industry providers to create relevant learning opportunities for students in the real world.

Stakeholders, especially students, stand to gain a great deal when symbiotic industry partnerships in fieldwork can be forged, and the WIL report cites these benefits throughout (Patrick et al. 2008). Hence, you have the opportunity to enhance your knowledge and skills in the authentic workplace; engage in activities that build strong curriculum vitae; develop professional networks for future employment; experience genuine practice opportunities in a supervised and 'controlled' environment; and test whether your chosen profession is really your occupation of choice.

Meanwhile, industry uses fieldwork partnerships as a means for strategic recruitment, gaining access to observe first hand the work of potential future recruits during the practicum. Workforce recruitment is an expensive exercise, with the advertising and appointment process of base grade health professionals costing in the region of thousands of dollars. Your fieldwork placement provides employers with the opportunity to observe the work of potential employees (you) over a lengthy period of time without commitment to hiring, thus providing both you and the employer time to assess each other's strengths and weaknesses. A good number of final year health students gain their first graduate positions in agencies where they have been on placement.

THINK AND LINK 19.2

Chapter 25 discusses workforce recruitment, and how recruitment can relate to fieldwork placements. Fieldwork placement provides opportunities for you to consider where you would like to work, and for agencies to observe your performance as a potential employee and set up a working environment you would like to return to.

Engaging students on placement also provides the means to promote professional development opportunities for agency staff through conducting student supervision and gaining access to university resources, such as the library and supervision training workshops. For these relationships to work, there needs to be a foundation of shared understanding about the purposes and expectations of each of the stakeholders. The importance of effective channels of communication between the parties cannot be underestimated. The coordination role of fieldwork arrangements should be acknowledged by all stakeholders as central to the success of the placement (Patrick et al. 2008). The legal and ethical responsibilities for fieldwork are generally acknowledged through formal contractual agreements between the health and human service industry sector and the tertiary education providers, with each discipline needing to adhere to the standards set down by its professional association for educating future professionals. Informally, the quality of the day-to-day communications between each of these parties greatly influences the degree to which reciprocity, respect and shared purpose for fieldwork placement can be developed. Not surprisingly, the informal networking and relationships between workers in organisations are frequently more powerful than the formally designated lines of accountability and control (Meads et al. 2008).

International fieldwork

Increasingly, Australian higher education institutions are partnering with industry and universities internationally to enable students to complete fieldwork placement abroad, while also hosting growing numbers of overseas students undertaking fieldwork in Australia. This developing trend is designed to keep pace with global changes in education and practice, to prepare graduates for working in the international context. While there is still debate about the pedagogical merits of international student placements at professional entry level, it is happening because of student demand.

Meanwhile, recent legislation developed out of concern for safeguarding the rights of international students visiting Australia (*Educational Services for Overseas Students Act* 2007) imposes severe restrictions on student visas, especially in regard to undertaking 'workplace training'. Also, employers have demonstrated reluctance to have international students on placement because of the limited potential for future recruitment and students' variable English skills and limited understanding of the Australian workplace culture (Patrick et al. 2008). Clearly more work is needed to develop mutually beneficial procedures and protocols between stakeholders to support this growing trend in undertaking international fieldwork. Partnerships are likely to include different stakeholders from those traditionally engaged, such as the Department of Immigration and Citizenship.

YOUR ROLE IN FIELDWORK PARTNERSHIPS

As mentioned above, you often gain access to your first graduate employment through a fieldwork placement. Being out in the field is your time to make a good impression, develop your professional networks and enhance the partnership arrangement for future cohorts of students. One of the significant findings from the recent WIL report was that an organisation's willingness to have students on placement was profoundly influenced by their experiences with earlier students (Patrick et al. 2008).

In your student role, you are clearly undertaking fieldwork to meet the requirements for your degree, but at the same time you are tacitly representing your discipline program and university. As such, you are central to building sustainable relationships between the industry and the learning institutions. Not all industry–university partnerships are robust; many can be tenuous, and experiences with students can either pave the way for future development between the parties, or result in ties between stakeholders being severed. Therefore you have a powerful role to play as a conduit between the university and workplace learning environment, with the potential to add great value to the ongoing education of your peers.

After graduating, you have the opportunity to develop your management skills and career prospects by supervising student fieldwork yourself. Most institutions offer training opportunities to graduates interested in taking on this role. In so doing, you will be contributing to both the ongoing growth and development of your chosen profession, while strengthening the partnership between your employing agency and educational institution. Students like to be supervised by alumni from their own degree program who are familiar with the curriculum and theory, fieldwork requirements and assignment expectations. Contributing to continuing education in this way will enable you to access ongoing learning opportunities from the education provider, while at the same time broadening your skills portfolio in the workplace. These proactive initiatives are in keeping with the ethos of lifelong learning and will demonstrate your willingness to accept professional responsibility.

THINK AND LINK 19.3

Promoting professional development of yourself as a new fieldwork educator is discussed in Chapters 23 and 24. You may not have thought this far yet, but as a graduated health professional there is opportunity for you to engage students on placement as their fieldwork educator.

Case Study 19.1	Forcefield analysis of the fieldwork enterprise

You are the director of an NGO (non-government organisation) with a staff of 25. The main focus of the work is in the area of aged care and disability. Your organisation has a small base in a regional town with several rural satellite offices. It has been hard to recruit qualified staff, and currently the budget is such that employees are overworked and stressed. The local university contacted you with a request to have two students on placement for a length of 70 days. The state government is offering a small funding incentive to rural agencies to support work-integrated learning for allied health students. Using forcefield analysis, consider if it is in the agency's interests to take on the students.

Forcefield analysis is a useful tool for weighing up pros and cons in decision-making. In conducting such an analysis, list all of the components integral to an issue and give each a weighting in terms of its impact on potential outcomes. Listed below are the factors that employers think about when considering having students on placement:

- funding arrangements for fieldwork
- risk management
- assessment of student performance
- insurance coverage
- workforce planning and policy
- staff development
- recruitment
- implications for service delivery
- agency capacity to support and oversee day-to-day student activity
- costs to the agency
- health and safety
- special requirements to meet students' personal circumstances (such as care of ageing parents or a disability)
- compatibility with organisation mission and other workers
- workload implications
- agency employment requirements (such as police checks or possession of a driver's licence).

Questions

Identify the likely positive and negative factors associated with each of the above items that need to be taken into account before making your decision whether or not to have students on placement.

SUMMARY

The aim of this chapter is to provide a practical introduction to the day-to-day dynamics of fieldwork education in the health and human services. In addition, we have encouraged you to think critically about partnerships in fieldwork placement. The perspectives of key stakeholders were introduced as a platform for discussing your role in fieldwork partnerships. You the student are a key contributor to (not just consumer of) fieldwork placement in health and human services. Issues of governance and sustainability are examined in relation to the delivery of fieldwork and the student role.

DISCUSSION QUESTIONS

1   What do you think some of the legal, political and economic tensions might be for government departments, professional associations and industry partners in developing long-term, sustainable fieldwork models for educating future practitioners?

2   Where does the power rest in negotiating fieldwork with students, the university, industry or government departments?

3   What are the synergies between your personal values and those of the stakeholders involved in your fieldwork education? Give an example of a contribution you're prepared to make that results in mutual benefit for yourself and another stakeholder.

References

Beddoe, L. & Maidment, J. (2009). *Mapping Knowledge for Social Work Practice: Critical Intersection*. Cengage Learning, Melbourne.

Courtney, M. (2008). *Inside My Job: Insider Information for Early Career Occupational Therapists*. Transition to Practice Project, Melbourne.

Etzkowitz, H. (2008). *The Triple Helix: University–Industry–Government Innovation in Action*. Routledge, Hoboken, NJ.

Hafford-Letchfield, T. (2006). *Management and Organisations in Social Work*. Learning Matters, Exeter.

Hirsch, W. & Weber, L. (eds) (1999). *Challenges Facing Higher Education at the Millennium*. American Council of Education. Oryx Press, Phoenix.

Meads, G., Ashcroft, J., Barr, H., Scott, R. & Wild, A. (2008). *The Case for Interprofessional Collaboration*. Wiley-Blackwell, Oxford.

Patrick, C., Peach, D., Pocknee, C., Webb, F., Fletcher, M. & Pretto, G. (2008). *The WIL Report. Work Integrated Learning. A National Scoping Study*. Australian Learning and Teaching Council (ALTC) Final Report. Queensland University of Technology, Brisbane <www.altc.edu.au and www.acen.edu.au>.

van Ginkel, H. (1999). 'Networks and Strategic Alliances within and between Universities and the Private Sector'. In W. Hirsch & L. Weber (eds), *Challenges Facing Higher Education at the Millennium*. American Council of Education. Oryx Press, Phoenix: 85–92.

CHAPTER 20
ETHICAL AND SUPPORTED DECISION-MAKING

Geneviève Pépin, Joanne Watson, Nick Hagiliassis and Helen Larkin

INTRODUCTION

Health professionals and other service providers have a legal and ethical responsibility 'to carry out their duties with sufficient care so that the service user does not suffer injury or loss as a consequence' (Baxter & Carr 2007: 7). This duty of care is informed through: professional codes of conduct; organisational policy and processes; state and federal statutes and standards; legal precedent; and national and international health and human rights charters. Much of the available literature (Ellis & Trede 2008; Villamanta Legal Service 1996) explores the interpretation of duty of care in everyday practice, and the need for health professionals to ensure that service users have the opportunity to exercise informed consent.

Implicit in the exercise of duty of care is that people understand the information and choices being presented, and the consequences that may arise from a particular intervention or approach. However, the obligation to exercise duty of care is further complicated when a person's competence is called into question; when health professionals are unsure as to the person's capacity to understand all of the issues and the potential consequences of either action or inaction.

This chapter does not address the processes and procedures surrounding the application of duty of care for people who would generally be regarded as competent decision-makers. Instead, it seeks to explore the application of these principles for people who are considered to be vulnerable decision-makers. *Vulnerable decision-makers* specifically refers to adults with disabilities, such as developmental disabilities, psychiatric disorders and psychosocial difficulties, or neurological deficit, for whom the characteristics associated with their condition can affect decision-making. These characteristics may include:

- difficulties understanding and communicating the available options and their advantages and disadvantages
- difficulties demonstrating judgment, reasoning and insight about certain choices
- presence of an interfering pathological perception, such as a delusional system, or interfering emotional state, such as severe depression or euphoria (adapted from Stebnicki 1997).

It is important for you to bear in mind that many people with disabilities are clearly and convincingly competent to make decisions. However, for some, particularly those with more severe or enduring disabilities, difficulties in making or communicating decisions can be present.

In such circumstances, health professionals often face dilemmas and uncertainty in relation to a person's health and wellbeing when attempting to reach agreement about his or her competence to make choices those health professionals may consider unwise or potentially dangerous. This uncertainty can result in negative and paternalistic practice 'in which assumptions are made by professionals about what is best for the service users in their care' (Baxter & Carr 2007: 7). This is often based on a fear of causing injury or other adverse event and the risk of consequent prosecution.

Baylies (2002: 736) recognised the need to develop tools that 'acknowledge the variability in the human condition and ensure, as far as possible, that all humans enjoy at least a basic level of functioning'. This chapter proposes tools that you can use to identify your role in decision-making processes and support vulnerable

REFLECTION 20.1

Duty of care
During your fieldwork placement, have you been involved with vulnerable clients or patients? What was your duty of care to the person? What decisions were made on their behalf? Was any consideration given to the person's preferences?

decision-makers so that the duty of care to protect the human rights and dignity of this group is not neglected.

SHOULD YOU BE INVOLVED OR NOT?

One of the most difficult but critical skills for anyone working in health and human services is creating clarity around roles and responsibilities. Do you have a *duty of care?* In which context do you have a professional duty of care? To whom do you have a duty of care? What is clearly within this duty and what falls outside of these obligations and responsibility? These questions start the exploration of the link between duty of care, *informed consent* and *risk* for those people who are considered to be vulnerable (McKenzie et al. 2001).

Charles Handy's *doughnut principle* (Handy 1994), although developed as a management tool, is also relevant for understanding the roles and responsibilities of those working in health and human services. Adapted by Michael Smull (1996) as a person-centred thinking tool, it can also be used by health professionals to determine their level of involvement when supporting someone with a disability through a decision-making process. The doughnut (Figure 20.1) has three concentric circles. The first, inner, circle is identified as core responsibilities. These are responsibilities that health professionals clearly have a duty of care to carry out, such as following applicable legislation, policies and procedures. The second, outer, circle refers to situations in which professionals have responsibility, but which require creativity and sound judgment; for example, assisting the person to try new things. Finally, the outer ring contains those aspects of a service user's life that are not the paid responsibility of health professionals, such as making moral decisions. This area is usually the domain of the person him- or herself in collaboration with those that know and love that person, such as family and friends.

Smull (1996) explains that the boundary between 'core responsibilities' and 'judgment and creativity' is usually well defined. In contrast, the boundary between 'creativity and judgment' and 'not paid responsibility' is more likely to be blurred. For example, prescribing a piece of equipment such as a wheelchair, which fits the person's needs, environmental factors and personal circumstances, could clearly be the duty of care of a health professional. However, it may not fall within his or her duty of care to oversee mobility in other areas of the person's life, such as a choice of leisure activities or travel plans.

The doughnut principle provides a useful framework for practitioners who are deliberating on their level of involvement around a decision, and conceptualising the difference between activities across these three zones.

Figure 20.1: The doughnut principle

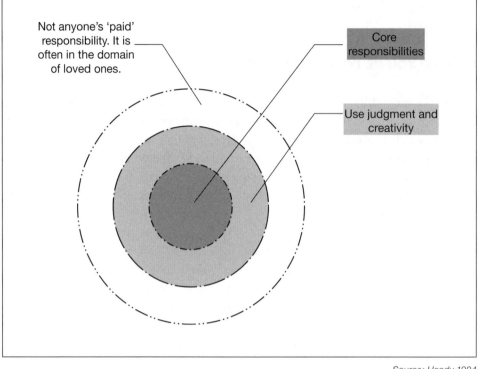

Not anyone's 'paid' responsibility. It is often in the domain of loved ones.

Core responsibilities

Use judgment and creativity

Source: Handy 1994

Risk or opportunity?

If the *doughnut principle* has helped you determine that you have some professional responsibility for the person in question, the next question to ask is: what is the level of risk involved? The *person-centred risk assessment* (Kinsella 2000), shown in Figure 20.2, has been developed to:

- explore the relationship between risk and the importance of an issue to the person
- problem solve around this relationship and identify strategies that balance safety within the context of the person's happiness.

Implicit in this approach is a strong collaboration between the person and the people who care for him or her, know that person well and have his or her best interests at heart.

Risk is multidimensional, and any risk assessment should reflect this. It is important to consider the consequences of the potential risk, not only on the person, but also on those supporting that person and on others within his or her community. In terms of the person taking the risk, it is important to consider the impact of the activity on the person's reputation and on how this person may be perceived. Just as important is consideration of whether there is any *risk of lost opportunities* for personal

Figure 20.2: The person-centred risk assessment

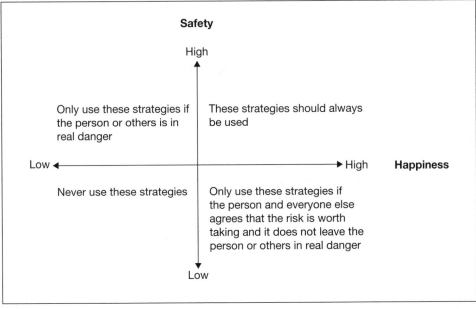

Source: Kinsella 2000

development if the person does not engage in the activity. Ask yourself if what you are assessing is a potential risk or a true opportunity.

As you move along the safety and happiness continuum of the *person-centred risk assessment*, you will be able to visualise and identify the impact of a specific scenario. What level of safety is involved in a specific scenario? How does it translate on the happiness continuum? Do the risks outweigh the happiness, or is it the contrary? Will the person's decision imply minimal risk and create a high level of happiness, or will it jeopardise his or her safety to the point of unacceptable risk to the person or others, where it 'may be necessary to intervene against the apparent wishes of clients in order to protect them from harm or unacceptable risk, particularly if their choice is not an informed one' (McKenzie et al. 2001: 29).

If you determine that you have a professional responsibility in relation to the person and there is an element of risk, the next question to ask is: is the person able to understand the consequences that may arise out of any action that he or she takes or is undertaken on his or her behalf? In this situation, discussion and intervention generally focus on an assessment of the person's competence to make a choice and to understand the consequences of these choices. The next section explores the concept of competence as it applies to vulnerable decision-makers.

COMPETENCE: A SNAPSHOT

Capacity and decision-making among certain vulnerable groups has seen much evolution. Historically, the approach adopted in this area has been somewhat paternalistic; that is, one in which decisions were made on behalf of people identified as vulnerable, underpinned by the attitude that people with disabilities do not possess the intellectual or personal capacity to contribute to decisions about their lives. This resulted in numerous injustices for people with disabilities, such as medical treatment and hospitalisation without consent, loss of control of finances and mass institutionalisation (Fennell 1996).

Over recent decades, there has been an emphasis on the rights of people with disabilities to make decisions for themselves, including those with severe and enduring disabilities. The right to make such decisions is enshrined in numerous pieces of legislation around the world (such as the *Adults with Incapacity Act* 2000, Scotland; the *Disability Act* 2006, Victoria, Australia; and the *Mental Capacity Act* 2005, England). Each of these is underpinned by principles of human rights and the right of self-determination of people with disabilities, recognising that a fulfilling life must include the right for people with disabilities to make choices and have control over their lives. These philosophical and legislative changes have seen a concurrent shift in the way health practitioners approach the issue of decision-making for people with disabilities. It is becoming increasingly recognised that duty of care includes the concepts of both minimising harm and facilitating individuals' rights and choices (O'Brien 1992, cited in McKenzie et al. 2001).

You therefore need to examine your attitudes, particularly with respect to the underlying belief that individuals with disabilities should not necessarily be protected, and that one's life can have an enhanced meaning through taking risks and making choices (Schalock 1997). You need to become more comfortable with the view that 'while the concept of duty of care exists for the protection of vulnerable clients it does not preclude risk-taking' (McKenzie et al. 2001: 30). This is not always easy, as it requires a recognition and objective interpretation of the belief systems and premises that underpin practice, but it is a critical element if one is to adopt a supported decision-making approach.

EVALUATING CAPACITY

Another major shift has been in the health professional's role in tests of *capacity*. Traditionally and currently, healthcare professionals are involved in assessing an individual's capacity to make a specific decision. This approach is often criticised on the grounds that it implies an all-or-nothing judgment; that is, one in which capacity is either all present, or all absent (Stebnicki 1997). Furthermore, it does not discriminate between the types of decisions, or the context or environment in which the decision would be implemented. As for everyone, capacity can fluctuate depending on the specific decision at hand, the specific moment in time and the environment and experiences of the individual who is making the decision. An all-or-nothing judgment does not capture these intricacies.

A finding of capacity is a legal decision made by the courts, or a legal mechanism of adult guardianship, as opposed to a 'medical decision' made by a health professional. However, health professionals are at times requested to provide opinions and formulations to inform decisions of capacity. The measurement of capacity is fraught with difficulties, as there is no single evaluation instrument or set of instruments to determine a person's capacity for decision-making, or even what such an instrument should comprise conceptually. For now, health professionals have access to functional assessment instruments (such as mental health and neuropsychological assessments, functional assessments and interview schedules) to evaluate factors that mediate a person's decision-making capacity. These tools are useful in informing decisions about a person's general decision-making status, but may be limited in assessing a person's capacity for decision-making in specific life areas (Iacono & Murray 2003). Information from these assessments should never be used in isolation, but rather alongside other systemic, interpersonal and contextual information. For the reason that capacity to make a choice is not simply dependent on a test score, functional assessments should inform, but not be the determinant of capacity for decision-making. Information about psychological assessment processes is summarised elsewhere (British Psychological Society 2006).

INFLUENCES ON COMPETENCE AND DECISION-MAKING

You have determined that you have a professional duty of care in relation to a specific person, and that there is a risk associated with a decision to be made. As a health professional and a member of a community of support for that person, you are interested in the factors that influence his or her own competence and decision-making. Therefore, one of your aims is to identify how and if a person has the ability to understand the issues and consequences related to a specific action or inaction. To do so, you need to explore the variety of characteristics associated with a range of health conditions, and the impact of these on individuals and on their capacity to make informed decisions.

The concept of capacity is complex, and emerges from the interplay of a range of factors. The International Classification of Functioning, Disability and Health (ICF) (see Figure 20.3) is a model developed by the World Health Organization (WHO), which addresses this complexity (WHO 2002). The ICF provides a framework to understand health and health-related issues, and uses a common language that transcends profession-specific terminology.

Figure 20.3: The International Classification of Functioning, Disability and Health

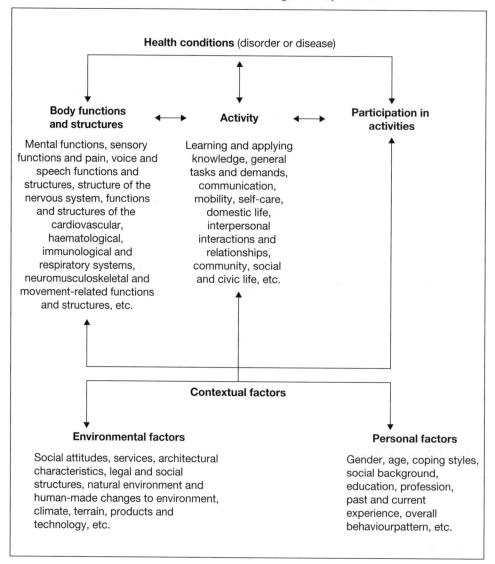

Source: WHO 2002

The ICF considers the notions of health and disability from a positive perspective; first by identifying different factors and influences related to the person's condition; and then, by looking closely at the interaction between these factors to explain a person's functioning. These factors pertain to body structure and body functions, activity and participation and contextual factors, including personal and environmental factors, that act either as facilitators or barriers to participation. Consider Case Study 20.1.

Case Study 20.1 | **Lillian**

Lillian is an 84-year-old woman with early-stage dementia, who has lived on her own since her husband died six years ago. She manages her personal self-care tasks independently, but in the last two years has received assistance from the local council with some domestic tasks. She attends church once a week, and does voluntary work at a local opportunity shop. Four weeks ago she fractured her hip, and is currently undergoing inpatient rehabilitation. She currently has acute confusion following surgery, and is disorientated in time and place; however, this is improving over time. Her adult children are anxious about her returning home, and are investigating residential care services, but Lillian is adamant that she wants to return home.

Question

What factors are influencing Lillian's competence and capacity to return home?

Using ICF terminology, Lillian's dementia, and hip fracture (*health conditions*) affect her memory, cognition and range of movement and pain experienced (*body functions and structures*). In turn, these have an impact on her ability to dress, shower and walk (*activities*) in the hospital setting, and will influence other activities into the foreseeable future. Her capacity to undertake her preferred recreational interests, manage her financial affairs and other necessary roles will affect her *participation*. The role of the healthcare team in assessing Lillian's capacity or competence to return home would need to include some deliberation in relation to the following factors:

- Lillian's competence, which will improve over time as her acute confusion and pain and range of movement (*body structure and function*) continues to improve
- rehabilitation, which will assist her to become more independent with her personal care tasks (*activities*)
- her capacity to undertake personal care and domestic tasks, best assessed in her own home (*environmental*)
- the attitude of her family to her return home (*environmental*)
- the home environment and need for modifications (*environmental*)
- the available community resources and supports (*environmental*)
- the available informal support networks (*environmental*)
- Lillian's determination to return home (*personal*)
- the organisational policy of the retirement village in relation to independence levels of residents (*environmental*).

By considering a variety of factors, the ICF provides a framework for the entire team, including the client, to understand the concept of competence of vulnerable decision-makers in different contexts. The ICF enables you to understand a person's unique circumstances, enablers and barriers in varied contexts. It helps identify appropriate interventions to eliminate or limit barriers, decrease risks and allow a person such as Lillian to make an informed and supported decision to maintain her participation in different meaningful activities. By exploring the various aspects of the environment, the ICF provides a context for the level of functioning and the decision-making process. It contributes to providing opportunities for actions and choices that would not otherwise be possible.

MODEL OF SUPPORTED DECISION-MAKING

This section presents a model developed by the second author, Joanne Watson, to promote choices and support decision-making with people who may be considered vulnerable decision-makers in some aspects of their daily life, as in Case Study 20.1. Although this model has been developed with the specific needs of people with significant disabilities in mind, its principles are applicable to all decision-makers, regardless of their vulnerability.

A *supported decision-making approach* has at its heart the principles that everyone is competent in making decisions, everyone communicates and we all seek support to make decisions from those we know and trust. The question that needs to be asked is not only about an individual's decision-making competence. Where there is uncertainty about a person's decision-making competence, our response must be based on the assumption that every human being is communicating, and that this communication will include preferences. With support, preferences can be built up into expressions of choice and into formal decisions. From this perspective, where someone 'lands' on a continuum of capacity is not half as important as the amount and type of support provided to build preferences into choices (Beamer 2001). Any supported decision-making process has as its foundation the need to truly listen to people in whatever mode they are using: words, objects, symbols, idiosyncratic body movements or other behaviours.

You need to listen to people not only in terms of what they *perceive* as important for them, but also what *is* important to them. There is a fine line between these two concepts, and it is a fundamental component of human service delivery. '*Important to*' is about what really matters to the person, while '*important for*' is about the health and support he or she needs to stay safe and well. Achieving balance between the two concepts is a challenge for many health practitioners. Unfortunately, for many vulnerable decision-makers it often comes down to *important for* them, the outcome being an imbalance between security issues and what makes life fulfilling.

The *supported decision-making model* (Watson 2009), illustrated in Figure 20.4, strives to provide a framework for truly reaching the heart of people's desires,

Figure 20.4: The supported decision-making model

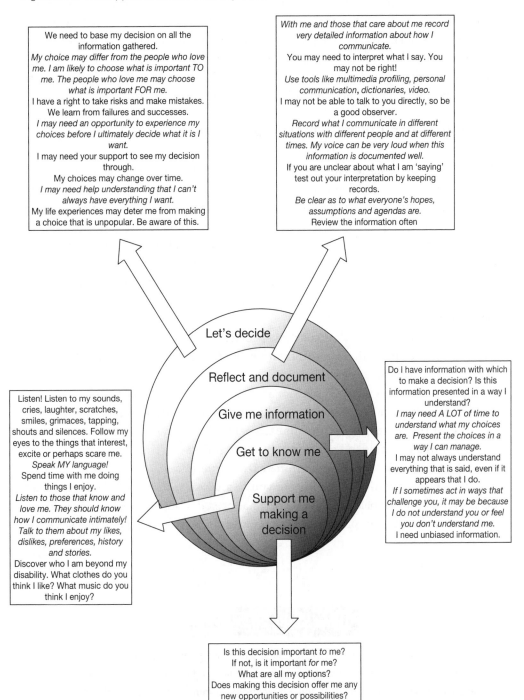

We need to base my decision on all the information gathered.
My choice may differ from the people who love me. I am likely to choose what is important TO me. The people who love me may choose what is important FOR me.
I have a right to take risks and make mistakes. We learn from failures and successes.
I may need an opportunity to experience my choices before I ultimately decide what it is I want.
I may need your support to see my decision through.
My choices may change over time.
I may need help understanding that I can't always have everything I want.
My life experiences may deter me from making a choice that is unpopular. Be aware of this.

With me and those that care about me record very detailed information about how I communicate.
You may need to interpret what I say. You may not be right!
Use tools like multimedia profiling, personal communication, dictionaries, video.
I may not be able to talk to you directly, so be a good observer.
Record what I communicate in different situations with different people and at different times. My voice can be very loud when this information is documented well.
If you are unclear about what I am 'saying' test out your interpretation by keeping records.
Be clear as to what everyone's hopes, assumptions and agendas are.
Review the information often

Listen! Listen to my sounds, cries, laughter, scratches, smiles, grimaces, tapping, shouts and silences. Follow my eyes to the things that interest, excite or perhaps scare me.
Speak MY language!
Spend time with me doing things I enjoy.
Listen to those that know and love me. They should know how I communicate intimately! Talk to them about my likes, dislikes, preferences, history and stories.
Discover who I am beyond my disability. What clothes do you think I like? What music do you think I enjoy?

Do I have information with which to make a decision? Is this information presented in a way I understand?
I may need A LOT of time to understand what my choices are. Present the choices in a way I can manage.
I may not always understand everything that is said, even if it appears that I do.
If I sometimes act in ways that challenge you, it may be because I do not understand you or feel you don't understand me.
I need unbiased information.

Let's decide

Reflect and document

Give me information

Get to know me

Support me making a decision

Is this decision important *to* me?
If not, is it important *for* me?
What are all my options?
Does making this decision offer me any new opportunities or possibilities?

Source: Watson 2009

preferences and dreams. It recognises a person's capacity to make a decision in a given context by including and considering contextual factors, as put forward by the ICF. It should be used in supporting vulnerable decision-makers to make choices and decisions. Supported decision-making should be a fluid, not a prescriptive process. It is a complex and multifaceted process. This model aims to provide health practitioners with guidelines and to inform decision-making processes.

A PATHWAY FOR GUIDING PRACTICE

This section presents a pathway that can be used to guide collaborative team thinking when in a situation where questions of professional duty of care, risks and competence may have an impact on decisions to be made about, with or for a person (see Figure 20.5). This pathway summarises, in diagrammatic form, the information contained in the previous sections of this chapter, and is designed to help you navigate through the decision-making processes. It highlights important questions that should be asked along the way, and provides strategies for implementation.

Case studies

This section presents the stories of three people. When you read Doug's, Sarah's and Sam's stories, keep in mind the information, strategies and tools presented earlier in this chapter. For each scenario:

- ask yourself if you have a professional duty of care in the context described
- reflect on the notion of risk potentially involved in the different scenarios
- consider the contextual factors for each person, and how they can enable or be a barrier to facilitating individual's rights and choices
- identify strategies to limit or eliminate the barriers.

These broad questions will prepare you to analyse each story from a supported decision-making perspective. A worksheet has been developed especially to help you apply the different concepts related to supported decision-making to Doug's, Sarah's and Sam's stories.

Case Study 20.2 | Doug

Doug is a 28-year-old man who experienced a head injury at 21 years of age. He uses speech to communicate, but sometimes this is difficult for others to understand, so he augments this using a text-to-speech electronic communication aid. His cognitive abilities have not been formally assessed, but it is estimated he has a mild learning disability. He is also observed to have limited literacy skills. At times he is impulsive in

---

Figure 20.5: The decision-making pathway

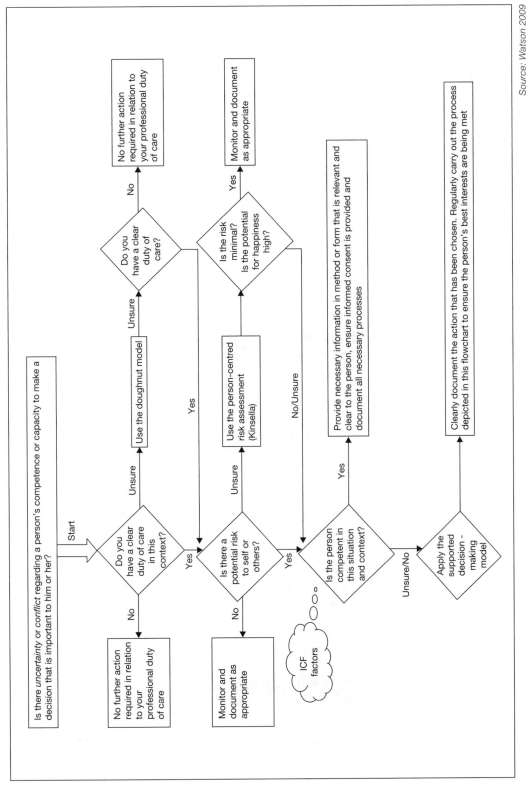

Source: Watson 2009

his actions, while he has been observed to be emotionally labile and easily agitated. He lives in supported accommodation. Through an informal arrangement, support staff assist him with most financial affairs, but he also has independent access to his money.

Recently, support staff have become concerned about frequent withdrawals from his bank account. When asked, he openly explained that he was using this money for gambling purposes, and that this was an activity that he enjoyed. He became agitated when it was suggested he should cease spending his money in this way. Further, he revealed that he was accessing these funds through ATM withdrawals at his local gaming venue, but was asking other patrons to perform these transactions on his behalf. Staff are concerned that his understanding of money is limited, and that he does not understand the financial implications of his actions. They are also concerned that, through having others withdraw money on his behalf, he may be placing himself in an unacceptably vulnerable position.

Case Study 20.3 Sarah

Sarah is 19 years old. She was diagnosed with anorexia nervosa when she was 16. Since then, she has been in and out of hospital several times. Sarah has said repeatedly that she does not have a problem, but while she was under age, her parents managed to get her to see different specialists. Sarah's parents are still very concerned about her health and wellbeing but now that she is an adult they feel there is little they can do but hope that she will realise she needs help. Recently, Sarah was hospitalised after fainting whilst waiting for the bus. At the hospital, Sarah was rapidly diagnosed with severe anorexia nervosa, and was transferred to the eating disorders unit in the psychiatric ward. Sarah refuses any type of intervention and wants to leave the hospital. The multidisciplinary team wants to start legal proceedings to demonstrate that she cannot make informed decisions about her medical treatment, and needs to stay in the hospital, even if it means staying as an involuntary patient. Sarah has decided to discharge herself despite her condition.

Case Study 20.4 Sam

Sam is a 64-year-old man with cerebral palsy. He has an intellectual disability and difficulties eating and drinking. Some of the people who know and love him, including his sister Beth, have indicated that one of Sam's greatest pleasures in life is drinking cool, fizzy lemonade. When the lemonade enters Sam's mouth he hums loudly, and rapidly moves his tongue in and out of his mouth. He also giggles when small quantities of lemonade are placed on his tongue. Although Sam receives most of his nutrition via a gastrostomy tube, Beth offers him a drink of lemonade each morning. Beth is a registered nurse with many years of experience in geriatrics, and she has also been appointed as Sam's legal guardian. The speech pathologist supporting Sam believes that thin fluids are dangerous as his swallowing difficulties are such that the fluid is highly likely to be aspirated into his lungs. Sam is currently living with Beth, and receives personal support and therapy services from a local disability agency. Sam is often hospitalised as a result of pneumonia, which is believed to be caused by the aspiration of food and drink. After these hospitalisations he usually receives services from district nursing for several weeks.

QUESTIONS

With reference to the *decision-making pathway* (Figure 20.5), work through the questions below. Complete one of these worksheets for each case study.
1 For Case Study 20.2/20.3/20.4 (circle the appropriate one), write briefly the issues contained in the case study where you think there is uncertainty or conflict about the person's decision-making capacity.
2 How many issues were you able to describe? _____
3 Using the *doughnut model*, locate each of the issues on the chart below.

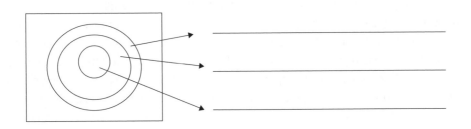

Do you have a clear duty of care in the context described in any of the issues listed above? Yes/No
4 If you answered Yes, locate these issue(s) on the *person-centred risk assessment (reference) grid* (Figure 20.2, page 267).

5 Using the ICF (Figure 20.3, page 270), describe the factors and the contextual barriers and facilitators that are influencing the person's decision-making capacity in this situation or context.

6 Using the *supported decision-making model,* describe the actions that you or the team could take to ensure that the person's best interests are being met.

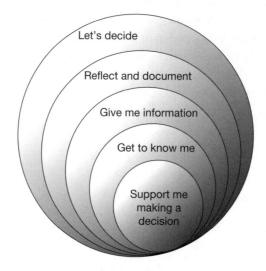

SUMMARY

In the case of vulnerable decision-makers, the role of the health professional is to share in the decision-making process with other people in the person's community of support, rather than to take on the role of substitute decision-maker. Such a community of support, composed of health professionals and others, collaboratively contributes opinions about enablers and barriers to a person's decision-making capacity and strategies for addressing these. Having a number of people involved offers a safeguard against any individual who might try to exert undue influence. The composition of a community of support should be led by the individual at the centre of the decision. This implies there will also be occasions when there is no role for a specific practitioner, either because his or her expertise is not relevant in that case, or because the individual has made a decision to that effect. This does not prohibit this health professional from challenging the decision made by the community of support if he or she feels that the decision of the group is not in the person's best interest. This chapter has outlined a process for you and others who support people who are considered to be vulnerable decision-makers or where a question arises in relation to a person's competence to make choices and decisions in everyday life. The tools described within this chapter are offered as one way forward by which health care professionals can bring together what may be differing professional and personal perspectives and life experiences to bring about solutions that are more rigorous, inclusive and respectful of every person's right to participate to their maximum potential in his or her chosen lifestyles and communities.

DISCUSSION QUESTIONS

1   Think about a time in your life where you felt you were taking a risk. How did you make your own decision? Who did you talk to? Who did you consult? What support did you get? What did you get out of this experience?

2   Reflect on your own attitude and belief system, and the impact these can have on the people to whom you provide service. Which attitudes and beliefs restrict the implementation of supported decision-making? Which attitudes and beliefs facilitate the implementation of supported decision-making?

3   Reflect on a past or current situation where you thought you had a duty of care. What are your thoughts on this situation now? What could or would you do differently?

References

Baxter, S. & Carr, H. (2007). 'Walking the Tightrope: The Balance Between Duty of Care, Human Rights and Capacity'. *Housing, Care and Support*, 10(3): 6–11.

Baylies, C. (2002). 'Disability and the Notion of Human Development: Questions of Rights and Capabilities'. *Disability and Society*, 17(7): 725–9.

Beamer, S. (2001). *Making Decisions. Best Practice and New Ideas for Supporting People with High Support Needs to Make Decisions*. Values Into Action, London.

British Psychological Society (2006). *Assessment of Capacity in Adults: Interim Guidance for Psychologists*. British Psychological Society, London.

Ellis, E. & Trede, F. (2008). 'Communication and Duty of Care'. In J. Higgs, R. Ajjawi, L. McAllister, F. Trede & S. Loftus. *Communicating in the Health Sciences* (2nd edn). Oxford University Press, Melbourne.

Fennell, P. (1996). *Treatment without Consent: Law, Psychiatry and the Treatment of Mentally Disordered People since 1845*. Routledge, London.

Handy, C. (1994). *The Age of Paradox*. Harvard Business School Press, Boston.

Iacono, T. & Murray, V. (2003). 'Issues of Informed Consent in Conducting Medical Research Involving People with Intellectual Disability'. *Journal of Applied Research in Intellectual Disabilities*, 16: 41–51.

Kinsella, P. (2000). *Person Centered Risk Assessment*. Paradigm, Liverpool.

McKenzie, K., Matheson, E., Paxton, D., Murray, G. C. & McKaskie, K. (2001). 'Health and Social Care Worker's Knowledge and Application of the Concept of Duty of Care'. *Journal of Adult Protection*, 3(4): 29–37.

Schalock, R. L. (1997). 'The Conceptualization and Measurement of Quality of Life: Current Status and Future Considerations'. *Journal of Developmental Disabilities*, 5: 1–21.

Smull, M. (1996). *Helping Staff Support Choice*. Support Development Associates, Kensington.

Stebnicki, M. A. (1997). 'A Conceptual Framework for Utilizing a Functional Assessment Approach for Determining Mental Capacity: A New Look at Informed Consent in Rehabilitation'. *Journal of Rehabilitation*, 63: 32–6.

Villamanta Legal Service (1996). *Duty of Care: Who's Responsible? A Guide for Carers Supporting People with Disabilities*. Villamanta Publishing Service, Geelong West.

World Health Organization (2002). *Towards a Common Language for Functioning, Disability and Health: ICF The International Classification of Functioning, Disability and Health*. World Health Organization, Geneva.

CHAPTER 21
THE THREE Rs: ROLES, RIGHTS AND RESPONSIBILITIES

Linda Wilson

LEARNING OUTCOMES

After reading this chapter you should be able to:
- identify key fieldwork stakeholders in successful industry placements
- understand a general overview of key fieldwork stakeholder roles, rights and associated responsibilities (three Rs)
- discuss the shifting boundaries between university, student and fieldwork placement agency, depending on the context.

KEY TERMS

Fieldwork
Fieldwork placement agency
Stakeholder
Three Rs (roles, rights, responsibilities)
Work-integrated learning environment

INTRODUCTION

This chapter aims to introduce you to the notion of the *three Rs (roles, rights and responsibilities)* for each stakeholder within a work-integrated learning experience. This information clarifies the three Rs, which may in turn assist in the successful completion of your placement. If needed, it may assist you with the wherewithal to address any inequities or other problems that might arise, allowing you to complete a course fieldwork requirement within an industry placement.

A very important and exciting phenomenon throughout universities is the increasing emphasis on fieldwork placement as a core component of entry-level courses. This increases the need for all stakeholders to understand the specific fieldwork placement requirements. For example, in some faculties, there are course rules stating that a fieldwork failure can be a reason to exclude a student from the course. This highlights how fieldwork, in some courses, can be treated differently from other core units (you may have the option of failing another core unit twice before you can be excluded). While not trying to scare you, this is why you need to have a greater understanding of the three Rs (roles, rights and responsibilities) as they pertain to fieldwork. Without this knowledge, a situation could arise where you are disadvantaged.

In the health and behavioural sciences disciplines there are considerable variations in fieldwork placement form and format. For example, fieldwork:

- can occur at different levels of courses; for example, expectations for fieldwork placement at first year are very different from those required in a final year placement
- occurs in a variety of settings that have differing expectations
- has specific requirements imposed by some professions; for instance, dictating which health professionals can supervise a student while on placement.

Many of these elements are profession specific, and lead into the university requirements for the fieldwork placement. Hence the approach in this chapter is a generic one, and you as a student should ensure that you have information specific to your course and discipline area.

KEY STAKEHOLDERS

There are *three key stakeholders* in the fieldwork process. They are the *student*, the *university* (represented by the fieldwork organiser or academic supervisor) and the *placement agency* (represented by the fieldwork educator or supervisor).

Broadly, the university is the placement instigator and has the major component of the organisational role and responsibilities. Students in some settings may contribute to the identification of fieldwork placement agencies, but primarily their role and responsibilities centre on engaging actively in learning, while the agency is the learning environment facilitator.

Even though a successful fieldwork is a partnership, each stakeholder has his or her own areas of interest, which at times can be in conflict with the interests of other stakeholders and the work-integrated learning objectives.

Table 21.1 provides examples of *stakeholder interests* as either *primary* or *secondary*. The interests under each heading (primary and secondary) are not prioritised, as these will vary between individuals and groups. A primary interest for the fieldwork placement agency is its core business; for the university its prime interest is placement organisation and students successfully completing placement. For most students the bottom line is passing. Some may scoff at this, and profess altruistic values, which is fine, but the reality is that a fieldwork placement experience can at one end be a successful learning partnership and at the other a massive conflict. Understanding what is important to other stakeholders aids clarity, and is a step to establishing a respectful working partnership. So it is best to be clear from the start what the bottom line is for all stakeholders.

THINK AND LINK 21.1

In Chapter 19, stakeholders are considered from a professional, government, university, health and human services and student perspective. This chapter and Chapter 19 reveal the complexity of practice that occurs when fieldwork placements are involved.

REFLECTION 21.1

A minute for priorities

As a student, it might be useful to take a minute to think about what are your priorities regarding your next fieldwork placement.

1 Identify what is the most important issue (bottom line) for you regarding your fieldwork.
2 What are your secondary interests concerning your fieldwork placement? i.e. 'It would be nice if ...'

Table 21.1: Examples of stakeholders' interests

Interest examples	Stakeholders		
	Student	**University**	**Placement agency**
Primary	• Passing the fieldwork	• Successful organisation • Academic rigour	• Service provision (core business) • Staff and service users
Secondary	• Positive learning experience	• Outcomes of the placement that are of benefit to the agency	• Student's learning experience

ROLES, RIGHTS AND RESPONSIBILITIES

As we clarify the key stakeholders' defined roles, embedded in each discussion are the rights and responsibilities of each stakeholder. The fieldwork placement relationship between each stakeholder is based on the recognition of mutual rights and responsibilities. This also includes the responsibilities to other parties outside the immediate fieldwork placement partnership.

The specifics of each stakeholder's responsibilities to other parties will vary depending on the initial situation. The following are some examples:

• students may have work or family responsibilities
• the university will have responsibilities to others; for instance, external professional registration bodies as well as other students. The university also has

responsibilities to the rest of the university, ensuring academic rigour and the university's reputation

- the fieldwork placement agency's responsibilities are related to its core business; for instance, service users and staff members. Agencies need to take several steps (for example, police checks) to protect their staff and service users. Agency responsibilities to clients also raise important issues for students regarding confidentiality and privacy.

The key agency person (fieldwork educator) regarding the fieldwork placement is the one who takes on the direct supervision of the student. The fieldwork educator in each agency may also be the key contact person for you and university staff. Universities rely heavily on the fieldwork educators, and value their contribution to your education. Ensuring that you have a good learning experience is a partnership between the agency, you and the university. All of these and many other elements contribute to a complex relationship within a fieldwork placement.

Table 21.2 has a summary of the three Rs and the three stakeholders.

Table 21.2: Outline of stakeholder three Rs

Three Rs	Stakeholders		
	University	**Agency**	**Student**
Role	• Placement parameter identifier and organiser	• Facilitator of student learning	• Active learner
Responsibility	• Ensure an appropriate agency is organised • Ensure academic rigour • Provide clear information regarding placement parameters • Ensure safety of students	• Orientate and induct student to agency • Provide learning opportunities • Provide feedback to the student and university regarding student performance	Students need to: • inform themselves of the placement parameters and the agency requirements • self-manage their own learning while on fieldwork placement • use initiative in learning • seek and utilise feedback on placement performance

Table 21.2: Outline of stakeholder three Rs (cont.)

Three Rs	Stakeholders		
	University	**Agency**	**Student**
Responsibility (*continued*)			• treat the fieldwork placement as if it were employment • observe university statutes, regulations and policies, and behave accordingly as a representative of the university
Rights		• to protect core business	• to ensure an appropriate, stimulating learning experience

Role of the university through its representatives

The role of the university can often be broken into several elements. They include:

- *identification of work-integrated learning parameters* including:
  - fieldwork objectives
  - requirements (hours)
  - set and mark assessment and evaluation requirements.
- *organisation of fieldwork*: for example, identifying appropriate agencies and liaising with them and the student, as well as initiating necessary screening processes
- *delivering administration requirements*: for example, ensuring course and university requirements
- *monitoring and supporting*: after having placed the student, the university's responsibilities continue through monitoring student progress and development, with a view to offering guidance or advice to assist the student and fieldwork educator in professional development.

PARAMETERS

Fieldwork parameters are what the placement must function within. They can take two forms: those imposed by the university and those originating from the field.

University parameters

Before a fieldwork placement even begins, university fieldwork parameters (such as the hours; objectives and assessment requirements; and whether it is a core course requirement) have gone through many stages in an approval process inside (*accreditation processes*) and outside (*external registration bodies*) the university. These processes contribute to ensuring the academic substance of work-integrated learning.

The aims and objectives will vary between fieldwork placements, with some being observational only, and others involving considerable interaction on your part. It is essential that all parties, particularly you, are very clear about what the fieldwork placement aims are. For example, if you are purely observing, and the placement agency expects you to be interactive and contribute to the environment, this could be the source of considerable angst.

After parameter development, the university is then responsible for the communication (to other stakeholders) and the meeting of these parameters.

Field-based parameters

Many fieldwork placements in the health and behavioural science field will provide services to individuals who are considered vulnerable clients (refer to the Part 3 checklist for a list of service users identified as vulnerable). In order to ensure client safety, a pre-placement police check (criminal history) of students is required: the relevant police department prepares an official historical report that covers all criminal information specific to an individual. The report is an official document that has several issues associated with it.

- In some organisations, the criminal history report requirement is policy based, and in others it is enshrined in legislation. An example of a policy-based requirement is the Department of Health in Victoria, which has incorporated its requirements in policy guidelines. A legislative example is the introduction of the *Working with Children (WWC) Act* 2005, which from 1 July 2006 requires all who volunteer or anyone who works with children to undergo a mandatory screening process. Funded organisations have the responsibility to ensure that employees or volunteers get a *Working with Children Check (WWCC)*, if required. For more information on the WWCC or the WWC Act 2005, visit the Department of Justice website at: <http://www.justice.vic.gov.au/workingwithchildren>.

- The upshot of the legislative or policy requirement is that agencies (particularly government-funded) *will not* allow students into the agency until they have seen the criminal history report. This creates the situation where all students enrolled in most health courses are required to have a police check if undertaking fieldwork placements. If you have any concerns regarding your criminal history, you are strongly advised to discuss these with the university at the earliest opportunity.

- There are two types of police checks, national and state. The process of gaining a police record check is state specific. If students are required to have a check from overseas, try the Australian Federal Police website: <http://www.afp.gov. au/business/national_police_checks.html#crim>. The university will usually have processes in place to facilitate applications for a 'police check', and will have information for students regarding how to go about this.

In relation to a criminal history report, the police department has very strict guidelines concerning the release of criminal history information to individuals and organisations outside the particular police departments.

The general requirements for a police check are as follows:

- a specific form available from the relevant police website (state-specific or federal)
- unless otherwise arranged, costs are met by the applicant (you); to access the student rate for the report you must have a personalised form that the university signs
- a new report is required every 12 months. This may mean that for a student enrolled in a three-year undergraduate course that has fieldwork each year, you may need to apply for three reports.

It is inappropriate for universities to be making final judgments about the appropriateness of students' criminal histories for a particular agency. While the student is on placement, the agency has the responsibility for the student, as well as its core business. As such, the agency will need to make the final decision regarding the appropriateness of the report content for the agency.

Another issue surrounding the criminal history report is its *ownership*. To *own a report*, students should have the report sent to them personally, because if the report is sent to the university, it is not allowed to give the student or anyone else a copy. The university should know what is in the report and sight it, but the agency will make the final decision.

In the event that an agency deems the report inappropriate, universities may attempt to find an alternative fieldwork placement. But there are many difficulties with this, as most funded agencies require an appropriate police check.

THINK AND LINK 21.2

Having a criminal history can make undertaking fieldwork placement extremely difficult. Other legal issues are discussed in Chapter 22.

Assessment and evaluation

Assessment and evaluation requirements are the critical endpoint for both the student and the university. From a student's perspective, this is often the most important information. The university needs to ensure the dissemination to all stakeholders of clear information before the placement. Aside from the actual tasks that must be done while on fieldwork placement, other issues need clarification before placement.

These issues include:

- Who does the responsibility for the final grade rest with? Is it the university or the agency?
- What are the assessment tasks, and what is the placement performance evaluation?
- In making judgments, does the university seek the advice of fieldwork educators who have close contact with students during the fieldwork experience, or is the evaluation based on observations?
- What is the process for dealing with the final assessment?

The importance of the assessment and fieldwork placement evaluation for students necessitates that considerable time is spent clarifying these issues, which is primarily a university responsibility.

THINK AND LINK 21.3

If you are interested in passing your fieldwork placement, you need to know the type of assessment used to evaluate whether you are successful or not. Chapter 14 is dedicated to assessment issues on fieldwork placement. Refer to this chapter if you want more information on assessment during fieldwork.

PLACEMENT ORGANISATION—PARTNERSHIP DEVELOPMENT

There are many organisational elements for which the university has total responsibility, including the identification of appropriate agencies, and preparing students and the agency for fieldwork placement. The responsibility for the organisation of the fieldwork placement and setting the tone regarding how the fieldwork placement proceeds rests with the university. Some placements may require student input into their organisation; for example, if a student is undertaking the fieldwork placement as a distance unit.

A successful fieldwork is an outcome of a partnership between the key stakeholders. The characteristics of a partnership include:

- mutual cooperation
- clear responsibility
- the achievement of a specified outcome.

Mutual cooperation is an essential element of many aspects surrounding fieldwork. For example, when organising a placement agency a university is bound by what is an appropriate and available venue. Sometimes this may conflict with a proximity issue for students. The solution is mutual cooperation.

Each stakeholder brings its individual perspectives on the issues, but in order for a placement to be successful the starting point must be common information between the stakeholders.

REFLECTION 21.2

Do I have to travel?
When you receive information about your placement from the university, have there been times when the placement meant you had to travel? Did you try to negotiate a different placement closer to home? If there were no suitable placements closer to home, what did you do? Was compromise a part of the solution?

Common information

Common information includes anything pertaining to the placement that, if disseminated, fosters transparency and accountability. This sharing of information needs to be orchestrated by the university. As outlined in Figure 21.1, an absolute necessity regarding a successful fieldwork placement is that fieldwork information is common to all stakeholders.

Each stakeholder contributes to the common information, which includes but is not exclusive to:

- the student:
  - any information that could impede placement completion; for example, a back injury
- the university:
  - general aim of the course
  - course structure information
  - how the fieldwork placement relates to the rest of the course
  - aim of the fieldwork placement: is it observational or participatory?
  - fieldwork organisation process
  - fieldwork assessment and evaluation requirements
- the fieldwork placement agency:
  - agency constraints
  - agency values
  - core business
  - organisation protocols for the placement.

The sharing of information should be done in an accessible manner that can be referred to as the need arises; for example, the university-prepared information should be provided to the agency and students, either in a hard copy in the form of a manual or contract, or from web sites with the appropriate information.

The dissemination of information to all stakeholders enables a clear starting point and eliminates surprises. It also creates an awareness of the other stakeholders' needs with a view to ensuring a successful placement for all stakeholders.

Figure 21.1: Integration of stakeholders into a common direction

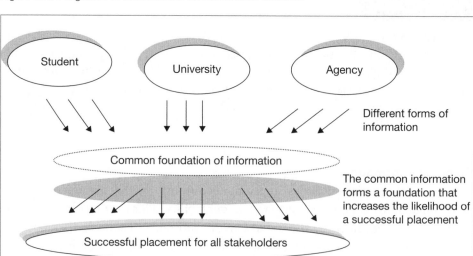

| Case Study 21.1 | What information is missing in this situation? |

The situation

A week into a full-time six-week fieldwork, a fieldwork placement agency has called the university wanting to discontinue a placement because Maree, a first year student, is not meeting agency expectations. Maree is not initiating any actions, and cannot undertake the tasks the agency needs her to do. The university rings Maree to organise a meeting. Maree is very distressed, and bursts into tears, saying that no one has explained anything (the toilet wasn't found till the second day), and it is not clear what tasks should be done and how. The language used is foreign and everyone in the agency is cliquey, and she does not know who to get information from.

Questions

What information from each stakeholder is missing in this situation?

1   The university
2   The fieldwork placement agency
3   The student.

Insurance

The university has an occupational health and safety responsibility to students regarding their safety and welfare. Most universities have insurance that covers public liability and professional indemnity, as well as personal accident insurance cover, for students not covered by WorkCover. Universities often have this information available on their websites. The policy usually provides insurance cover for compensation to a third party in respect of physical injury and/or property damage caused by a student. This includes the student as well as others. The university should provide the student and agency with a certificate of currency, as well as explain the process for putting in a claim.

Confidentiality and privacy

Because of the nature of service provision and the collection and storage of intimate information in the health and behavioural science field, confidentiality and privacy are major considerations.

As with other aspects of fieldwork placement, each stakeholder has specific responsibilities. The university has a responsibility to develop in students an awareness of the issues surrounding confidentiality and privacy. The agency has a responsibility to inform students of its policies. You have a responsibility to ensure you are informed about and adhere to agency policies.

In general terms, someone who is bound by the rules of confidentiality must not pass onto anyone else information concerning individuals, unless:

- the individual consents or agrees; or
- it's the only way a job can be completed properly. For example, a health worker can pass on information about individuals without getting permission first, if it's necessary to ensure that an individual receiving services (patient, client, service user) will get access to the best treatment needed; or the law says there is an exception to the general rule. The exceptions usually permit the release of confidential information without an individual's consent if it is in the public interest.

Students and the university need to take all reasonable and necessary steps to maintain confidentiality, and protect and advance the reputation of the agency and its clients.

THINK AND LINK 21.4

Confidentiality is an important issue when working in health and human services. Chapter 22 has further information on confidentiality from a legal perspective.

Non/payment of students

Before fieldwork placement finalisation, the issue of payment to you for tasks performed by you during hours on fieldwork placement needs to be clarified. Where you and the agency enter into agreement for you to be employed on a casual or part-time basis, such agreement must operate outside the student fieldwork placement, and should not operate to the detriment of your or the agency's performance of the fieldwork placement. You do not get paid for undertaking fieldwork.

Placement costs

Sometimes within agencies there are established protocols regarding such things as parking, meals and refreshments. The university needs to clarify meeting these costs before fieldwork placement commences. It is usual that you will either pay the going rate or make other arrangements for yourself. Universities are not usually liable for these types of costs.

General control and discipline

Students and staff of a university, although within a fieldwork placement, are bound by the rules, regulations, protocols, procedures and by-laws of the agency. Discipline and control of students and staff of a university is a university responsibility. The person in charge of the agency or department is entitled to issue instructions to university students and staff on matters affecting client–patient–service user care, and such instructions should be complied with fully and promptly. Students are also bound by university rules regarding their behaviour while on fieldwork placement, and should ensure that they are aware of what is expected of them while on placement.

REFLECTION 21.3

Another file!
As a student in your final year placement, you have been placed in a small understaffed community organisation. The first 20 hours of the placement have been spent filing and photocopying. What do you do?

Role and responsibilities of the placement agency as represented by the fieldwork educator

The agency and fieldwork educator play a vital role in your fieldwork placement and professional preparation as they provide you with relevant field-based practical guidance, stimulation, encouragement and advice, as well as constructive criticism.

There are many issues surrounding placement organisation and associated individual responsibilities that need to be clear at the onset. For example, you need to have the name of the contact person for all correspondence from the university, and whether it is the fieldwork educator's responsibility to complete the relevant assessment and evaluation requirements. Contact processes with the university need to be established in case there are any concerns about your progress or competence.

Areas in which the fieldwork educator can assist the student are:

- creating an environment where the student feels at ease and is a participant rather than observer
- treating the student as a professional colleague
- orientating the student to the organisation (for example, explaining the day-to-day issues, such as parking), and inducting the student to the agency through providing information on procedures and discussing agency philosophy, policies and occupational health and safety issues
- discussing student expectations, and any written university requirements for the student during the placement
- demonstrating various instructional techniques and discussing methods and materials relevant to particular service users
- providing opportunities for the student to observe and become familiar with as many aspects of the agency as possible
- providing the student with continuous comprehensive and constructive performance critiques, identifying specific strengths, weaknesses and strategies for improving the student's competence
- providing continuing liaison and consultation with the university coordinator of student placements
- discussing agency expectations
- completing the relevant evaluations and assessments of the student in conjunction with the student.

Role of the student

The role of the student while undertaking a fieldwork placement is that of an active learner. The agency is responsible for facilitating the learning and the university, for its organisation. You are responsible for your own learning.

While undertaking a fieldwork placement, you are accepted by courtesy of the agency and staff, and are expected to conduct yourself in a professional manner, accepting responsibility in your role as student. The activities undertaken while on fieldwork placement will vary depending on the type of agency and the placement parameters. An important point for you to note is that many fieldwork placements are organised without payment to the agency.

Even though your role is unpaid, it is preparation for future workplaces, therefore associated workplace behaviour is expected from you. Including the following:

- Punctual and regular attendance at the placement venue.
- If you are absent during the fieldwork placement, it is expected that you will notify the agency as early as possible and negotiate with their fieldwork educator how this lost time will be made up. If the agency does not know when you are coming, it makes it difficult to plan, which could have a negative impact on the opportunities afforded to you. You will also need to identify a communication

strategy with the agency; for example, an exchange of contact details between you and the agency's fieldwork educator.

- It is also your responsibility to notify the fieldwork educator of any circumstances likely to pose a risk to either you or any of the agency's clients or staff; for instance, the presence of any infection or an inability to perform a certain task, such as lifting.
- Identification of appropriate attire should be done pre-placement. Individual requirements vary according to the agency, the task and settings. A dress code would be based on industry standards; for example, if you are working with children, then appropriate attire might be neat casual, yet if you were working in the head office of an organisation, business attire would be more appropriate. In some environments there may be certain safety concerns requiring specific attire. Some settings require students to wear uniforms. You should identify the dress requirements before commencing the fieldwork placement.
- While on fieldwork placement you are expected to locate and familiarise yourself with local policies and procedures relevant to your role within the agency.
- You must negotiate with the fieldwork educator, client or client advocate acceptable access to confidential client records in order to complete placement tasks. You are to maintain confidentiality at all times.
- You are to communicate with staff and/or the fieldwork educator any incidents or issues that may be significant to the wellbeing of clients, patients or service users.
- Injury on fieldwork placement or an accident must be reported to the immediate fieldwork educators, and appropriate action taken within the organisation. You are also expected to notify the university as soon as possible, and lodge a report with the university.
- You should communicate with the university regarding any issues that may be significant regarding the fieldwork placement.
- During the placement, you are expected to initiate discussions regarding your placement performance with the fieldwork educator, identifying strengths and areas to focus on for improvement. This can be done in a formalised review at specified times or in an ad hoc manner. Often a good fieldwork educator will initiate these conversations, but it is your responsibility to obtain feedback.
- It is also your responsibility to ensure you and the fieldwork educator complete the required evaluation and assessment requirements.

Before undertaking fieldwork placements, you will need discipline-specific information, but there are some general issues that are relevant across professions. Aside from the course-related information, other areas of information and skill development you need include:

- processes to clarify personal values: there are often situations that will challenge your values
- clarification of what you are responsible for and to whom you are accountable

- time management
- professional issues, including:
  - duty of care
  - occupational health and safety: self
  - occupational health and safety: others
  - occupational health and safety: environment; for example:
    - infection control
    - lifting
    - emergency situations
- communication issues: written or verbal communication with:
  - professionals and other team members
  - service users, patients and clients
  - the university
- privacy and confidentiality: your responsibility is to ensure you are informed about the issues and adhere to the policies; further information regarding the legislative requirements can be found on <www.privacy.vic.gov.au>.

THINK AND LINK 21.5

Reflective practice will help you cope with your responsibilities. Chapter 13 provides some practical exercises to help you reflect about how you perform.

ADDRESSING PLACEMENT CONCERNS

Sometimes concerns arise regarding a fieldwork placement for one of the stakeholders. There are mechanisms in place that are enshrined in the rights and responsibilities afforded to each stakeholder. These mechanisms are context specific, and will vary between placement agencies as well as from university to university. Agencies have mechanisms to address concerns as well as the universities.

Student concerns

From your perspective, problems can arise concerning placement from two perspectives. The first is in relation to university actions, and the second is events at the agency. The processes to deal with both of these perspectives are hierarchical and evidence based. You may need an external party to assist in either process. A useful resource is the local student union.

First, if you have concerns regarding the actions of a university's representative, the steps to go through are outlined in Figure 21.2. At any point you can approach any level of the university hierarchy with your concerns. For example, if the concerns are with the fieldwork organiser or academic supervisor, it would be appropriate to

Figure 21.2 University mechanisms to address student concerns

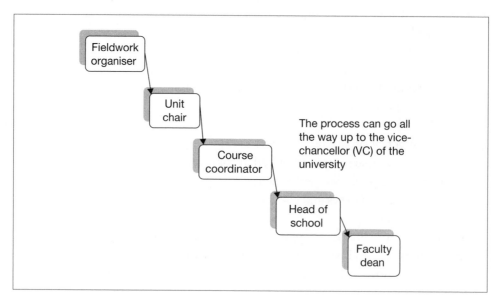

approach the unit chair. If the issue is not resolved to your satisfaction, you could approach the course coordinator or the head of school.

Concerns regarding an issue or event at an agency require a different process. It is the university's responsibility to monitor and support fieldwork placements, and you should contact your university fieldwork organiser or academic supervisor. This person will talk you through your options and help you to identify strategies to deal with the scenario as appropriate. Also within the agency there should be specific complaint protocols. These processes are all evidence based. You should ensure that you are familiar with the agency policies. You can discuss these with the university academic supervisor, who can support you through the process as appropriate.

Agency concerns

To address agency concerns regarding a student while on placement, there need to be clear communication processes identified between the agency, student and university. It is presumed that the agency will, where possible, attempt to address any concerns directly with the student. There needs to be clarity about the processes involved where a student needs guidance. If advice provided does not bring the desired result, or where serious concerns exist about the student's competence, it would then become a university responsibility. The agency has the right to deny the student access to the agency, thus ending the student's fieldwork placement. This can occur if the student's actions or behaviours are inconsistent with the agency's expectations. For example the student may not be performing patient- or client-based actions competently; the agency's primary responsibility is to its clients or patients, and on that basis denies the student access to the agency. The university needs to have clearly outlined processes in place to deal with this if it occurs.

The university has the responsibility to ensure that there are support mechanisms in place for the agency and for you. Sometimes students can be intimidated by what is occurring and may find it difficult to initiate any action, but as with other stakeholders, students have rights as well as responsibilities. To access your rights, you may need to speak to a party outside the placement: an appropriate choice would be a student union representative.

Case Study 21.2 | Three scenarios

Scenario A

You are working with people who frequently exhibit aggressive behaviour. You are unsure of the best way to handle the situations as they arise. You ask your fieldwork educator, and she says, 'Don't worry; you will soon pick it up.'

1   What do you do?
2   Who should you consult?

Scenario B

You have been asked to undertake a risky complex task that you have only seen described in your textbook. Your fieldwork educator is being called away by an emergency. She asks, 'Will you be all right if left alone?'

1   What do you say?
2   Who is principally responsible for the outcomes in this situation?

Scenario C

In your role as a student you have witnessed the mistreatment of clients, patients or service users. An experienced staff member with whom you are working continues to verbally abuse clients, stating that this is the only language that they understand. This staff member will have input into your evaluation.

1   What do you do?
2   What information do you need?
3   With whom should you discuss the issue?

SUMMARY

A successful fieldwork placement results from clarity of the three Rs (roles, rights and responsibilities). This, in conjunction with discipline-specific information, forms the core information that must be communicated between the three key stakeholders.

As with all partnerships, if one stakeholder fails to meet its responsibilities, this could have a negative impact on the rights of other stakeholders. If this occurs, the processes to address this imbalance should be outlined, and accessible to all parties, at the beginning of the fieldwork.

From a student perspective, awareness of your role, rights and responsibilities is a foundation for a successful fieldwork placement.

DISCUSSION QUESTIONS

1   What are the key elements to facilitate a successful fieldwork placement?
2   As a student, what are your responsibilities regarding your fieldwork placement?
3   How do you address problems in your fieldwork placement?

Useful Websites
Australian Federal Police: www.afp.gov.au/business/national_police_checks.html#crim
Australian Government: www.aifs.gov.au/nch/resources/police/policechecks
Department of Health: www.dhs.vic.gov.au
Department of Justice: www.justice.vic.gov.au/workingwithchildren
New South Wales Government: www.police.nsw.gov.au
Office of the Victorian Privacy Commissioner: www.privacy.vic.gov.au
Queensland Police: www.police.qld.gov.au
South Australia Police: www.sapolice.sa.gov.au
Tasmania Police: www.police.tas.gov.au
Victoria Police: www.police.vic.gov.au
Western Australia: www.police.wa.gov.au
www.checkwwc.wa.gov.au

CHAPTER 22
LEGAL ISSUES

Richard Ingleby

LEARNING OUTCOMES

After reading this chapter, you should be able to:
- understand the university's obligations to students
- discuss the legal issues surrounding fieldwork placement
- discuss the meaning of confidentiality.

KEY TERMS

Community-based healthcare
Confidentiality
Negligence
Obligation
Vicarious liability

INTRODUCTION

This chapter discusses three legal issues arising out of the relationship between fieldwork placement students and the university at which they are studying:

1 the obligation of the university as an employer to provide a safe workplace
2 the liability of the university for acts of negligence committed by fieldwork placement students
3 the confidentiality of information obtained by and about placement students.

These issues are discussed in the context of placements in:

a hospitals
b community-based service provision
c client-health student interaction.

The purpose of the discussion is to make you and those responsible for you aware of potential legal issues relating to fieldwork placements, so as to reduce the risk of illegal and/or inappropriate behaviours and improve the quality of the fieldwork placement experience.

THE OBLIGATION OF THE UNIVERSITY AS AN EMPLOYER TO PROVIDE A SAFE WORKPLACE

Universities are employers of people. Employers have many legal duties towards their employees. Most of those duties are now part of legislation. In Victoria, section 21(1) of the *Occupational Health and Safety Act* 2004 (Vic) ('the Act'), which has equivalents in other jurisdictions, provides that:

> An employer must, so far as is reasonably practicable, provide and maintain for employees of the employer a working environment that is safe and without risks to health.

The definitional section of the Act provides that an employer is a person who employs one or more other persons under contracts of employment or contracts of training. The combination of these sections means that a university has a responsibility to make sure that its fieldwork placement students have a safe working environment.

Obviously the lack of any precise definition of concepts such as 'so far as is reasonably practicable' and 'safe and without risks to health' means that the interpretation of the duty is a practical problem from the perspective of the university. The High Court has held, in *Miletic* v *Capital Territory Health Commission* (1995) 130 ALR 591 per Brennan, Deane, Dawson, Gaudron and McHugh JJ at 594, that:

> the question whether a reasonable person would take steps to avoid a foreseeable risk of injury to another is to be answered by balancing 'the magnitude of the risk and the degree of the probability of its occurrence, along with the expense, difficulty and inconvenience of taking alleviating action and any other conflicting responsibilities' which may exist.

The university therefore needs to consider:
- the risks of harm to which its fieldwork placement students might be exposed
- how likely it is that such harm will occur
- the expense, difficulty and inconvenience of preventing the harm
- other conflicting responsibilities.

Clearly this is not a straightforward balancing act to achieve. One of the university's 'conflicting' responsibilities is to ensure the quality of the students whom it accredits by the award of a degree. If a university is going to accredit a social work student with a qualification, this necessarily imports a component of real-life experience. In social work, as in other health professions, there are vital training elements which can only be derived from experience of the real world.

Because books and lectures are not enough to provide practical experience, fieldwork placement students need real-life experience if their studies are to be of practical value. But the very reality of the real world includes exposure to danger. In taking the student to a setting other than, and less protected than, the university, fieldwork placement students will necessarily be exposed to risks, and also exposed to risks whose management is less susceptible to the control of university processes. Indeed, one of the most important purposes of fieldwork placements is to give students experience in relation to such risks.

If a fieldwork placement student suffers injury while on a placement, then a legal question might arise as to whether the university has fulfilled its duties:
- to take reasonable care to provide a safe system of work
- not to expose the student to an unnecessary risk of injury.

THINK AND LINK 22.1

Risk is an important issue for you on placement in terms of yourself, but also in terms of the clients or patients you may encounter. Chapter 20 puts forward some ways to think about unacceptable risk to vulnerable clients. Chapter 21 also discusses responsibility of the university to fieldwork placement, as well as your responsibilities as a student.

HOSPITAL SETTINGS

In a hospital there are risks of infection. It would clearly be unreasonable to expect a university to ensure that a hospital fieldwork placement student was only brought into contact with healthy people. But the duty to prevent harm would cover the need to ensure that a fieldwork student was properly educated as to the nature of the risks and preventive measures before entering the hospital setting.

REFLECTION 22.1

Hospital
1   What are the most likely events to occur in a hospital that will put you, the student, in a position where your physical safety is at risk?
2   What can be done to reduce the likelihood that such events occur?
3   What can be done to reduce the harm caused by such events if they do occur?
4   Who is the person in the hospital the student should contact as a first resort in the event of any emergency?
5   What are the hospital's processes for dealing with an emergency?
6   What has been the experience of previous students in this hospital?

THINK AND LINK 22.2

Chapter 5 introduces the student to placements in acute hospital settings. That chapter describes the emergency codes used in such a setting. As a student in a hospital setting, you need to know what those codes mean, and how to act in each situation.

COMMUNITY-BASED SERVICE SETTINGS

With *community-based service* provision, students will be brought into contact with people who may have psychiatric conditions and/or issues relating to drug and alcohol abuse. Here there is a risk of the student being physically attacked. In order to fulfil its duty to prevent harm, the university might require that fieldwork placement students not be left alone with clients of such services. The university might also require the community-based service to have protocols in place to reduce the risk of such harms and to provide strategies in the event that such harms eventuate. Even if the university does not require the community-based service to have protocols, the community-based service is itself the employer of its own employees, and as such has a duty to provide a safe workplace. This duty would extend to fieldwork placement students, because it is clearly foreseeable that such persons would come into contact with the clients of the service. The community-based service could hardly argue that it was unaware of the risks posed by the nature of its clients, as these risks are likely to be the rationale for the existence of the service in the first place. If the community-based service program's protocols were more stringent than university requirements, this would hardly be a cause for concern; but if they were less so, then the university should be reluctant to allow students to spend time in such fieldwork placements.

As is the case with hospital-based placement, the existence of procedures designed to minimise risk would impose a duty on the university to ensure that students were aware of them.

REFLECTION 22.2

Community
1 Taking into account the particular purposes and clients of the community-based service in which your fieldwork placement is to take place, what are the:
   a possible causes of your physical safety being at risk?
   b most likely causes of your physical safety being at risk?
2 What can be done to reduce:
   a the likelihood that such events occur?
   b the harm caused by such events if they do occur?
3 What should you do in the event of an emergency?
4 What has been the experience of previous students in this community-based service?

CLIENT–HEALTH PROFESSIONAL INTERACTIONS

In the setting of client–health professional interaction, the risk of physical attack remains, although the likelihood of the harm might be lower. However, settings that involve more intimate and one-on-one interactions involve risks of sexual and racial harassment in a context of power imbalance between the professional and the fieldwork placement student. The key point here is not so much that the university would be liable for every such incident; rather, if the university ever became aware of any particular professional's propensity for harassing behaviour or comments, there would be a duty to ensure that students were not exposed to that behaviour. So if a student reported that a particular health professional made comments about 'some sort of Asian thing' or seemed too intimate in his or her interactions with the student, then the university would be negligent if it exposed subsequent students to that sort of behaviour, even if it were not liable for the first incidents.

REFLECTION 22.3

Inappropriate behaviour

1 What is it that makes a comment inappropriate for sexual or racist comment?
2 What should you do if a professional to whom you are assigned makes a comment that is inappropriate because of its sexual or racial nature?
3 What should you do if you are the subject of an inappropriate sexual advance by a professional to whom you are assigned?

THE LIABILITY OF THE UNIVERSITY FOR ACTS OF NEGLIGENCE COMMITTED BY FIELDWORK PLACEMENT STUDENTS

The university may be legally liable for acts committed by students who are on fieldwork placements. A student who is on a placement can be seen either as the agent of the university or the employee of the university. By reason of the doctrine of *vicarious liability*, the university will be liable for the losses to a third party caused by the negligence of a student. It is immaterial whether the third party is a client of or a representative of the fieldwork placement setting. The doctrine of vicarious liability imposes a legal obligation on the university, even if the university is not implicated in or even aware of the act that gives rise to the action in negligence against the student. All that is required (although there is much uncertainty at the outer limits of the meaning of the phrase) is that the negligence be in the course of the student's fieldwork placement.

One practical implication of the doctrine of vicarious liability is that a person who suffers loss by reason of a fieldwork placement student's negligence may well prefer to pursue legal action against the university, because the university has 'bigger pockets' from which to fund an award of damages and costs.

In hospitals, fieldwork placement students are unlikely to be directly involved in the provision of treatment. This means that they are unlikely to be in a position where they can cause damage by the negligent provision of treatment. But a university which wants to ensure that it minimises the risk of vicarious liability should ensure that its fieldwork placement students are aware that they should confine their activities to the sphere of their placement.

In community-based service fieldwork placements, the student is perhaps equally unlikely to cause loss to the clients of the service. But an issue of vicarious liability could easily occur if, for example, the student drove a client from one place to the other and in the course of that journey caused loss to the client and to other members of the public by negligent driving. In such circumstances the victims of the negligent driving would have a claim against the university.

In the case of a fieldwork placement with a client–health professional, perhaps the likeliest act of negligence is a negligent disclosure by the student (as discussed in the next section of the chapter) that breaches the confidentiality of the client–health professional setting. In such circumstances, the client would have an action in negligence against the university.

The existence of vicarious liability is an incentive for universities to ensure that its fieldwork placement students are properly briefed before their placements.

REFLECTION 22.4

Negligence
1   What are the most likely situations where a third party might be caused loss by the negligence of a placement student?
2   What strategies can be introduced to reduce the risk of such losses occurring?

THE CONFIDENTIALITY OF INFORMATION OBTAINED BY THE STUDENT ON PLACEMENT

There are various legal ways in which an obligation of *confidentiality* may attach to information obtained by a student in the course of their fieldwork placement. The principles of vicarious liability discussed in the previous section obviously mean that the breach of the obligations may create legal consequences for the university as well as the student.

Of most direct relevance for students who are in hospital fieldwork placements are statutory provisions that make information confidential. For example, section 141(2) of the *Health Services Act* 1988 (Vic), which has equivalents in most other Australian jurisdictions, creates a statutory obligation of confidentiality by making it a criminal offence for a 'relevant person' (which would include a fieldwork placement student) to divulge information that would identify a patient or recipient of health services, unless the disclosure falls within a narrowly prescribed band of exceptions. This statutory provision was not completely new, as there were longstanding provisions of the *Evidence Act* precluding doctors from giving evidence about their patients without the patient's consent. The Victorian Supreme Court has given section 141(2) an interpretation to protect patients. In *PQ* v *Australian Red Cross Society* [1992] 1 VR 19 at 29, McGarvie J held that the intention of the section was:

> to confer on patients a legal protection of the nature of that which in ordinary speech would be referred to as 'patient confidentiality' ... To render a protection of confidentiality to a patient real, what needs to be protected from disclosure in the vast majority of cases is the information that has been obtained in respect of the patient, not merely the information that the person was a patient.

The *Health Records Act* 2001 (Vic), as its title suggests, makes specific provisions which are designed to

> promote fair and responsible handling of health information by—
> (a) protecting the privacy of an individual's health information that is held in the public and private sectors; and
> (b) providing individuals with a right of access to their health information; and
> (c) providing an accessible framework for the resolution of complaints regarding the handling of health information.

These provisions include the power to order 'that the complainant is entitled to a specified amount, not exceeding $100,000, by way of compensation for any loss or damage suffered by the complainant, including injury to the complainant's feelings or humiliation suffered by the complainant, by reason of the act or practice the subject of the complaint'.

The *Health Act* 1958 (Vic) contains a specific provision in relation to the privacy of an HIV-infected person by stating that (in section 128):

> A person who, in the course of providing a service, acquires information that a person has been or is required to be tested for HIV or is infected with HIV, must take all reasonable steps to develop and implement systems to protect the privacy of that person.

There are equivalent provisions in the *Mental Health Act* 1986 (Vic).

Students with community-based services may be on fieldwork placement pursuant to a contractual arrangement. It may well be that the terms of this contract include an obligation of confidentiality within other terms, such as those making provision for matters such as insurance and regulation of mutual responsibilities.

If such a contract also contains a requirement that fieldwork placement students maintain the confidentiality of information derived by them in the course of their placement, then the fieldwork placement student's breach of confidentiality will be a breach of the contract. Such a breach of contract could give rise to a claim for damages (against the student and the university), in addition to other forms of relief to limit the disclosure of the confidential information.

Students who are in client–therapist fieldwork placements are perhaps less likely to have a contractual source of an obligation of confidentiality. But the laws of equity might create a 'breach of confidence' action against the student and the university if a student discloses confidential information without the authorisation of the client/patient. As mentioned in the previous section, another possible source of an obligation of confidentiality is the law of negligence. If, as would normally be the case, the fieldwork placement student owes the client a duty to keep information confidential, then the disclosure of such information will be a breach of that duty of care which could give rise to an action for damages (against the student and the university) if the client suffers foreseeable harm by the disclosure.

It is not difficult to conceive of circumstances in which a fieldwork placement student makes a negligent disclosure or breaches a confidence deriving from his or her experience in the client–health professional setting. I say this because of personal experience, and also because I am confident that my personal experience is not atypical. The extent to which passengers on public transport (and invariably this means crowded public transport where notions of privacy are fanciful) engage in the practice of:

- reading documents to which obligations of confidence applies
- discussing 'interesting' features of their day

might be reduced if the people whose confidences were being breached became aware of the breaches and took legal action in relation to them.

As a barrister I once agreed to the briefing solicitor's request to send along a work experience student. When I informed this student that it was very important that everything she saw or heard remained confidential, she assured me that she was aware of how important that was. She was less assured when I told her that I had heard her talking to her friend about her previous day's experiences when we were travelling on the same train the previous evening. I have also heard people on trains discussing their legal proceedings in circumstances where they cannot possibly have known whether the people around them were acting for the other parties to the proceedings. Confidentiality means confidentiality. Students need to be aware of this. You cannot go wrong if you simply adopt the practice that you do not discuss your professional practice except in the course of your professional interactions.

Case Study 22.1 | Julie

For her last fieldwork placement, Julie was assigned to a psychiatric ward in a large metropolitan hospital. She had had training in document storage and confidentiality, both at university and at the hospital. During the placement, a personality from a local TV channel was admitted. Julie was smitten. She was excited to be so close to this person that she started telling her family about this person and the admission to the psychiatric ward. She told her university friends, one of whom had a family member who worked as crew at the same TV channel as the TV personality admitted for treatment. Julie had no idea that her friend had family involved in television. The TV personality filed an action for damages against Julie and the university.

Questions

1   What aspect of duty of care had Julie failed to keep?
2   Did she knowingly breach confidentiality?
3   What course of action can the university take if Julie is guilty?
4   What has Julie learnt?

SUMMARY

This chapter has discussed the legal issues that arise from students undertaking fieldwork placements in hospital, community-based and client–health professional settings. Three issues were the focus of the chapter. These were the obligation of the university to provide a safe workplace or learning place for students on fieldwork placements; the liability of the university for negligence of a student; and confidentiality. There are areas where you could have legal action taken out against you: such as, discussing cases outside of your fieldwork placement and being negligent in your behaviour with clients. Learning professional behaviour on your placement also covers taking into account ramifications of your actions towards clients and other professionals.

DISCUSSION QUESTIONS

1   What would your reaction be as a health student if you were travelling home on the train and heard two people discussing a research assignment that you had submitted three weeks ago? What would you do about it?

2   On placement, how aware are you of your own personal safety?

3   What has been your experience of safety procedures when on fieldwork placement? (For example, two staff are asked to attend home visits; visits are forbidden after 5 p.m.?)

References and Further Reading

For an organised statement of relevant legal principles see Halsbury's *Laws of Australia* (2008). LexisNexis, Sydney.

In relation to occupational health and safety more specifically, see Johnstone, R. (2004). *Occupational Health and Safety Law and Policy: Texts and Materials*. Law Book, Sydney.

In relation to principles of the law of negligence see Luntz, H., Hambly, D., Burns, K., Dietrich, J. & Foster, N. (2008). *Torts: Cases and Commentary*. LexisNexis, Sydney. See also Mendelson, D. (2007). *The New Law of Torts*, Oxford University Press, Melbourne.

PART 3 CHECKLIST
ETHICS, LAW AND RESPONSIBILITIES

FOSTERING PARTNERSHIPS WITH ACTION

As a student you are an important stakeholder in your fieldwork education. To understand the role of the other stakeholders:

- access and read the fieldwork agency's or facility's annual report
- go to the home page of your discipline's professional association and search for documents, policies and working party activities related to fieldwork placement
- mindmap (using an illustrative diagram) the key real-world issues for each of the stakeholders involved in your fieldwork placement
- access a copy of the contract (if there is a current document of this kind) that your university has with a major provider of fieldwork placement. Identify your responsibilities and those of the other stakeholders.

ETHICAL DECISION-MAKING

In considering your duty of care, the following tools could be considered:

- The doughnut model (Handy 1994) (Figure 20.1): is the presenting issue a core responsibility or one for which I need to use my judgment?
- The person-centred risk assessment (Kinsella 2000) (Figure 20.2): what are the risks involved?
- The International Classification of Functioning, Disability and Health (WHO 2002) (Figure 20.3): what do the issues look like when analysed by the ICF?
- The supported decision-making model (Watson 2009) (Figure 20.4): how do I balance the person's wishes and happiness with risk and health wellness? What are 'important for' and 'important to'?
- Decision-making pathway (Watson 2009) (Figure 20.5): I can use this when professional duty of care, risks, and competence may have an impact on decisions to be made about, with or for a person.

THE THREE Rs: ROLES, RIGHTS AND RESPONSIBILITIES

If I am working with any of the groups listed below, I require a pre-placement police check and a Working with Children Check (WWCC).

- Do I have mine?

I require such a check because the following groups are the categories of clients or patients where an unacceptable level of risk may exist if these clients are exposed to inappropriate persons:

- any person under the age of 21 years who is subject to an order of the court that relates to their welfare
- any person under the age of 18 years who is subject to a protective service notification, investigation or involvement
- any person who is subject to an order of the Children's Court or subject to guardianship, following a protection application
- any person under 18 years to be placed for adoption
- any person under 18 years who receives a residential or home-based care or other service funded through Protection and Care and/or Supported Accommodation and Assistance Program (SAAP)
- any person who is deemed an eligible person under the *Intellectually Disabled Persons' Services Act* 1986
- any person who receives a facility-based or inhome accommodation service funded under the *Disabled Persons' Services Act* 1986
- any person who receives services for care or treatment of a mental illness, under the *Mental Health Act* 1986
- any person who receives services through an early childhood intervention program
- any person who receives services under the Home and Community Care (HACC) program
- any person who receives treatment through the School Dental Health Program, the School Nurses Program, the Tuberculosis (TB) Program and by a Sexual Health Centre
- any person defined as a patient under the *Alcohol and Drug Dependent Persons Act*
- any aged or infirm person who receives inhouse services
- any person who receives public rental housing services
- any other such client or patient who receives direct care services and where in the view of the relevant manager, there may exist an unacceptable level of risk by exposing these clients or patients to inappropriate persons.

I am aware of my responsibilities on placement, which are:

Punctual and regular attendance at the placement venue.

If absent during the fieldwork placement, I will notify the agency as early as possible, and will negotiate with their fieldwork educator how this lost time will be made up.

I have identified a communication strategy with the agency; for example, an exchange of contact details between me and the agency's fieldwork educator.

I will notify the fieldwork educator of any circumstances likely to pose a risk to either me or any of the agency's clients or staff; for instance, the presence of any infection or an inability to perform a certain task, such as lifting.

I understand and will adhere to the dress code.

I will locate and familiarise myself with local policies and procedures relevant to my role within the agency.

I understand about maintaining confidentiality at all times.

I am to communicate with staff and/or my fieldwork educator any incidents or issues that may be significant to the wellbeing of clients, patients or service users.

I will report any injury on fieldwork placement or an accident to the immediate fieldwork educators. I will also notify the university as soon as possible, and lodge a report with the university.

I will communicate with the university regarding any issues that may be significant regarding the fieldwork placement.

I realise it is my responsibility to obtain feedback on my performance.

I will ensure that the fieldwork educator completes the required evaluation and/or assessment requirements.

I also need to include:

processes to clarify personal values: there are often situations that will challenge my values

clarification of what I am responsible for and to whom I am accountable

time management

professional issues, including:

duty of care

occupational health and safety: self

occupational health and safety: others

occupational health and safety: environment; for example:

infection control

lifting

emergency situations.

I will also need to develop my written and verbal communication with:

professionals and/or other team members

service users, patients or clients

the university.

LEGAL ISSUES

As a student there are aspects of my behaviour that could end up in legal action. Such actions are:

breaches of confidentiality

negligence with clients

I am also aware that the university has legal responsibility to provide me with a safe working environment.

PART 4
TRANSITION TO PRACTICE

Chapter 23: You Become the Supervisor   **315**

Chapter 24: Starting Out in Supervision   **329**

Chapter 25: Health Workforce Recruitment   **345**

In Part 4 we assume that you are now making the transition from student to health professional. Not only are we assuming that you are a health professional, but we are assuming that you will now be taking on the role as a new fieldwork educator.

The chapters in this section give you information on transition from student to a fieldwork educator (Chapter 23) and on issues involved in supervision of a student (Chapter 24). The final chapter (Chapter 25) is about recruiting students back to your workplace. This may be particularly important if you work in a rural or remote area, or if your workplace is short staffed and looking for staff.

We wish you all the best in your career as you now venture as a newly graduated health professional into the new role of fieldwork educator.

CHAPTER 23
YOU BECOME THE SUPERVISOR

Jennifer Pascoe, Uschi Bay and Michelle Courtney

LEARNING OUTCOMES

After reading this chapter, you should be able to:
- put in practice useful strategies from your fieldwork placement experience to assist you with making the transition into working as a qualified health professional
- develop a framework for taking active steps for your continuing professional development
- use the conceptual links between your own supervision experiences and your professional development, and how these can inform your role as a fieldwork educator.

KEY TERMS

Clinical education or placement
Continuing professional development
Fieldwork education supervisor
Fieldwork education
Fieldwork placement
Fieldwork supervisor
Lifelong learning
Line management
Mentoring
Reflection
Transition

INTRODUCTION

This chapter aims to encourage you to reflect on your experiences of working in your field of practice as a student, and to explore the implications for you in relation to your professional role of fieldwork educator. It is very important for newly qualified health professionals to identify continuing professional development opportunities to support current and future work roles. *Continuing professional development* may be a source of support and satisfaction for you as you move into your professional work. We encourage you to plan actively and pursue various kinds of professional development opportunities. One stimulating form of continuing professional development is becoming a fieldwork educator to students in your field undertaking their first qualification in their chosen profession.

The term *transition* often implies that we journey from one destination to another and somehow arrive at an endpoint. However, we feel that we are always in the process of 'becoming' as health professionals, because we are continually learning, relearning and/or unlearning old assumptions to develop new ways of working with people. Hence the notion of *continuing professional development* or *lifelong learning* reflects the dynamic engagement with ideas, practices and people that practitioners enjoy throughout their working life.

We aim to support your reflections, conceptualisation and planning for these transitions by outlining various strategies that may assist you with this vital aspect of your ongoing professional practice.

This chapter is divided into three sections, each containing information and suggested reflection guides to help you make the progression from student to beginning fieldwork educator.

WORKING IN THE FIELD—AS A STUDENT

Reflection on your fieldwork placement

Moving from fieldwork placements as a student into your first qualified professional practice position is an important milestone. This time is recognised as challenging and exciting in the human services and health literature. It is common to feel both eagerness and readiness to go into the workplace to take up your role, but to also be filled with trepidation about how little you feel you actually know. You may be wondering how the skills and knowledge that you have learnt at university and during your fieldwork placement will transfer to new workplace settings and your new job.

One important strategy is to reflect systematically (Schon 2003) on your fieldwork experience, your positive and negative feelings, and what moving into the workplace as a qualified health professional means to you.

REFLECTION 23.1

Your fieldwork experience
1 What skills and knowledge do you feel you have gained through your fieldwork placement?
2 What were the joys and sources of satisfaction for you during fieldwork placement?
3 What does this mean to you and your approach to seeking a job in a particular workplace?

4   What were the frustrations and sources of dissatisfaction during your fieldwork placement?

5   What was the value of supervision for you during fieldwork education?

6   What aspects of your fieldwork experience do you seek to take with you into your workplace learning?

7   How has your work-integrated learning influenced your choice of workplaces for practising in your specific field?

8   What areas of professional work in your field would you like to develop further?

9   What workplaces or opportunities are available for expanding and exploring these interests?

From your reflections, what can you learn to inform your career goals? Writing down your responses to these questions may be useful in evaluating and reflecting on your work-integrated learning to inform your choice of job, workplace and continuing professional development priorities.

Reflecting on your responses to these questions can be undertaken in a number of ways; for example, as part of your evaluation (both formally and informally) of the fieldwork placement experience with fellow students or staff at the university, and with your fieldwork educator(s) at the placement organisation. Discussions with fellow students about their fieldwork education experiences can help you find out more about a number of practice settings; for example, a large acute city hospital; a community-based placement; experience from a rural and remote site; someone who had no onsite profession-specific supervisor; or in a private practice setting. What were their reflections? What can you learn from this for your own career goals? These reflections can feed into your preparation for your first job as a qualified practitioner.

THINK AND LINK 23.1

Section 1, Chapters 2 to 11, plus Chapter 15, discuss a variety of settings and experiences that you may encounter. If, during your discussions with fellow students, there are practice settings where no one in your group has had experience, refer back to these chapters to find the placement setting about which you want more information.

Preparing for your first professional job

As you begin applying for your first professional job and preparing for job interviews, use the reflection process to identify the skills and experiences that you wish to use to promote yourself to potential employers. Acknowledging that you may not have had work-integrated learning experience in the specific type of job for which you are applying, look to identify transferable skills and/or skills that you have been developing and may be related to the potential job; for example, having experience in administering standardised assessments; attention to following instructions and procedures; and ability to interpret accurately and record the results of the assessment. You can also promote your ability to work in teams, effective communication with a range of clients and their families and other similar skills which you may have developed during fieldwork placements.

Collating material from your studies and fieldwork placement experiences that enable you to demonstrate your skills to your employer is not only self-affirming, but also conveys your knowledge and ability to learn from experience. You may develop a portfolio as a method of presenting samples of key skills and experiences from your fieldwork placement.

Case Study 23.1 | **Jane's fieldwork experiences**

Jane has recently completed her final fieldwork placement before completing her physiotherapy course. She is concerned that she may not have the specific required and desirable attributes and skills that are listed in some of the interesting job advertisements. After spending time reflecting on her fieldwork placements, Jane identified some skills and experiences that she felt comfortable in promoting to potential employers, even though they may not necessarily be specific to the job:

- 'I have worked with a wide range of clients, and I am comfortable with developing intervention strategies to meet various needs of clients according to age, abilities, lifestyles and cultures.'
- 'I spent some time in a large rehabilitation centre, working with a number of health professionals from a range of disciplines. I feel that I have developed a good understanding of what the various professions can bring to the team and patient care.'
- 'I worked in a rural community setting where there was no physiotherapist. In this situation, I gained experience in problem-solving and communicating with other professionals, clients and the community. I used my initiative to establish a professional support network by contacting a physiotherapist in a nearby town, and the local chapter of the professional association.'

Questions
1   Reflect on your fieldwork experiences to develop your own examples.
2   Do your examples differ from Jane's, or are they similar?

Use the job interview process as a professional development activity in its own right. You can learn more about yourself and your expectations of your professional career, by reflecting on the content and outcomes of each job application and interview that you attend. Use this reflection and learning process to update and target your portfolio for each new interview.

Moving from being a student to a new health professional can be facilitated by reflecting particularly on your fieldwork placement experiences, gaining perspectives from fellow students and using the job application and interview process as a learning experience. This will enable you to identify a repertoire of relevant experiences, skills and attitudes that you can adapt responsibly to promote yourself to potential employers. As you move on to become a new professional, you can develop and consolidate many of these skills.

WORKING IN THE FIELD—AS A NEWLY QUALIFIED PRACTITIONER

At last—you have started your first job in your chosen profession! In this first year of practice, you may experience both elation and fear, great expectations about the workplace and some coming to terms with the realities of many settings (Tryssenaar & Perkins 2001).

We will now explore some of the key issues and strategies for you in this early phase of your career, with a focus on reflecting on your experiences as a fieldwork placement student.

Orientation strategies

Orientation to your workplace and your role are important early steps for the new health professional, just as it was when you were a student. Induction or orientation programs are important in the transition process, and provide initial pertinent information about the specific job requirements, such as time and place of attendance, use of office space and equipment, resources and client access to resources. Information about communication processes in the organisation is also helpful (Hummell & Koelmeyer 1999). Developing professional support systems, good personal self-care and informal family and friendship networks are also important orientation strategies (Cusick et al. 2004).

Reflect on your fieldwork experiences. What strategies did you use to become familiar with new environments? Did you need a map to help you find your way around your workplace? How did you remember the names of all the staff who were in your immediate and wider working environments? Did you write them down in a notebook? Was carrying a staff contact list with you helpful for remembering names? Did you use a computer-based calendar or reminder system to help you keep appointments, schedule sessions and so forth? If these and other strategies worked for you when you were a student, use them again in your first job.

You may wish to refine or develop these strategies, or you may find new ones, but it is important that you know what has worked for you in the past and is likely to work for you again in the early stages of your new job. This is important not only in the context of starting your new job, but is also important to remember when you begin working with fieldwork placement students; for example, your experience and strategies may be used when developing an induction or orientation program.

Continuing professional development

Your fieldwork placements were a starting point for your continuing professional development. Your university fieldwork liaison person, along with clinicians and others in your fieldwork placement settings, were key factors in shaping your early professional development activities. As you enter the workforce, undertaking continuing professional development should be embedded in your role as a professional. In conjunction with your workplace supervisor, you can identify a range of continuing professional development needs and opportunities for your development as a professional. It is important that you plan and target your continuing professional development activities, so that you can maintain focus in relation to achieving your career goals. However, there may also be an opportunistic element in your continuing professional development; for example, taking advantage of a presentation by a visiting academic.

Think about how you learned new skills, and how you responded to the challenges of the workplace during your fieldwork experiences. What is your preferred learning style? Do you learn best by having a skill demonstrated first by a more experienced professional, and then trying it out for yourself? Do you prefer a trial-and-error approach? Do you prefer to try to develop many skills at once, or is your learning style more suited to focusing on gaining confidence in a few skills at a time before moving on to other areas? Are networks in your workplace or wider professional community helpful in giving you the support and feedback that you may require? This may be particularly relevant if you are working as a sole practitioner and/or have a position in a rural or remote location.

You may find that you learn better from some people rather than others. Think back to your fieldwork placements: what strategies did you develop for situations in which the teaching style, for example of your fieldwork educator, did not facilitate your learning? Did you negotiate to learn from other professionals? Was co-teaching available to you? Did you resolve to learn as much as possible from the individual, and then seek additional learning from another source? These strategies will also apply in your new workplace.

Mentoring is another way in which professionals in all fields are encouraged to identify and develop their ongoing learning in the workplace. The focus with mentoring is usually on career planning and personal development, rather than learning specific practitioner skills or competencies. Some mentoring schemes are formalised, so that an active process is in place for various new workers to be allocated or matched with a mentor. As with best practice in supervision, it is recommended that you establish a contract with your mentor regarding the purpose, process and outcomes of the mentoring relationship.

By reflecting on many of the situations you encountered during your fieldwork placement, you will be able to identify how you can best develop the skills required for your new job. Take responsibility for learning in a style that best suits you. Your understanding of the need for using learning and teaching styles that best suit an individual will be of great value when you work with fieldwork placement students.

As you move on to supervising fieldwork placement students, you will be modelling a professional behaviour: that of being committed to and actively involved in a planned continuing professional development program.

Supervision as a tool for continuing professional development

Your fieldwork experiences contained the key element of supervision. This was a structured process, and you may have felt that the focus was on enabling you to achieve the requirements of the fieldwork placement; that is, passing. As you move into your career as a professional, supervision will take on the focus of being a tool for continuing professional development to develop your skills as a health professional.

In this period of transition, as you begin your new career, you should look for all available opportunities for formal and informal supervision, mentoring and continuing professional development. However, while having a mentor and/or supervisor at this stage is extremely important, you should not assume that you will have access to a supervisor in your workplace (Tryssenaar & Perkins 2001). Do not limit your idea of professional supervision to *line management*; that is, your immediate supervisor or boss. There is a difference between line management and professional supervision, which focuses mainly on the development of your professional skills and competencies.

Reflect on the style of supervision that you valued most during your fieldwork experiences. Do you prefer direct feedback, with constructive criticism? Do you have difficulty in receiving negative feedback? What type of feedback and learning from the supervision process enables and inspires you to learn and develop your skills?

Be proactive in working with your supervisor to ensure that your learning needs are addressed, by wherever possible using your preferred learning style. This may not always be possible, and will require some flexibility from all involved; however, it is your responsibility to bring these issues to the attention of your workplace supervisor. Reflect on this experience as you begin to work with fieldwork placement students, so that you can best meet their learning and development needs.

Managing expectations

Professional practice is rewarding and challenging partly because it is unpredictable and requires ongoing learning. The pressure you may place on yourself and perceive from others is that you should be able to 'hit the ground running': you expect yourself to know everything and be able to do the work required straight away. However, it is important to remind yourself and others that it takes time to learn your job, understand the organisation, establish relationships with people and identify all the key stakeholders. Plan actively to learn these various aspects of your work.

Case Study 23.2 | Sri at work

Sri is a newly qualified social worker employed in an education facility for troubled young people. A young woman disclosed a current situation of sexual abuse to Sri during a one-to-one interview. Sri expected that she, as a qualified social worker, could respond on the spot to this situation, both to assist the troubled student and validate her role in the organisation. Sri negotiated with the young woman for several hours to gain information and consult with relevant agencies before taking action.

Questions

1 As a newly qualified social worker, how stressed do you think Sri may have been in this interview?
2 Were Sri's self expectations realistic?
3 If you were Sri, what would you discuss about this situation with your mentor next time you met?

 THINK AND LINK 23.2

Sri had encountered a vulnerable client. Chapter 20 discusses working ethically with vulnerable clients. Information from this chapter may help you answer the questions to the Sri case study.

If you are overextending yourself, you are likely to miss some of these learning processes. This is why self-care is very important in professional practice. Be mindful too that your co-workers will also be experiencing varying degrees of stress in the work environment. As a team member, understand that your priorities need to be considered along with those of the whole team, so you may need to be patient at times when seeking advice and assistance from others.

It is really important for your ongoing personal and professional development to find suitable supervision of your professional practice that allows you to reflect on your experiences, and also to reflect on this process critically as you move into becoming a fieldwork educator.

REFLECTION 23.2

What type of supervision do you prefer?

1 What type of supervision did you most value as a student?
2 Is a formalised supervision program available to you in your workplace? Is the supervision practice specific?
3 In your workplace, is your line manager also your supervisor? Is this the right arrangement for you?
4 Are you considering your overall career planning?
5 How can your supervisor and line manager contribute? Would a mentor be helpful?
6 What are your short- and long-term goals for your ongoing professional development?
7 Does your workplace meet your learning needs?
8 What other professional development opportunities are available to you outside your workplace?
9 Are you keeping a reflective diary as a learning tool?

As you move into the next phase of your early career, you should have consolidated some key areas that are essential for a beginning fieldwork educator. You will have a good understanding of the values, expectations and services of your employing organisation. You will demonstrate a range of work skills, including self-management, management in the workplace and profession-specific skills. You will be committed to, and actively engaged in continuing professional development, supervision and/or mentoring and being a reflective practitioner. You are now prepared for the next phase in the transition process.

WORKING IN THE FIELD—AS A BEGINNING FIELDWORK EDUCATOR

Becoming a first-time fieldwork educator is a significant step, as you experience the transition through various phases of your career. It may seem a daunting role to undertake, but there are benefits, which we will explore briefly in this section, along with some of the key elements of best-practice supervision.

The benefits of becoming a fieldwork educator are many. In the fieldwork educator role you will be required to articulate your professional practice, explain your conceptual maps of the interrelations between theory and practice and explain your organisational setting and policy environment, as well as demonstrating various professional skills and attributes. Your ability to demonstrate competence in these areas will be reassuring as you advance in your career and move on to other roles and positions.

Another benefit of becoming a fieldwork educator is the relationship with university fieldwork education liaison and other academic staff. These connections could lead to other opportunities, such as being engaged as a sessional tutor, marker or deliverer of guest lectures, serving on university committees and providing input to university curriculum and school policy. These are all potential opportunities that would contribute to your career development.

Your professional association or peak body will probably have specific definitions for the different levels of job classification related to expectations about when you should take on supervisory responsibilities. Contact your professional body for guidelines, so that, in conjunction with your employer, you can have a realistic picture of what is expected, and the benefits for you in relation to undertaking student supervision.

The university that has arranged the fieldwork placement is responsible for providing information about the purpose of the placement, including required learning experiences for the student; documentation and assessment requirements; contracts; and all other information that will clearly guide you and the student during the fieldwork experience.

Your role as a fieldwork educator

The fieldwork educator's role comprises three elements: managing, educating and supporting the student in a one-to-one relationship. The management or administrative function of the fieldwork educator's role includes pre-screening interviews, informing agency staff of the student's placement, consulting and negotiating duties, arranging organisational orientation, establishing a learning contract, attending field educators' professional development seminars, liaising and meeting with university staff and scheduling time for supervision and evaluation of the placement.

When you are planning for the arrival of your first fieldwork student, as a beginning fieldwork educator, it is timely to reflect on all the administrative functions, including induction and orientation to assist the student to learn about your workplace.

Case Study 23.3	**Leah as a fieldwork educator**

Leah is waiting today to meet Chris, her first fieldwork placement student. Leah is feeling excited, challenged and a little apprehensive about how she will perform in this new role as fieldwork educator. In preparation, Leah has completed the following list of actions:

- met with the university fieldwork education liaison person and discussed the work-integrated learning requirements and assessments, and read the relevant documents prepared by the university
- conducted a pre-screening interview with Chris, and gained some idea of the learning objectives that Chris and the university have for the fieldwork placement
- gained organisational support for her new role as fieldwork educator through her own supervisor. Leah's agency provides fieldwork placements for a range of health, social work and human services students
- informed the staff in her immediate team of the arrival of Chris and gained approval from staff for Chris to observe their day-to-day work
- made time available this morning to take Chris on a tour of the agency to introduce him to relevant staff, and has arranged an informal morning tea to welcome Chris
- arranged a desk for Chris to use while attending the workplace, as well as access to the organisation's intranet, and provided a list of times when formal organisational inductions are being conducted for new staff—Leah aims to encourage Chris to attend
- arranged that, on their tour of the organisation, Leah will show Chris the professional library the team has been collating—it should provide some valuable professional reading material
- collected a number of key documents about the organisation for Chris, such as the annual report, the policy and procedures manual and the internal phone directory
- arranged to attend the fieldwork educator workshops offered by her local university for fieldwork educators, to extend her learning about this new role.

Question

What sort of experience do you think Chris will have with Leah as the fieldwork educator?

The teaching role of the fieldwork educator requires attending to the learning style and needs of the student, and being aware of your own learning styles. There is some evidence that a match of learning styles between supervisor and student is advantageous for student learning on placement (Razack 2002). This is an exciting area of learning for new fieldwork educators: Fernandez (2003) argues that the new fieldwork educators should seek awareness of relevant concepts of teaching and learning in preparation for becoming a fieldwork educator. Many universities provide professional development for fieldwork educators as part of their fieldwork placement programs.

Your reflections on your learning and the kind of discussion and supervision that has assisted you to understand learning in the workplace will again assist you in becoming alert to the fieldwork placement learning and supervision needs of your fieldwork placement students.

The key qualities of a good fieldwork educator include being able to identify a range of appropriate theoretical and intervention approaches; the ability to manage anxiety (of both the supervisor and the supervisee); the appropriate use of professional power; a sense of humour; and patience (Hawkins & Shohet 2006).

The third aspect of the fieldwork educator relationship is about supporting the self-awareness of the fieldwork student. Razack (2002) advises that some caution in handling emotional difficulties is required. Only those emotional difficulties that pertain to the student's learning should be included in supervision.

As part of your preparation for this new and exciting role as a fieldwork education supervisor, it is important to read some accounts by people like Pereira (2008), who shares the experience of supervising students early in his career. Pereira provides suggestions for making the experience positive for both the student and the new fieldwork educator. Some of the aspects that he emphasises include having clear learning goals and expectations for the fieldwork placement; providing feedback (formal and informal); facilitating self-directed learning opportunities; and under-taking an evaluation before the final evaluation to enable monitoring of progress.

Your reflections on the strategies that facilitated positive experiences for you, both as a fieldwork education student and a newly qualified professional, may assist you with planning your process as a fieldwork education supervisor.

REFLECTION 23.3

Your new role
1 Do you have sufficient information from the relevant university to guide you?
2 Do you have support for your new role from your workplace; for example, time allowed for meeting with students as part of the fieldwork education process?
3 Are you able to access support from others in your service setting; for example, in areas of practice in which you feel less competent?
4 Do you understand the learning style of the fieldwork placement student?
5 How can you learn more about being a fieldwork educator? What are your support networks?

Becoming a fieldwork educator is a significant transition phase in your professional career. You are moving to a higher level in your profession, that of contributing to the education of future professionals. Your competence in professional skills, understanding of the key factors in a successful fieldwork education program and involvement in related continuing professional development will enable you to facilitate the fieldwork education of students. Undertaking this role will benefit your future career goals.

SUMMARY

Work-integrated learning is a key factor in the preparation and development of future health professionals in the human services and health professions. This chapter has explored the phases in career transition from student to entry-level practitioner to beginning fieldwork educator, within the framework of continuing professional development, as being crucial for your career.

Strategies for developing your skills for this role have been presented, including resources for your professional development, your own supervision and mentoring and networking with colleagues. The importance of reflecting on your own experience of fieldwork placements, supervision and practice has been highlighted as a key element in your professional development for the role.

DISCUSSION QUESTIONS

1 How can your reflection on your experience as a student involved in fieldwork placement inform your plans for your career, including becoming a fieldwork educator?
2 What is the role of reflection on your student fieldwork supervision experience in preparing you to become a fieldwork educator?
3 What skills, knowledge and attitudes do you need to develop to become an effective fieldwork educator?
4 What professional development activities can you undertake to enable you to become a fieldwork educator?

References

Courtney, M. & Farnworth, L. (2003). 'Professional Competence for Private Practitioners in Occupational Therapy'. *Australian Occupational Therapy Journal*, 50: 234–43.

Cusick, A., McIntosh, D. & Santiago, L. (2004). 'New Graduate Therapists in Acute Care Hospitals: Priorities, Problems and Strategies for Departmental Action'. *Australian Occupational Therapy Journal*, 51: 174–84.

Fernandez, E. (2003). 'Promoting Teaching Competence in Field Education: Facilitating Transition from Practitioner to Educator'. *Women in Welfare Education*, 6: 103–29.

Hawkins, P. & Shohet, R. (2006). *Supervision in the Helping Professions* (3rd edn). Open University Press, Berkshire.

Hummell, J. & Koelmeyer, K. (1999). 'New Graduates: Perceptions of their First Occupational Therapy Position'. *British Journal of Occupational Therapy*, 62(8): 351–8.

Pereira, R. B. (2008). 'Learning and Being a First-Time Student Supervisor: Challenges and Triumphs'. *Australian Journal of Rural Health*, 16: 47–8.

Razack, N. (2002). *Transforming the Field: Critical Antiracist and Anti-oppressive Perspectives for the Human Services Practicum*. Fernwood Publishing, Halifax.

Schon, D. A. (2003). *The Reflective Practitioner*. Ashgate, Aldershot, Hants.

Tryssenaar, J. & Perkins, J. (2001). 'From Student to Therapist: Exploring the First Year of Practice'. *American Journal of Occupational Therapy*, 55: 19–27.

Further Reading

Best, D. (2005). 'Exploring the Roles Of The Clinical Educator'. In M. Rose & D. Best (eds), *Transforming Practice through Clinical Education, Professional Supervision and Mentoring*. Elsevier, Sydney: 45–9.

Courtney, M. (2008). *Inside my Job: Insider Information for Early Career Occupational Therapists*. Department of Human Services, Victoria, Melbourne.

Etheridge, S. A. (2007). 'Learning to Think Like a Nurse: Stories from New Nurse Graduates'. *Journal of Continuing Education in Nursing*, 38: 24–30.

Kilminster, S. M. & Jolly, B. C. (2000). 'Effective Supervision in Clinical Practice Settings: A Literature Review'. *Medical Education*, 34: 827–40.

Lee, S. & Mackenzie, L. (2003). 'Starting Out in Rural New South Wales: The Experiences of New Graduate Occupational Therapists'. *Australian Journal of Rural Health*, 11: 36–43.

Miller, P. A., Solomon, P., Giacomini, M. & Abelson, J. (2005). 'Experience of Novice Physiotherapists Adapting to their Role in Acute Care Hospitals'. *Physiotherapy Canada*, 57: 145–153.

Rugg, S. (1996). 'The Transition of Junior Occupational Therapists to Clinical Practice: Report of a Preliminary Study'. *British Journal of Occupational Therapy*, 59(4), 165–8.

Sweeney, G., Webley, P. & Treacher, A. (2001). 'Supervision in Occupational Therapy, Part 2: The Supervisee's Dilemma'. *British Journal of Occupational Therapy*, 64(8): 380–6.

Thomas, Y., Penman, M. & Williamson, P. (2005). 'Australian and New Zealand Fieldwork: Charting the Territory for Future Practice'. *Australian Occupational Therapy Journal*, 52: 78–81.

CHAPTER 24
STARTING OUT IN SUPERVISION

Liz Beddoe

LEARNING OUTCOMES

After reading this chapter, you should be able to:
- reflect on becoming a supervisor: the next step in your journey
- know the purpose of field supervision and the supervisor's key tasks
- discuss fieldwork supervision
- reflect on working with power and difference.

KEY TERMS

Fieldwork education
Levels of student supervision
Personal authority
Placement contract
Professional authority
Reflection
Role authority

INTRODUCTION: BECOMING A SUPERVISOR

As a new graduate you will be busily involved in establishing yourself as a competent health professional, fully engaged in the tasks that process entails: you may be working towards meeting competency goals or logging hours to meet the requirements established by your profession before you can be fully registered. Sooner or later you will be asked to take on supervising a student for a fieldwork placement in your workplace. Pereira (2008: 247) acknowledges the challenge of taking on student supervision of occupational therapy students in a busy rural setting:

> My own apprehension was further challenged by supervising two students at the same time. How was I going to manage my very busy caseload demands, supervising students and maintaining quality in my assessments and interventions?

Supervising students is often a precursor to taking on clinical supervision of other health professionals. This chapter focuses mainly on the provision of supervision for fieldwork placement students, but also offers many ideas that will assist you as starting health professionals. So what is the purpose of supervision and what are the main tasks and responsibilities of the fieldwork educator?

Professional (or clinical) supervision is a practice that is gaining strength within professions, linked to quality assurance efforts to ensure that health professionals are fit and competent to practise. The components of such legislation have led to professions developing requirements for ongoing professional education and development. Ferguson (2005: 294) provides a broad definition of supervision that applies across disciplines:

> Professional supervision is a process between someone called a supervisor and another referred to as the supervisee. It is usually aimed at enhancing the helping effectiveness of the person supervised. It may include acquisition of practical skills, mastery of theoretical or technical knowledge, personal development at the client/therapist interface and professional development.

In student supervision, the primary purpose is to ensure that students have the opportunity to reflect on the direct service they observe, practise specific skills, learn about assessing service user needs, understand the challenges of practice and develop self-management skills in real clinical settings, as shown in Figure 24.1.

THE FOCUS OF SUPERVISION

Supervision within fieldwork education is a structured, interactive and collaborative process that takes place within a purposeful professional relationship. Supervision involves observation, monitoring, coaching and supporting students during their fieldwork placement. Supervision will focus on all four aspects of the student's

Figure 24.1: The focus of supervision

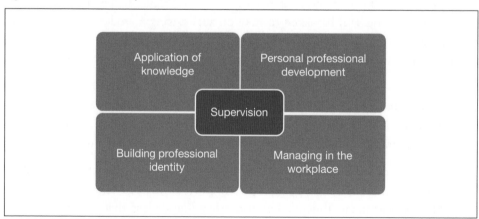

Source: Beddoe 2009

professional development, as shown in Figure 24.1, and may include examination and exploration of the elements shown in Figure 24.2.

As you can see in Figure 24.2, there are some fairly weighty matters to be addressed in supervision, and all this in the context of an exciting but often stressful fieldwork placement. It is in part because of this complexity that the supervisory relationship between the student and fieldwork educator is of major importance. The fieldwork educator has a dual role within this relationship (Beddoe 2000). She or he must simultaneously motivate the student's professional development while managing a busy clinical practice load. There are issues of service user safety and organisational administrative imperatives to be completed. An effective relationship must be established between the student and the fieldwork educator to provide a vehicle for learning, with a strong focus on the tasks of building professional identity and managing the demands of the workplace in professional practice.

The other major contribution of the supervision relationship is to your student's learning, both about the nature of supervision and about managing oneself in professional relationships and developing reflective practice, both as an individual health professional and a member of a team. As health professionals, we manage many relationships with supervisors, managers and co-workers, those in other disciplines as well as the service users. In these professional relationships we give and receive feedback, advocate for service user and patient needs and deal with tensions and conflict. The supervision relationship provides a safe place in which

Figure 24.2: The focus of the fieldwork placement supervision

1 Application of knowledge	• Applying theory in practice • Practising clinical skills • Identifying cultural, social, technical, ethical and emotional aspects of practice
2 Personal professional development	• Building skills for self-management and self-care • Making effective use of supervision • Growing awareness of personal values, attitudes and beliefs
3 Building professional identity	• Articulating professional roles and boundaries • Fostering inquiry • Developing critical thinking • Applying ethical principles
4 Managing in the workplace	• Managing service delivery tasks • Meeting agency requirements • Becoming a good colleague • Learning to work in multidisciplinary teams

Source: Beddoe 2009

these interpersonal skills can be developed. As the fieldwork educator, you need to balance support and advocacy functions with teaching and assessment.

As the fieldwork educator, you stand in the middle of a 'tangle of relationships and face the demanding task of being both an assessor and an advocate for the student', often in the organisational context (Beddoe 2000: 44). Three phases of the field supervision relationship and the key tasks in each can be identified, as summarised in Table 24.1. Each phase is discussed in detail below.

Phase 1: Building the supervision relationship

One of the immediate tasks facing the new fieldwork educator is the application of discipline-specific skills in a new dimension of practice. There are four main elements to this process of translation:

- the ability to work with the service user or patient at arm's length instead of hands on, meanwhile addressing the perceptions and reactions of the student
- the recognition of the centrality of teaching and learning in supervision if it is to be effective in supporting students and health professionals to achieve their learning goals
- thoughtful planning of activities to promote confidence
- developing an understanding of the separation of the *process* of supervision from the *role* of fieldwork educator.

The process of becoming a fieldwork educator involves developing the ability to stand back from using one's own knowledge and skills actively with service users or patients, and instead taking a role one step back in order to facilitate development in the student. There are benefits for both fieldwork educator and student in this process.

Table 24.1: The course of the supervision relationship

Phase	Key tasks
Relationship building	<ul><li>Pre-placement planning</li><li>Orientation to workplace</li><li>Building rapport</li><li>Clarifying mutual expectations of supervision</li><li>Exploration of practice styles and theoretical orientations</li></ul>
Consolidation of learning and development	<ul><li>Managing anxiety and emotions</li><li>Managing the dependence–autonomy continuum</li><li>Exploring the professional environment</li><li>Strengthening the feedback process</li><li>Reviewing learning goals and achievement</li></ul>
Review and ending	<ul><li>Evaluating the relationship</li><li>Managing impacts of assessment and endings</li><li>Reviewing placement learning and achievement of goals</li><li>Saying farewell</li></ul>

Urdang (1999) studied the experience of a group of social work practitioners as they began to supervise students on placement. A key finding was that fieldwork educators' self-esteem increased, both through mastery of a new skill and the validation, through teaching and supervising the student, of their own knowledge base and practice. Most fieldwork educators indicated that work as a fieldwork educator increased both their self-awareness and capacity to analyse their work, much of which had become automatic (Urdang 1999).

Nothing influences the effectiveness of supervision more than the quality of the supervision relationship (Bond & Holland 1998: 77). When you begin to prepare for your fieldwork educator role, it is very useful to explore your own development and consider what it is you have to offer a student. New fieldwork educators often feel ambivalent, as they 'simultaneously relish the opportunity to influence a new health professional, whilst fearing the student's critical gaze' (Beddoe 2000: 45). You will also be evaluated during field education: by the student, by the educational institution and by your senior colleagues in your workplace. You may suddenly feel less confident about your own practice, and be worried that you are not good enough for the task of supervision. In your own supervision you can reflect on your personal experience as a student and the aspects of good supervision you want to emulate, and the things you might want to improve upon or even avoid. You may wish to write about this experience in a reflective way (see Reflection 24.1).

REFLECTION 24.1

Reflection for the fieldwork educator

> Far from beginning with a clean slate, the new supervisor will be a blend of all that has gone before in their personal and professional lives (Brown & Bourne 1996: 19).

Write a brief personal professional biography. Describe your motivation to enter your profession; your key personal values; the theories and intervention that have shaped your practice; the model(s) of practice you most favour; and your personal perspective on the nature and direction of your profession.

Add to this a brief description of your experiences in your own fieldwork placements, noting the successes and challenges you faced, and how you managed your anxieties.

Then either on your own, or with your supervisor, address the following questions:

1 What worked best in your fieldwork placement supervision when you were a student?
2 If there were difficulties for you, what were they, and how might you avoid them in providing supervision for a student?
3 What are your worries or fears about the student supervision?
4 What are your hopes for this new aspect of your professional career?
5 How will you go about building an effective, enjoyable relationship in supervision?

THINK AND LINK 24.1

Reflecting on your experience of fieldwork placement when you were a student is a good starting point to understanding yourself as a fieldwork educator. Together with the reflection above, refer also to Chapter 23. Chapter 23 discusses and provides reflections about the transition from student to fieldwork educator.

A student in one of my courses once asked, 'When does it stop? Should my supervisor get supervision too? And her supervisor ...?' This may seem absurd as long as we are influenced by an image of a hierarchy. Instead, it may be more attractive to see the process as a chain of supervision relationships by which health professionals are linked to each other to nurture safe and effective practice in health and social care.

Seek ongoing professional education for your role as a fieldwork educator, including attending seminars, studying formal and higher qualifications in supervision or fieldwork education or refresher courses. Shared activities with other health professionals who also work with students can provide additional learning opportunities for fieldwork educator and student alike. Learning to work alongside other professionals in healthcare settings is an important aspect of fieldwork education. As a fieldwork educator, you can play a significant part in ensuring your student has opportunities to work alongside other disciplines and learn how each has a role, perspective and, often, professional culture and expectations about how to relate to service users and others. This provides rich opportunities for learning, both from other bodies of knowledge and from the experience of teamwork (Smith & Anderson 2008).

THINK AND LINK 24.2

Continuing professional education is important to all health professionals. Chapter 23 discusses continuing professional education from your learning needs. Learning to work alongside other professionals is also important for service delivery. Chapter 16 considers working in teams and interprofessional learning.

The Leicester model of interprofessional education suggests these important aspects of working together: the immersion into patient and professional experiences; developing understanding of different professional perspectives, theory and policies; and joint work to find solutions to problems identified (Smith & Anderson 2008: 769).

It is important to remember that students are not all the same; many will be young and still developing their personal skills and belief systems; some will be mature students and some may be training in a new profession and having to adjust to being a novice again. Students may also feel anxious that their fieldwork education experience will contain challenges, especially from service users and other professionals. Students are often very anxious about exposing their lack of

> ### Case Study 24.1 | Let's do this together
>
> Ashwaq and Miranda are your two social work students. Their placement coincides
> with the fieldwork placement of Robert and Philippa, who are nursing students. The
> setting is a busy community health team attached to a children's hospital. You and
> Christina, the nurse educator, are both relatively new to your fieldwork education role,
> and feel there will be benefits in sharing ideas and even planning to bring the students
> together. You get together before the students arrive and plan some joint activities.
>
> At the halfway stage, you and Christina decide to compare notes about how your
> fieldwork education roles are going. You find that you have one student who is hard
> to engage in one-to-one supervision. You use your peer supervision relationship
> to rehearse some ideas, and agree to try a joint supervision session to see if this is
> helpful. In this session some discussion of patients known to all the students results in
> an interesting and lively debate about roles and approaches. At the end of the session
> the students agree to meet without you to discuss their projects.
>
> #### Questions
>
> 1   Would you consider this to be a successful supervision session?
> 2   What outcomes are positive from your point of view? Are there any negative
>   outcomes?

experience and skill as they test out their skills in new situations, and even very
confident students may approach the practice environment feeling uncertain about
their abilities. It can be helpful for you as a new fieldwork educator to share some of
your thoughts and feelings, and perhaps to share some of your own journey from
student to professional to fieldwork educator. Being open to an exploration of mutual
hopes and concerns will help build a constructive and trusting relationship.

Clarifying expectations

The *placement contract* in fieldwork education addresses the specific expectations
between the student, the supervisor and the education institution. This agreement
will have addressed practical matters, the timeframe of the placement, agency
conduct rules, arrangements for supervision and backup during the absence of the
fieldwork educator. An additional discussion of the boundaries of the supervision
relationship itself, especially the role of support, will be needed. Remind your
student that old and new personal issues may be triggered by stressful situations
encountered in practice, and that you can support her or him when seeking
appropriate professional help elsewhere. It may be useful to discuss specific
examples of such possibilities and how they would be dealt with in supervision.

In checking out your students' understanding of the role and purpose of supervision, you could direct your student to some reading about how to make the most of supervision. Davys (2007) suggests that the critical success factors include: understanding the purpose of supervision; knowing what you want from your fieldwork educator; taking an active role in negotiating a contract; and preparation, active participation and willingness to be open and reflective in each supervision session (Davys 2007: 28–39).

Phase 2: Consolidation of learning and development

Once the supervision relationship is established and you have started to work together, there is a period of consolidation when you build on the good foundations laid down earlier. One of the many differences between student supervision and supervision of qualified practitioners is that all the work of relationship building and beginning the practice learning process needs to happen very quickly because of the short timeframe of the fieldwork placement. Several key elements contribute to the consolidation of a positive relationship to support student learning (see Figure 24.3).

Figure 24.3: Student and practitioner supervision: key differences

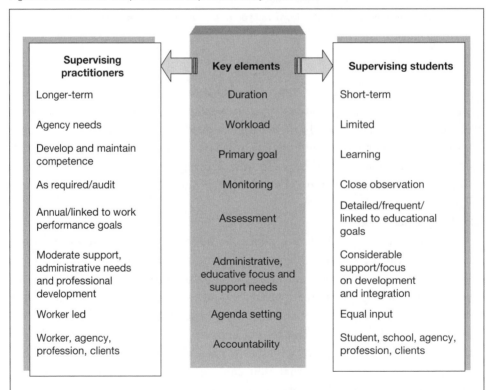

Supervising practitioners	Key elements	Supervising students
Longer-term	Duration	Short-term
Agency needs	Workload	Limited
Develop and maintain competence	Primary goal	Learning
As required/audit	Monitoring	Close observation
Annual/linked to work performance goals	Assessment	Detailed/frequent/ linked to educational goals
Moderate support, administrative needs and professional development	Administrative, educative focus and support needs	Considerable support/focus on development and integration
Worker led	Agenda setting	Equal input
Worker, agency, profession, clients	Accountability	Student, school, agency, profession, clients

Source: Davys & Beddoe 2000

Table 24.2: Supervisee levels of independence

Level	Dependency to autonomy	Features of level
1	Dependency	*Anxiety:* the supervisee needs structure, rehearsal of tasks, encouragement and supportive feedback
2	Fluctuation between dependency and greater independence	*Initial anxiety reduced:* the supervisee may undertake some tasks with confidence, but lacks flexibility. Focus improved, and may start to question practices and the supervisor's authority
3	Proficiency and confident independence	*Greater confidence and proficiency in most professional tasks:* some flexibility and creativity in unexpected situations. More self-directed and reflective without prompting
4	Professional autonomy	*Greater insight:* deepening awareness of self-in-action in practice. Uses supervision to explore ideas to extend repertoire of treatment ideas and interventions

The themes of the middle phase of supervision include consolidation of learning; experiencing feedback; and managing self in the workplace. During this phase, some students may experience conflict between their need for their fieldwork educator to be in charge and their emerging sense of professional competence. Therefore some will seek greater autonomy. For others, lack of confidence may mean they require considerable support to undertake even relatively simple tasks. Good preparation for undertaking discipline-specific activities, with clear parameters, opportunities for reflection and regular review are all essential components in building student confidence. Continuous opportunities for feedback and student-led reflection can contribute to a growing sense of accomplishment and personal development. Ideally, during this phase students can experience some independence while appreciating constructive input and oversight of their work.

A *stages model of supervision* utilises a developmental approach to these issues. Hawkins and Shohet (2006: 70–5) have described four levels of supervisee development to map the learning journey. Table 24.2 outlines the stages of supervision in relation to a dependency–autonomy continuum as students learn to become more autonomous.

It is, however, important to remember that a limitation of developmental models is that they can impose generalised expectations. Each student will be unique. A mature student such as Nita (Case Study 24.2) will build her own pathway. Initially anxious in a new role, she finds her voice, and draws on old skills to show initiative, even if a little prematurely from her fieldwork educator's point of view.

Case Study 24.2	Nita

Nita is a mature physiotherapy student on fieldwork placement with Mary, who has been registered for five years. Nita has changed course at the age of 40, having practised as a registered nurse. Mary works in a very busy outpatient service in a large teaching hospital. One of the features of this setting is that, as well as seeing 'booked' patients, it also admits urgent assessments at very short notice when there is pressure to achieve early discharge. Initially Nita, who lacks confidence, is a very anxious student, and in the first two weeks of her fieldwork placement checks everything three times with Mary. Every time Mary turns around Nita is there with a new question, some days with so many competing demands that Mary feels overwhelmed and thinks, 'Why did I agree to take a mature student?'

She perseveres, and through a process of trial and error finds that Nita's confidence grows through having a step-by-step written plan for even simple activities. In the last week of the fieldwork placement, Mary is very surprised to return from her lunch break to find Nita has independently started an assessment with a patient referred from a ward. She is motivated by a wish to be helpful and prove herself, but without waiting for Mary's approval, she has changed the appointment board in the clinic and liaised with the nurse managers about the rescheduling of appointments. Mary acknowledges Nita's enthusiasm and initiative, and gently reminds Nita of her role and the limits of her autonomy. Nita laughs and says, 'Oops! My inner staff-nurse just popped up!'

Question

The line between autonomy and dependency can clash with role boundaries about what is the student role. In Nita's case, was it autonomy, dependency or role boundaries that were the issue when she organised a patient assessment independently?

Managing authority and power

A key to the effective and non-oppressive use of power and authority in supervision is the clear understanding of the differences between the *role* and the *process* of supervision. The supervisory role is imbued with authority and power. Both fieldwork educators and students bring to this new relationship their ideas, beliefs and the 'baggage' of previous experiences of authority. Both may fear being 'found out' as having less knowledge than they should. Both need to be able to create a place where it is all right not to know: 'both supervisee and supervisor need to feel that they can occupy this place. Paradoxically, it is from this place that deep understanding and fresh insight can come' (Pickvance 1997: 141). Case Study 24.2 could have ended badly, if (a) Nita had been offended and had retreated to anxiety, or (b) Mary had not addressed the issues but had still felt uncomfortable.

Hughes and Pengelly (1997: 168–9) distinguish between three sources of authority in supervision: *role authority*, conferred by the organisation and the university; *professional authority*, earned through credible practice of knowledge and skill; and *personal authority*. Personal authority stems from the individual's demeanour and ability within professional relationships to exercise the other two forms. Too much reliance on any of these sources of authority leads to conflict in supervision. Too little exercise of legitimate authority can lead to collusion and the collapse of safe practice. Students need to know that their fieldwork educator has the confidence to exercise authority if needed in order to challenge unsafe practice. Coming to terms with the authority and influencing power in your new role can produce tensions that might still need to be resolved. In the new role there is a partial shift away from direct discipline-specific work toward changed relationships that need to be forged with colleagues, managers, educators and students. New fieldwork educators often feel that they are exposed to a critical gaze from all sides.

THINK AND LINK 24.3

Chapter 12 discusses models of supervision. It may be relevant to you to review this chapter now.

Emotional awareness

Supervision is part of the constellation of resources that health professionals can call upon to manage the anxiety and uncertainty generated by clinical practice, especially because of the current emphasis on risk management. In many professions there are contradictory trends: on the one hand, health professionals may feel pressure to undertake evidence-based practice; on the other, they are urged to trust their feelings and listen to hunches. Supervision provides a space in which these competing voices can be heard and attended to, thus allowing room for the safe expression of feelings. If supervision provides opportunities for the safe expression and exploration of these feelings, they may contribute to growth and provide a rich source of information about service users' strengths and vulnerabilities. Supervision that recognises health professionals' emotional responses as valid and significant may provide a key to safe practice. If students can tolerate experiencing and thinking about their emotional responses to service users, they will find in them a rich source of information about some of the themes and issues in the lives of their service users and patients (Hughes & Pengelly 1997: 79–91).

Many barriers prevent the exploration of feelings in supervision:
- fieldwork educators may be too busy and task focused to take time to listen and reflect

- fieldwork educators may think that feelings are messy and unwelcome, and should be minimised in discussion of cases, especially if they wish to be perceived as scientific and objective
- feelings may be perceived as a sign of weakness, making fieldwork educators feel uncomfortable about negative feelings about their clients or patients; we are supposed to respect people unconditionally, but we may be fearful about facing unpleasant and abusive service users
- fieldwork educators fear their 'hunches' might prejudice service users' rights.

Hughes and Pengelly (1997: 176) note that containment in supervision is often used as if it were a means of control: 'keeping the lid on'. They prefer to think of it as 'the process in which authority becomes translated into effective interaction'. Most students want more from supervision than empathetic hand-patting. In reflective supervision, taking the lid off is essential, not to expose or treat the student, but in order to explore the impact and the implications of strong feelings on practice. In dealing with the emotional content of supervision, feelings may be subject to *accommodation* or, in a contrasting approach, the *exploration* of feelings may lead to more reflective practice, as shown in Table 24.3. In an exploratory process, feelings can be both accepted and valued as a rich source of information and ideas. It is possible to experiment widely with a range of strategies that can be constructed, challenged and rehearsed within a safe space. If feelings are merely accommodated, then the fieldwork educator may rely on prescriptive approaches to avoid too many difficult questions.

Where does the professional boundary finish and stray over into the personal? A general rule of thumb recommended by most is that supervision should focus on personal things only when they have a direct impact on the work. Supervision can bring into focus all the key elements of interaction with clients: our feelings and use of self in our work, our understanding of and reactions to the experiences of others, our skills, our knowledge base and our ability to manage all of these in a helping relationship. A brief case scenario may illustrate this point.

Table 24.3: Coping with uncertainty

Accommodation supervision style	Exploration supervision style
<ul><li>Seeking for 'known' things</li><li>Rules for action</li><li>Prescriptive interventions</li><li>Task-orientated practice</li><li>Blueprints to determine action</li><li>Obsession with predetermined outcomes</li><li>Low tolerance of feelings</li><li>Feelings to be tidied away and minimised</li></ul>	<ul><li>Accepting there is no absolute known</li><li>Seeking more questions</li><li>Exploration of uncertainty</li><li>Reflective practice and willingness to experiment</li><li>No fixed expectations of outcome</li><li>Open exploration of feelings</li><li>Feelings as evidence for practice</li></ul>

Case Study 24.3 | **Josie**

Josie is a 28-year-old social work student who has just started a 16-week placement in a busy surgical service. Today she comes to supervision with a very difficult issue to talk about. At your suggestion, Soli, a senior practitioner, has invited her to co-work in a new case just referred to the service. The patient is Lucy, a 49-year-old woman with four children aged between five and fifteen, who has just been given a diagnosis of breast cancer with an uncertain prognosis. Josie's mother had surgery for breast cancer just one year ago. She is currently well, but the family is still fearful about the future. Josie is dreading going to meet Lucy. She really wants the opportunity to co-work with Soli, but her eyes filled with tears when she read the referral. She wonders whether she'll cope. She's frightened that when she sees Lucy she'll be reminded of her mother, and that her grief will come to the surface.

Josie is faced with painful issues. First, she needs to be supported for being open about her distress in her supervision session. Being able to be honest and vulnerable is important for learning. In this situation it's really important that Josie is able to talk about her feelings and shed some tears if necessary. It is equally important that her fieldwork educator has the ability to listen, hold her distress and let her express her feelings.

The second part of this supervision encounter will be working out with Josie whether she can work with Lucy and her family in a support role alongside Soli, or whether it is too soon for her to deal with a situation so close to her own heart. Her fieldwork educator has the responsibility to help her talk through this situation, and together to come up with an approach that affirms Josie's emerging self-management skills.

Key supervision questions for you as Josie's fieldwork educator

1   What do you need to focus on in the exploration of this issue in supervision?
2   What strengths does Josie's personal experience give her in working with Lucy? What can make her vulnerable?
3   What are similar aspects in Josie's story, and what are different?
4   How might Lucy's practical and emotional support needs be different from those of Josie, because of her culture, her socioeconomic situation and her family structure?
5   What steps do you take next? What support do you need to give Josie? What resources do you need?

Ethical practice in complex contexts

Supervision is often seen as the site for ethical teaching. This would be fine if ethics were a simple matter. However, as you may already have learned in your professional journey, they are more likely to be messy and confusing. Some recent changes have further challenged how professionals operate (Bagnall 1998):

- professionals are more subject to the scrutiny of regulators, a critical media and the public
- there is greater acceptance of social and cultural diversity in our society
- there is greater tolerance of contradictions in the moral dimensions of our professional and personal lives
- rigid rule books have in part been replaced by contextualised ethics
- situational ethics take cognisance of specific cultural contexts.

As a consequence, new supervisors may feel a deep sense of insecurity about what the rules are. To some extent, this may leave individuals without a protective cloak of clear unequivocal ethical rules (Bagnall 1998: 83). The diversity of perspectives may be confusing, and values that seemed unimpeachable may be contested. Fieldwork educators can provide guidance by fostering the following attributes: valuing diversity; providing empathetic responsiveness to the lived realities of others; recognising that each professional encounter is unique; and teaching skills for negotiating complex and contested decisions. Students need to be 'able to accept and deal with uncertainty and ambiguity, and the absence of cookbook solutions' and to 'learn that when moral conflicts or ethical dilemmas arise, they can only be resolved through dialogue and a process of moral reasoning' (Gray & Gibbons 2007: 224).

THINK AND LINK 24.4

Chapter 20 discusses working ethically in context. This chapter will add more information to ethical questions which may arise in supervision.

Phase 3: Review and ending

The final phase of the student supervision relationship involves tasks of closure and evaluation. The process of assessment may dominate all other considerations at this phase. During this phase, you as the fieldwork educator need to assess honestly and report on the student's achievement according to the formal requirements of the fieldwork placement, while continuing to facilitate learning in a supportive environment. Anxiety about this can be reduced by continuous feedback and review throughout the placement. It may be useful for you, as the fieldwork educator, to make an effort to balance this preoccupation with some attention to locating the assessment as a milestone in the student's development. While the assessment may be, in the placement context, summative, the student is engaged in continuous learning, and will ultimately take this experience into a professional career in which he or she will experience many appraisals.

THINK AND LINK 24.5

Assessment is a key aspect of fieldwork placements from the student's perspective. Chapter 14 discusses assessment in fieldwork settings, and Chapter 17 discusses what happens when students fail.

Two further tasks complete the fieldwork placement. The first task is to review how well the supervision relationship has assisted the student's learning. This should include feedback from both participants about the achievement of the learning outcomes and the experience of supervision itself. The second task is to undertake farewells, with attention to both formal and informal processes. The fieldwork placement, often a major experience for students, will shape some of their perceptions of the profession and how it is conducted.

SUMMARY

Becoming a fieldwork educator is more than a rite of passage for a health professional. It requires the management of some key tasks in re-visioning practice with a different focus. It requires individual consideration of identity, culture and the processing of your own relevant personal experience; for example, the experience of being supervised, the experience of power and authority and the development of complex teaching and learning skills.

DISCUSSION QUESTIONS

1   Have you thought of activities to support interprofessional learning?
2   Do you have a plan for your own support?
3   Are there potential benefits from working with fieldwork educators from other disciplines to the benefit of your students and your own practice?

References

Bagnall, R. (1998). 'Professional Codes of Conduct: A Critique with Implications for Continuing Professional Education'. In D. Dymock (ed.), *CPE 98: Meeting the Challenge of Change*. Department of Administration and Training, University of New England: 81–91.

Beddoe, L. (2000). 'The Supervisory Relationship'. In L. Cooper & L. Briggs (eds), *Fieldwork in the Human Services*. Allen & Unwin, Sydney: 41–54.

Bond, M. & Holland, S. (1998). *Skills of Clinical Supervision for Nurses*. Open University Press, Buckingham.

Brown, A. & Bourne, I. (1996). *The Social Work Supervisor*. Open University Press, Buckingham.

Davys, A. (2007). 'Active Participation in Supervision: A Supervisee's Guide'. In D. Wepa (ed.), *Clinical Supervision in Aotearoa/New Zealand: A Health Perspective*. Pearson Education, Auckland: 26–42.

Davys, A. & Beddoe, L. (2000). Supervision of Students: A Map and a Model for the Decade to Come. *Social Work Education*, 19(5): 438–49.

Ferguson, K. (2005). 'Professional Supervision'. In M. Rose & D. Best (eds), *Transforming Practice through Clinical Education, Professional Supervision and Mentoring*. Elsevier Churchill Livingstone, Edinburgh: 293–307.

Gray, M. & Gibbons, J. (2007). 'There are No Answers, Only Choices: Teaching Ethical Decision Making in Social Work'. *Australian Social Work*, 60(2): 222–38.

Hawkins, P. & Shohet, R. (2006). *Supervision in the Helping Professions* (3rd edn). Open University Press, Maidenhead.

Hughes, L. & Pengelly, P. (1997). *Staff Supervision in a Turbulent Environment: Managing Process and Task in Front-line Services*. Jessica Kingsley, London.

Pereira, R. (2008). 'Learning and Being a First-Time Student Supervisor: Challenges and Triumphs'. *Australian Journal of Rural Health*, 16: 247–8.

Pickvance, D. (1997). 'Becoming a Supervisor'. In G. Shipton (ed.), *Supervision of Psychotherapy and Counselling: Making a Place to Think*. Open University Press, Buckingham: 131–42.

Smith, R. & Anderson, L. (2008). 'Interprofessional Learning: Aspiration or Achievement?' *Social Work Education*, 27(7): 759–76.

Urdang, E. (1999). 'Becoming a Field Instructor: A Key Experience in Professional Development'. *Clinical Supervisor*, 18(1): 85–103.

CHAPTER 25
HEALTH WORKFORCE RECRUITMENT

Adrian Schoo and Karen Stagnitti

LEARNING OUTCOMES

After reading this chapter, you should be able to:
- understand some of the links between fieldwork placement and workforce recruitment
- discuss the uniqueness of rural workforce recruitment and rural fieldwork placements
- understand fieldwork placements in view of future recruitment of staff.

KEY TERMS

Fieldwork educator supervision
Final fieldwork placements
Graduate
Orientation
Rural health settings
Workforce recruitment

INTRODUCTION

This chapter outlines the links between fieldwork placements that you have undertaken and the jobs that you apply for. *Workforce recruitment* is when you apply for a position and hope to be recruited to the position. Workforce recruitment is important in both metropolitan and rural settings. However, rural settings have a unique set of considerations, which are highlighted in this chapter. The objectives of the chapter are to establish the influence of the fieldwork placement in graduates' choice of workplace setting; the issues around rural placement and workforce recruitment; and what workplaces can do to encourage students to return as graduates to work in their institutions or centres.

FIELDWORK AND STUDENTS' CHOICE OF WORKPLACE SETTING

Fieldwork placement and the timing of the placement have been associated with students' choice of workplace setting after graduation. A study by Doherty and colleagues (2009) found that occupational therapy graduates' decisions to apply for particular positions were strongly related to their fieldwork placement experiences. For example, they found that a student's experience in a nontraditional placement was significant in a student's choice of a community-based career (Doherty et al. 2009). The connection between where students undertake fieldwork placement and their strong preference to practise in a particular area is not a new concept. Crowe and Mackenzie (2002) also reported fieldwork placements to be the most important factor influencing a student's decisions to pursue an area of practice upon graduation. Of particular note, fieldwork placements completed in the latter part of a student's degree are most influential in persuading the student to choose a certain area of practice. Fieldwork placements undertaken near the end of a degree, together with a positive experience at the fieldwork placement, effective partnerships between the placement and university and a student's sense of effectiveness in the area are the most influential factors determining speciality choice of graduates (Ezersky et al. 1989; Frank 2008). The evidence that fieldwork placements have the potential to strongly influence practice preference of new graduates provides opportunities for work settings to attract new staff to their establishment. The conditions for a positive learning experience in fieldwork placements have been covered elsewhere in this book.

THINK AND LINK 25.1

Preparing for your fieldwork placement was covered in Chapter 1. Students who prepare well for a placement begin in a less stressed state. Chapter 13 presents valuable activities for the students to enable them to get the best out of their placement.

REFLECTION 25.1

The last placement
Consider your last fieldwork placement undertaken as a student.
1 Was the placement a positive experience?
2 Did you feel effective in the work you undertook at the fieldwork placement?
3 Was the fieldwork placement influential in where you work now? Why?

RURAL PLACEMENTS AND WORKFORCE RECRUITMENT

Since a student's positive experience of a fieldwork placement can influence practice choice, one strategy that is used to encourage students to consider a career in a rural or remote area is for students to undertake a rural fieldwork placement. For students undertaking a rural fieldwork placement, the conditions that contribute to an effective placement differ from placements carried out within the student's familiar geographical region.

THINK AND LINK 25.2

Rural and remote settings can be challenging for some students. Chapter 10 discusses what to prepare for in rural and remote fieldwork settings. Refer to Chapter 10 for more information about these settings.

Students who experienced a rural placement, and who were surveyed after their fieldwork placement (Burch & Newman 2007), listed the top five most important points that had an impact on their overall experience as:

- the skill of the fieldwork educator in giving a positive learning experience
- the experience of combining a variety of work, including patient access, assessment and treatment, with a variety of clinical conditions
- fieldwork educators and mentors who were professional, gave peer support and were friendly
- the presence of infrastructure support, such as affordable and available accommodation
- the opportunity to see a variety of parts of Australia while learning about rural health issues within the local context.

In Burch and Newman's (2007) survey, positive aspects of the rural fieldwork placement were counterbalanced by concerns raised by the students. Students' concerns included:

- the quality and costs of accommodation, because rural fieldwork placements require a student to relocate for a short period of time. The experience of accommodation can be positive or negative. For some students, paying for accommodation during the fieldwork placement was an onerous burden
- the expenses incurred during fieldwork placement, together with loss of income and being unable to work
- isolation and separation from family and friends and usual sources of social support
- commitments of family and partner, partner's needs and housing commitments
- isolation and distance from the university or teaching site, with the student sometimes missing lectures (the sense of isolation was exacerbated if the student experienced a poor learning experience)
- students requiring clarification of what they should expect, with more information on the caseload they would be working with (Burch & Newman 2007).

A government strategy to help encourage health professionals into rural and remote areas has been established by the university departments of rural health. There are 11 UDRHs in Australia at the time of writing. While each UDRH offers a variety of activities and supports within its student placement program, there are common elements between them, including placement coordination; facilitating accommodation; orientation, welcome and preparation; cultural training; clinical experience; supervisor support; student support and access to resources (Burch & Newman 2007).

UDRHs in Australia use students' fieldwork placement as a way to attract health professionals to rural areas to address the maldistribution of personnel between metropolitan and rural areas. Some professionals in the field have raised concern about whether young graduates are provided with professional support and career options to keep them working in rural areas (Schoo et al. 2008). Consequently, the challenge is to provide rural professional support and career options that are comparable to those offered in urban areas.

In an endeavour to establish whether rural placements actually translate into graduates seeking jobs in rural areas, a study of 429 allied health and nursing students showed that, after controlling for rural background, the value and duration of rural fieldwork placement were significantly associated with rural employment after graduation (Playford et al. 2006). Although having a rural background influences graduates' choices of commencing careers in a rural area, rural fieldwork placement is an important strategy that can be used to influence students' intention to take up a rural position. Several universities have started to recruit from and train in rural areas, and so far the effects are very positive. For example, more than 70 per cent of the pharmacists trained at Charles Sturt University remain practising in rural townships (Barton 2006).

Survey results for nursing students' pre- and post-rural fieldwork placement found a 12 per cent increase in the number of graduates intending to seek rural employment (Courtney et al. 2002). Interestingly, more than 30 per cent of the nursing students who opted for rural placement had no previous experience of a rural lifestyle, and more than 50 per cent of this subgroup indicated their intention to seek rural employment after their rural fieldwork placement (Courtney et al. 2002). In medicine, positive rural fieldwork placement and education have been shown to increase interest in rural health practice (Australian Medical Workforce Advisory Committee 2005; Eley & Baker 2005). For a rural fieldwork placement to be positive, it must be matched with a positive fieldwork environment in order to increase interest in rural practice (Eley & Baker 2005). Hence, equipping rural health professionals with adequate supervisory skills is an essential strategy to increase the chance that students have a positive rural experience.

THINK AND LINK 25.3

For a new fieldwork educator, supervising his or her first student can be daunting. Chapters 23 and 24 discuss different aspects of the transition from student to fieldwork supervisor, with Chapter 24 discussing in detail the three phases of supervision.

WHAT WORKPLACES CAN DO TO ENCOURAGE STUDENTS TO RETURN AFTER FIELDWORK PLACEMENTS

A good work-integrated learning experience is underpinned by the opportunities provided by the fieldwork placement, as well as the skills of individual fieldwork educators and relationships between the university and the placement (Burch & Newman 2007; Frank 2008). The role of the fieldwork educator, orientation to the setting and specific placement characteristics, such as caseload, are aspects of a placement that may encourage students to return. Consider John's story below.

Case Study 25.1	John leaves home for the country

John had never left home before. He had never been out of the city, so commencing his final fieldwork placement in a small rural town 100 kilometres from his home filled him with trepidation. He had many misgivings. He would have to take leave from his permanent part-time job, he wouldn't see his friends each week, he had no family support where he was going and he didn't even have a photograph of the building where he would be working.

When John arrived on his first day, his fieldwork educator welcomed him. He was introduced to all the staff, he was orientated to the procedures, policies and routines of the service, and he was also invited to join the local basketball team while he was on placement. The team was called the Good for You. John's fieldwork educator structured supervision sessions so that he could build on his knowledge and extend his clinical reasoning skills.

After several weeks, John finished his fieldwork placement and it was time to return home. To his surprise, he was sad to leave. During his placement he had made some real bonds with the staff, he was the star of the basketball team, he was never lonely and he had had exposure to a wide variety of clients. When he finished his degree, he rang the service in the small rural town to see if there were any positions available.

Questions

1 List the factors that may have influenced John to apply for a job in this small rural town.

2 What could have happened during John's rurual placement that might have turned him against the experience? If John had had a negative experience, do you think he would have considered going back to the small town?

The fieldwork educator

Optimising the skill of the fieldwork educator is one way a workplace can influence a student to return as a graduate. Training health professionals to be a fieldwork educator is of double benefit: it assists both the professionals themselves (particularly new recruits who are inexperienced in student supervision) and the students they supervise. Rural health professionals who are supervising students:

- value the contribution they make to students' knowledge and skills
- take the opportunity to promote rural practice as a career option to their students
- enjoy the teaching role as a fieldwork educator
- are stimulated by being a supervisor and keeping up with professional development
- tend to increase their time reviewing their discipline-specific knowledge (Shannon et al. 2006; Frank 2008).

Supervision training needs are generic across the health professions, and can be taught in a multiprofessional training program (Hook & Lawson-Porter 2003). Supervisors who encourage graduates to become competent in performing routine tasks before moving them on to complex tasks requiring a high level of clinical reasoning are valued by new graduates (McInstry 2005).

Fieldwork educators should be provided with basic training, then supported and given access to specific workshops or seminars in their region. Web-based training programs exist in Australia. In Victoria, a government-funded support network for clinical supervisors with online training, which is relatively cheap, can be accessed at any time by the clinician. The Victorian support network for clinical supervisors organises in each region regular workshop meetings that are accessible by video conference (VC). It records presentations and makes it available for viewing online and facilitates discussion online.

THINK AND LINK 25.4

Chapter 23 discusses continuing professional education as important for the health professional, and that supervision of a student can also be seen as professional continuing development. Chapter 18 expands on the online technology that is available for students and fieldwork educators.

Orientation and support networks

For a previous fieldwork student returning to a workplace as a graduate, supervision and support from experienced health professionals and orientation to the workplace can help them make the transition to practice (Stagnitti et al. 2005). Frank (2008) gave an example of a university where academic nursing staff were partnered with a health service and assisted in orientation of students and new staff, which resulted in students gaining employment from their fieldwork placement as well as remaining employed by the service one year later.

Orientation is important both for fieldwork experience and for beginning a new position as a new graduate. When health professional students are orientated to the new fieldwork placement, they experience low levels of stress. New graduates have been found to adapt to the workplace more quickly if well orientated to the new workplace (Frank 2008). During John's fieldwork placement (Case Study 25.1) he was both well orientated and integrated socially by being invited to join the basketball team. Fieldwork educators who have good support networks in place are well suited to student recruitment from their regions.

Variety of caseloads

John (Case Study 25.1) also enjoyed a varied caseload on his fieldwork placement. Seeing a variety of clients is one way to introduce to John the possibilities that his health profession could offer service opportunities as well as a career path if he wants to specialise in any particular area or client condition. For example, improving rural population health outcomes requires educating professionals, particularly new graduates, as well as students from different disciplines in the prevention, detection and management of common chronic diseases (Dade Smith et al. 2006), and the need to work together as a team (Albert et al. 2004). Understanding health issues prepares students for their clinical experience and for the need to work with other professionals after graduation (Albert et al. 2004). Developing a strong interest in a particular area also adds to the excitement of going to work.

FINAL WORD

While the workplace can encourage students to return through well thought-out orientation, social networks, variety of client caseload, opening students' eyes to the possibilities of their profession, not all factors can be controlled. For students who have family nearby or partners to consider, returning to work at a previous fieldwork placement is made much easier if they know what to expect. However, students without any previous connection to an area, geographically or socially, can be encouraged to return as health professionals in practice if the fieldwork experience has been enjoyable.

REFLECTION 25.3

What would you do?

1 What factors could you build into your fieldwork educator role to encourage students to return?
2 What would you do if you had a student, who you knew you would not employ as a graduate, but who starts to ask about possible future positions?

SUMMARY

The student's experience of placements in the latter part of their degree can be very influential as to where that student chooses to practise. Rural placements have been used as a strategy to provide a positive experience to students and to encourage them to consider choosing a practice setting in a non-metropolitan region. The quality of the fieldwork experience, and hence the potential influence on student choices of where to work as a new graduate, is strongly influenced by the quality of the supervision and the fieldwork experience during the placement. Supervisor training is recommended as a way not only to build capacity in the health professions of a region but also to strengthen the possibility of a positive student experience on fieldwork.

DISCUSSION QUESTIONS

1 What influenced my choice of practice setting?
2 Which fieldwork placement experience was the most influential on my decision on where to practise?

References

Albert, E., Dalton, L., Spencer, J., Dunn, M. & Walker, J. (2004). 'Doing It Together: The Tasmanian Interdisciplinary Rural Placement Program'. *Australian Journal of Rural Health*, 12: 30–1.

Australian Medical Workforce Advisory Committee (2005). 'Doctors in Vocational Training: Rural Background and Rural Practice Intentions'. *Australian Journal of Rural Health*, 13: 14–20.

Barton, D. (2006). 'The Path to Rural Dentistry'. *PartyLine*, 27: 4.

Burch, J. & Newman, V. (2007). *University Department of Rural Health Student Placement and Satisfaction Project: Final Report*. Australian Rural Health Education Network, Canberra <http://www.Burch & Newman, 2007.org.au>

Courtney, M., Edwards, H., Smith, S. & Finlayson, K. (2002). 'The Impact of Rural Clinical Placement on Student Nurses' Employment Intentions'. *Collegian*, 9(1): 12–18.

Crowe, M. J. & Mackenzie, L. (2002). 'The Influence of Fieldwork on the Preferred Future Practice Areas of Final Year Occupational Therapy Students'. *Australian Occupational Therapy Journal*, 49(1): 25–36.

Dade Smith, J., O'Dea, K., McDermott, R., Schmidt, B. & Connors, C. (2006). 'Educating to Improve Population Health Outcomes in Chronic Disease: An Innovative Workforce Initiative across Remote, Rural and Indigenous Communities in Northern Australia'. *Rural and Remote Health*, 6(606): 1–15.

Doherty, G., Stagnitti, K. & Schoo, A. (2009). 'From Student to Therapist: Follow-up of the First Cohort of Students'. *Australian Occupational Therapy Journal*, 56: 341–9.

Eley, D. & Baker, P. (2005). 'Does Recruitment Lead to Retention? Rural Clinical School Training Experiences and Subsequent Intern Choices'. *Rural and Remote Health*, 6(511): 1–11.

Ezersky, S., Havazelet, L., Hiller Scott, A. & Zettler, C. L. (1989). 'Speciality Choices in Occupational Therapy'. *American Journal of Occupational Therapy*, 43(4): 227–33.

Frank, B. (2008). 'Chapter 2. Enhancing Nursing Education through Effective Academic–Service Partnerships'. *Annual Review of Nursing Education*, 6: 25–43.

Hook, A. D. & Lawson-Porter, A. (2003). 'The Development and Evaluation of a Fieldwork Educator's Training Programme for Allied Health Professionals'. *Medical Teacher*, 25(5): 527–36.

McInstry, C. (2005). 'From Graduate to Practitioner: Rethinking Organisational Support and Professional Development'. In G. Whiteford & V. Wright-St Clair (eds), *Occupation and Practice in Context*. Elsevier, Sydney, 129–42.

Playford, D., Larson, A. & Wheatland, B. (2006). 'Going Country: Rural Student Placement Factors Associated with Future Rural Employment in Nursing And Allied Health'. *Australian Journal of Rural Health*, 14(1): 14–19.

Schoo, A. M. M., McNamara, K. & Stagnitti, K. E. (2008). 'Clinical Placement and Rurality of Career Commencement: A Pilot Study'. *Rural and Remote Health*, 8: 964.

Shannon, S. J., Walker-Jeffreys, M., Newbury, J. W. Cayetano, T., Brown, K. & Petkov, J. (2006). 'Rural Clinician Opinion of Being a Preceptor'. *Rural and Remote Health*, 6(490).

Stagnitti, K., Schoo, A., Reid, C. & Dunbar, J. (2005). 'Retention of Allied Health Professionals in the South-West of Victoria'. *Australian Journal of Rural Health*, 13: 364–5.

Further Reading

Adamson, B. J., Hunt, A. E., Harris, L. M. & Hummel, J. (1998). 'Occupational Therapists' Perceptions of their Undergraduate Preparation for the Workplace'. *British Journal of Occupational Therapy*, 61(4): 173–9.

Bourke, L., Sheridan, C., Russell, U., Jones, G., De Witt Talbot, D. & Liaw, S.-T. (2004). 'Developing a Conceptual Understanding of Rural Health Practice'. *Australian Journal of Rural Health*, 12: 181–6.

Christie, B., Corcoran Joyce, P. & Moeller, P. (1985). 'Fieldwork Experience, Part I: Impact on Practice Preference'. *American Journal of Occupational Therapy*, 39(10): 671–4.

Hummell, J. & Koelmeyer, L. (1999). 'New Graduates: Perceptions of their First Occupational Therapy Position'. *British Journal of Occupational Therapy*, 62(8): 351–8.

Lee, S. & Mackenzie, L. (2003). 'Starting Out in Rural New South Wales: The Experiences of New Graduate Occupational Therapists'. *Australian Journal of Rural Health*, 11(1): 36–43.

Lincoln, M. A., Adamson, B. J. & Cant, R. V. (2001). 'The Importance of Managerial Competencies for New Graduates in Speech Pathology'. *Advances in Speech-Language Pathology*, 3(1): 25–36.

McKenna, K., Scholtes, A., Fleming, J. & Gilbert, J. (2001). 'The Journey through an Undergraduate Occupational Therapy Course: Does It Change Students' Attitudes, Perceptions and Career Plans?' *Australian Occupational Therapy Journal*, 48(4): 157–69.

Paterson, M. L., McColl, M. & Paterson, J. A. (2004). 'Preparing Allied Health Students for Fieldwork in Smaller Communities'. *Australian Journal of Rural Health*, 12: 32–3.

Veitch, C., Underhill, A. & Hays, R. B. (2006). 'The Career Aspirations and Location Intentions of James Cook University's First Cohort of Medical Students: A Longitudinal Study at Course Entry and Graduation'. *Rural & Remote Health*, 6(537): 1–8.

PART 4 CHECKLIST
TRANSITION TO PRACTICE

- [ ] Reflect on your own fieldwork experiences.
  - [ ] What was helpful to you?
  - [ ] What was not helpful to you?
- [ ] Action: From this reflection I have listed what I have gained in knowledge and skills from my fieldwork experiences.

ORIENTATION TO MY FIRST JOB

- [ ] I have reflected on what I did to orientate myself to my fieldwork placements:
  - [ ] What strategies did I use to become familiar with new environments?
  - [ ] Did I need a map initially to help me find my way around?
  - [ ] How did I remember the names of all the staff who were in my immediate and wider working environments?
  - [ ] Did I write these down in a notebook?
  - [ ] Did I carry a staff contact list, and was this helpful for remembering names?
  - [ ] Did I use a computer-based calendar or reminder system to help me keep appointments, schedule sessions and so forth?
- [ ] Action: If these and other strategies worked for you when you were a student, use them again in your first job.

BEING A FIELDWORK EDUCATOR

- [ ] Reflect on what learning and teaching style best suits you.
- [ ] Action: Plan your continuing professional development around your own identified learning needs.
- [ ] Action: Your understanding of the need for using learning and teaching styles that best suit an individual will be of great value when you work with fieldwork placement students. You will be aware that each student has his or her own learning style.
- [ ] As a new fieldwork educator, you will be required with your student/s to:
  - [ ] articulate your professional practice
  - [ ] explain your conceptual maps of the interrelations between theory and practice
  - [ ] explain your organisational setting and policy environment
  - [ ] demonstrate various professional skills and attributes.
- [ ] Action: I can do this.

As a new fieldwork educator you can help your student to:

- understand the purpose of supervision
- know what they want from you as their fieldwork educator
- take an active role in negotiating a contract with you
- prepare for sessions
- engage in active participation and be willing to be open and reflective in each supervision session.

As a fieldwork educator I am becoming aware of the different phases of supervision:

- establishing the relationship
- consolidating the relationship
- closure and evaluation

In terms of recruiting students to my workplace, my role as a fieldwork educator is important to:

- orientate the student
- connect the student to social networks (such as sports teams) if needed
- check on accommodation (if needed)
- provide a variety of clients
- support the student in the student's learning.

REFERENCES

Adams, M., Aylward, P., Heyne, N., Hull, C., Misan, G., Taylor, J. & Walker-Jeffreys, M. (2005). Integrated Support for Aboriginal Tertiary Students in Health-Related Courses: The Pika Wiya Learning Centre. *Australian Health Review*, 29(4): 482–8.

Adamson, B. J., Hunt, A. E., Harris, L. M., & Hummel, J. (1998). 'Occupational Therapists' Perceptions of their Undergraduate Preparation for the Workplace'. *British Journal of Occupational Therapy*, 61(4): 173–9.

Adamson, L. (2005). 'Inspiring Future Generations of Occupational Therapists'. *Australian Occupational Therapy Journal*, 52: 269–70.

Adler, N. J. (2007). *International Dimensions of Organizational Behavior* (5th edn). South-Western, Cincinnati, OH.

Albert, E., Dalton, L., Spencer, J., Dunn, M. & Walker, J. (2004). 'Doing It Together: The Tasmanian Interdisciplinary Rural Placement Program'. *Australian Journal of Rural Health*, 12: 30–1.

Arhin, A. O. & Cormier, E. (2007). 'Using Deconstruction to Educate Generation Y Nursing Students'. *Journal of Nursing Education*, 46(12): 562–67.

Alford, C. L., Miles, T., Palmer, R. & Espino, D. (2001). 'An Introduction to Geriatrics for First-Year Medical Students'. *Journal of the American Geriatric Society*, 49(6): 782–7.

American Psychiatric Association (2002). *Diagnostic and Statistical Manual of Mental Disorders, 4th Edition, Text Revision*, American Psychiatric Association, Washington, DC.

Arrington, M. (2008). *Facebook No Longer The Second Largest Social Network*. <http://www.techcrunch.com/2008/06/12/facebook-no-longer-the-second-largest-social-network/> accessed 18 February 2009.

Australian Bureau of Statistics (2006). *Deaths, Australia, 2005*. ABS Catalogue No. 3302.0. Commonwealth of Australia, Canberra.

Australian Bureau of Statistics (2007). *Work-Related Injuries*. Commonwealth of Australia, Canberra, 2005–06.

Australian Bureau of Statistics/Australian Institute of Health and Welfare (2008). *The Health and Welfare of Aboriginal and Torres Strait Islander Peoples*. ABS Cat. No. 4704.0, Australian Bureau of Statistics, Canberra.

Australian Institute of Health and Welfare (2001). *Health and Community Services Labour Force*. Cat. No. HWL 27. AIHW, Canberra.

Australian Institute of Health and Welfare (2002). *Australia's Health*. Canberra. AIHW Cat. No. Aus 25.

Australian Medical Workforce Advisory Committee (2005). 'Doctors in Vocational Training: Rural Background and Rural Practice Intentions'. *Australian Journal of Rural Health*, 13: 14–20.

Australian Nursing and Midwifery Council (2006). *RN Competency Standards* <http://www.anmc.org.au/professional_standards/index.php> accessed 27 January 2009.

Australian Physiotherapy Council (2006). *Australian Standards for Physiotherapy* <http://www.physiocouncil.com.au/file_folder/AustralianStandardsforPhysiotherapySummary> accessed 27 January 2009.

Australian Psychological Society (2009). <psychology.org.au/.../organisational/ workplace.gov.au> accessed 24 January 2009.

Aveling, N. (2001). '"Where Do You Come From?" Critical Storytelling as a Teaching Strategy within the Context of Teacher Education'. *Discourse: Studies in the Cultural Politics of Education*, 22(1): 35–48.

Baerlocher, M. O. & Detsky, A. S. (2008). 'Online Medical Blogging: Don't Do It!' *Canadian Medical Association Journal*, 179(3): 292.

Bagnall, R. (1998). 'Professional Codes of Conduct: A Critique with Implications for Continuing Professional Education'. In D. Dymock (ed.), *CPE 98: Meeting the Challenge of Change*. Department of Administration and Training, University of New England: 81–91.

Baird, B. N. (2008). *The Internship, Practicum and Field Placement Handbook: A Guide for The Helping Professions* (5th edn). Pearson Prentice Hall, NJ.

Barney, T., Russell, M. & Clark, M. (1998). 'Evaluation of the Provision of Fieldwork Training through a Rural Student Unit'. *Australian Journal of Rural Health*, 6: 202–7.

Barr, H., Freeth, D. Hammick, M., Koppel, I. & Reeves, S. (2006). 'The Evidence Base and Recommendations for Interprofessional Education in Health and Social Care'. *Journal of Interprofessional Care*, 20, 75–8.

Barton, D. (2006). 'The Path to Rural Dentistry'. *PartyLine*, 27: 4.

Baum, F. (2002). *The New Public Health*. Oxford University Press, Melbourne.

Baxter, S. & Carr, H. (2007). 'Walking the Tightrope: The Balance Between Duty of Care, Human Rights and Capacity'. *Housing, Care and Support*, 10(3): 6–11.

Baylies, C. (2002). 'Disability and the Notion of Human Development: Questions of Rights and Capabilities'. *Disability and Society*, 17(7): 725–9.

Beamer, S. (2001). *Making Decisions. Best Practice and New Ideas for Supporting People with High Support Needs to Make Decisions*. Values Into Action, London.

Beddoe, E. (2000). 'The Supervisory Relationship'. In L. Cooper & L. Briggs (eds). *Fieldwork in the Human Services: Theory and Practice for Field Education, Practice Teachers and Supervisors*. Allen & Unwin, Sydney: 41–54.

Beddoe, E. & Maidment, J. (2009). *Mapping Knowledge for Social Work Practice: Critical Interactions*. Cengage Learning, Melbourne.

Best, D. (2005). 'Exploring the Roles of the Clinical Educator'. In M. Rose & D. Best (eds), *Transforming Practice through Clinical Education, Professional Supervision and Mentoring*. Elsevier, Sydney: 45–9.

Biggs, J. & Tang, C. (2007). *Teaching for Quality Learning at University* (3rd edn). McGraw-Hill Education, Berkshire.

Birth Matters, Autumn 2009.

Blair, S., Hume, C. & Creek, J. (2007). 'Occupational Perspectives on Mental Health and Well-being'. In J. Creek & L. Lougher (eds) *Occupational Therapy and Mental Health*. Churchill Livingstone Elsevier, Philadelphia, PA.

Bogo, M., Regehr, C. & Power, R. (2002). *Competency-Based Evaluation (CBE) Tool*. Faculty of Social Work, University of Toronto.

Bogo, M. & Vayda, E. (1986). *The Practice of Field Instruction*. University of Toronto Press, Toronto.

Bond, M. & Holland, S. (1998). *Skills of Clinical Supervision for Nurses*. Open University Press, Buckingham.

Boud, D. (2000). 'Sustainable Assessment: Rethinking Assessment for the Learning Society'. *Studies in Continuing Education*, 22(2): 151–67.

Boud, D. & Edwards, H. (1999). 'Learning for Practice: Promoting Learning in Clinical and Community Settings'. In J. Higgs & H. Edwards (eds), *Educating Beginning Practitioners*: Butterworth Heinemann, Oxford: 173–9.

Bourke, L., Sheridan, C. M., Russell, U., Jones, G. I., Dewitt Talbot, D. & Liaw, S. (2004). 'Developing a Conceptual Understanding of Rural Health Practice'. *Australian Journal of Rural Health*, 12(5): 181–6.

Boyd, D. M. & Ellison, N. B. (2007). 'Social Network Sites: Definition, History, and Scholarship'. *Journal of Computer-Mediated Communication*, 13(1): 210–30.

Braithwaite, J., Westbrook, J. I., Foxwell, A. R., Boyce, R., Devinney, T., Budge, M., Murphy, K., Ryall, M., Beutel, J., Vanderheide, R., Renton, E., Travaglia, J., Stone, J., Barnard, A., Greenfield, D., Corbett, A., Nugus, P. & Clay-Williams, R. (2007). *An Action Research Protocol to Strengthen System-wide Interprofessional Learning and Practice*. BMC Health Service Research, 7: 144. <www.pubmedcentral.nih.gov/articlerender.fcgi?artid=2212639> published online 13 September; accessed 8 February 2009.

British Psychological Society (2006). *Assessment of Capacity in Adults: Interim Guidance for Psychologists*. British Psychological Society, London.

Brown, A. & Bourne, I. (1996). *The Social Work Supervisor*. Open University Press, Buckingham.

Burch, J. & Newman, V. (2007). *University Department of Rural Health Student Placement and Satisfaction Project: Final Report*. Australian Rural Health Education Network, Canberra <http://www.arhen.org.au>.

Burchfield, J. A., Marenco, A., Dickens, D. & Willock, K. (2000). 'An Anti-Smoking Project Instituted by Senior Nursing Students in a Rural Community'. *Issues in Comprehensive Pediatric Nursing*, 23(3): 155–64.

Carson, B., Dunbar, T., Chenall, R. D. & Bailie, R. (2007). *Social Determinants of Indigenous Health*. Allen & Unwin, Sydney.

Chermiss, C. (2000). 'Social and Emotional Competence in the Workplace'. In R. Bar-On and J. D. A. Parker (eds), *The Handbook of Emotional Intelligence: Theory, Development, Assessment, and Application in the Home, School and in the Workplace*. Jossey-Bass, San Francisco: 433–58.

Christie, B., Corcoran Joyce, P. & Moeller, P. (1985). 'Fieldwork Experience, Part I: Impact on Practice Preference'. *American Journal of Occupational Therapy*, 39(10): 671–4.

Cleake, H. & Wilson, J. (2007). *Making the Most of Field Placement* (2nd edn). Thomson, Melbourne.

Commonwealth Department of Health and Ageing (2000). *The Australian Healthcare System: An outline*. <http://www.health.gov.au/internet/main/publishing.nsf/Content/EBA6536E92A7D 2D2CA256F9D007D8066/$File/ozhealth.pdf> accessed 12 January 2009.

Connelly, F. M. & Clandinin, D. J. (1990). 'Stories of Experience And Narrative Inquiry'. *Educational Researcher*, June–July: 2–14.

Cooper, L., Gooding, J., Gallagher, J., Sternesky, L., Ledsky, R. & Berns, S. (2007). 'Impact of a Family-centered Care Initiative on NICU Care, Staff and Families'. *Journal of Perinatology*, 27: S32–S37.

Courtney, M. (2008). *Inside My Job: Insider Information for Early Career Occupational Therapists*. Transition to Practice Project, Melbourne.

Courtney, M., Edwards, H., Smith, S. & Finlayson, K. (2002). 'The Impact of Rural Clinical Placement on Student Nurses' Employment Intentions'. *Collegian*, 9(1): 12–18.

Courtney, M., & Farnworth, L. (2003). 'Professional Competence for Private Practitioners in Occupational Therapy'. *Australian Occupational Therapy Journal*, 50: 234–43.

Courtney, M. & Wilcock, A. (2005). 'The Deakin Experience: Using National Competency Standards to Drive Undergraduate Education'. *Australian Occupational Therapy Journal*, 52: 360–2.

Couzos, S. & Murray, R. (1999). *Aboriginal Primary Health Care: An Evidence-Based Approach*. Oxford University Press, South Melbourne.

Crawford, M. W. & Kiger, A. M. (1998). 'Development through Self-assessment: Strategies Used during Clinical Nursing Placements'. *Journal of Advanced Nursing*, 27: 157–64.

Cresswell, A. (2009). '"Killing Season" a Dangerous Time to be in Wards'. *The Australian*, October 15, accessed 11 January 2010 at www.theaustralian.com.au/news/killing-season-a-dangerous-time-to-be-in-wards/story-e6frg6o6-1225786864229.

Crowe, M. J. & Mackenzie, L. (2002). 'The Influence of Fieldwork on the Preferred Future Practice Areas of Final Year Occupational Therapy Students'. *Australian Occupational Therapy Journal*, 49(1): 25–36.

Cusick, A., McIntosh, D. & Santiago, L. (2004). 'New Graduate Therapists in Acute Care Hospitals: Priorities, Problems and Strategies for Departmental Action'. *Australian Occupational Therapy Journal*, 51: 174–84.

Dade Smith, J., O'Dea, K., McDermott, R., Schmidt, B. & Connors, C. (2006). 'Educating to Improve Population Health Outcomes in Chronic Disease: An Innovative Workforce Initiative across Remote, Rural and Indigenous Communities in Northern Australia'. *Rural and Remote Health*, 6(606): 1–15.

Davys, A. (2007). 'Active Participation in Supervision: A Supervisee's Guide'. In D. Wepa (ed.), *Clinical Supervision in Aotearoa/New Zealand: A Health Perspective*. Pearson Education, Auckland: 26–42.

Davys, A. & Beddoe, L. (2000). Supervision of Students: A Map and a Model for the Decade to Come. *Social Work Education*, 19(5): 438–49.

Department of Health and Ageing. (2009). *Improving Maternity Services in Australia: The Report of the Maternity Services Review*. Commonwealth of Australia, Canberra.

Department of Veterans Affairs (2008a). *Stigma.* <http://at-ease.dva.gov.au/www/html/88-stigma.asp> accessed 30 January 2009.

Department of Veterans Affairs (2008b). *Debunking the Myths.* <http://at-ease.dva.gov.au/www/html/87-debunking-the-myths.asp> accessed 30 January 2009.

Diener, M. (2006). Deakin University's Occupation, Wellness and Life Satisfaction Centre: working locally to achieve diverse competencies. 14th Congress of the World Federation of Occupational Therapists, 23–28 July 2006. WFOT Congress Abstracts.

DiMicco, J. M. & Millen, D. R. (2007). Identity management: multiple presentations of self in Facebook. Proceedings of the 2007 International ACM Conference on Supporting Group Work. <http://portal.acm.org/citation.cfm?id=1316624.1316682> accessed 20 February 2009.

Doherty, G., Stagnitti, K. & Schoo, A. (2009). 'From Student to Therapist: Follow up of a First Cohort of Bachelor of Occupational Therapy Students'. *Australian Occupational Therapy Journal,* 56: 341–9.

Donen, N. (1999). 'Mandatory Practice Self-Appraisal: Moving towards Outcomes Based Continuing Education'. *Journal of Evaluation in Clinical Practice,* 7: 297–303.

Doubt, L., Paterson, M. & O'Riordan, A. (2004). 'Clinical Education in Private Practice: An Interdisciplinary Project'. *Journal of Allied Health,* 33, 47–50.

Dunst, C. J. & Trivette, C. M. (1996). 'Empowerment, Effective Help-Giving Practices and Family Centred Care'. *Pediatric Nursing,* 22(4), 334–7, 343.

Eley, D. & Baker, P. (2005). 'Does Recruitment Lead to Retention? Rural Clinical School Training Experiences and Subsequent Intern Choices'. *Rural and Remote Health,* 6(511): 1–11.

Ellis, E. & Trede, F. (2008). 'Communication and Duty of Care'. In J. Higgs, R. Ajjawi, L. McAllister, F. Trede & S. Loftus. *Communicating in the Health Sciences* (2nd edn). Oxford University Press, Melbourne.

Etheridge, S. A. (2007). 'Learning to Think Like a Nurse: Stories from New Nurse Graduates'. *Journal of Continuing Education in Nursing,* 38: 24–30.

Etzkowitz, H. (2008). *The Triple Helix: University–Industry–Government Innovation in Action.* Routledge, Hoboken, NJ.

Ezersky, S., Havazelet, L., Hiller Scott, A. & Zettler, C. L. (1989). 'Speciality Choices in Occupational Therapy'. *American Journal of Occupational Therapy,* 43(4): 227–33.

Fennell, P. (1996). *Treatment without Consent: Law, Psychiatry and the Treatment of Mentally Disordered People since 1845.* Routledge, London.

Ferguson, K. (2005). 'Professional Supervision'. In M. Rose & D. Best (eds), *Transforming Practice through Clinical Education, Professional Supervision and Mentoring.* Elsevier Churchill Livingstone, Edinburgh: 293–307.

Fernandez, E. (2003). 'Promoting Teaching Competence in Field Education: Facilitating Transition from Practitioner to Educator'. *Women in Welfare Education,* 6: 103–29.

Fineout-Overholt, E., Melnyk, B. M. & Schultz, A. (2005). 'Transforming Health Care from the Inside Out: Advancing Evidence-Based Practice in the 21st Century'. *Journal of Professional Nursing,* 21(6): 335–44.

Fook, J. (2002). *Social Work: Critical Theory and Practice.* Sage, London.

Fook, J. & Gardner, F. (2007). *Practising Critical Reflection: A Resource Handbook.* Open University Press, Maidenhead.

Fook, J., Ryan, M. & Hawkins, L. (2000). *Professional Expertise: Practice, Theory and Education for Working in Uncertainty.* Whiting & Birch, London.

Frank, B. (2008). 'Chapter 2. Enhancing Nursing Education through Effective Academic–Service Partnerships'. *Annual Review of Nursing Education,* 6: 25–43.

Gandy, J. S. (2002). Preparation for Teaching Students in Clinical Settings. In K. F. Shepard, & G. M. Jensen (eds). *Handbook of Teaching for Physical Therapists* (2nd edn). Butterworth-Heinemann, New Jersey: 211–53.

Gibbs, T. (2004). 'Community-based or Tertiary-based Medical Education: So What Is the Question?' *Medical Teaching,* 26(7): 589–90.

Gobelet, C., Luthi, F., Al-Khodairy, A. T. & Chamberlain, M. A. (2007). 'Vocational Rehabilitation: A Multidisciplinary Intervention'. *Disability and Rehabilitation,* 29(17): 1405–10.

Gray, J., Smith, R. & Homer, C. (2009). *Illustrated Dictionary of Midwifery.* Butterworth Heinemann Elsevier, Sydney.

Gray, M. & Gibbons, J. (2007). 'There are No Answers, Only Choices: Teaching Ethical Decision Making in Social Work'. *Australian Social Work,* 60(2): 222–38.

Gwozdek, A. E., Klausner, C. P. & Kerschbaum, W. E. (2008). 'The Utilization of Computer Mediated Communication for Case Study Collaboration'. *Journal of Dental Hygiene*, 82(1): 1–10.

Hafford-Letchfield, T. (2006). *Management and Organisations in Social Work*. Learning Matters, Exeter.

Haggerty, J., Reid, R., Freeman, G., Starfield, B., Adair, C. & McKendry, R. (2003). 'Continuity of Care: A Multidisciplinary Review'. *British Medical Journal*, 327: 1219–21.

Haller, G., Myles, P. S., Taffe, P., Perneger, T. V. & Wu, C. L. (2009). 'Rate of Undesirable Events at Beginning of Academic Year: Retrospective Cohort Study'. Accessed 11 January 2010 at BMJ; 339: 3974 doi:10.1136/bmj.b3974.

Halsbury's Laws of Australia (2008). LexisNexis, Sydney.

Handbook for Field Educators in Social Work and Social Welfare (1991). Charles Sturt University, Albury–Wodonga.

Handy, C. (1994). *The Age of Paradox*. Harvard Business School Press, Boston.

Hatem, M., Sandall, J., Devane, D., Soltani, H. & Gates, S. (2008). *Midwife-led Versus Other Models of Care for Childbearing Women*: Cochrane Database of Systematic Reviews, 4.

Hawkins, P., & Shohet, R. (2006). *Supervision in the Helping Professions* (3rd edn). Open University Press, Berkshire.

Hayes, R. (2002). 'One Approach to Improving Indigenous Health Care Is through Medical Education'. *Australian Journal of Rural Health*, 10(6): 285–7.

Healey, J. & Spencer, M. (2008). *Surviving Your Placement in Health and Social Care: A Student Handbook*. McGraw Hill, New York.

Hendron, J. G. (2008). *RSS for Educators: Blogs, Newsfeeds, Podcasts, and Wikis in the Classroom* (1st edn). International Society for Technology in Education, Washington, DC.

Hicks, P. J., Cox, S. M., Espey, E. L., Goepfert, A. R., Bienstock, J. L., Erickson, S., Hammoud, M. M., Katz, N. T., Krueger, P. M., Neutens, J. J., Peskin, E. & Puscheck, E. E.. (2005). 'To the Point: Medical Education Reviews Dealing with Student Difficulties in the Clinical Setting'. *American Journal of Obstetrics and Gynecology*, 193(6): 1915–22.

Higgs, J. & Jones, M. (2000). *Clinical Reasoning in the Health Professions*. Butterworth Heinemann, Oxford.

Higgs, J. & Titchen, A. (2000). 'Knowledge and Reasoning'. In J. Higgs & M. Jones (eds), *Clinical Reasoning in the Health Professions* (2nd edn). Butterworth Heinemann, Oxford: 22–32.

Hirsch, W. & Weber, L. (eds) (1999). *Challenges Facing Higher Education at the Millennium*. American Council of Education, Oryx Press, Phoenix.

Holland, J. & Henriot, P. (1995). *Social Analysis: Linking Faith and Justice*. (12th edn). Dove Communications, Melbourne.

Hook, A. D. & Lawson-Porter, A. (2003). 'The Development and Evaluation of a Fieldwork Educator's Training Programme for Allied Health Professionals'. *Medical Teacher*, 25(5): 527–36.

Hughes, L. & Pengelly, P. (1997). *Staff Supervision in a Turbulent Environment: Managing Process and Task in Front-line Services*. Jessica Kingsley, London.

Hummell, J. & Koelmeyer, K. (1999). 'New Graduates: Perceptions of their First Occupational Therapy Position'. *British Journal of Occupational Therapy*, 62(8): 351–8.

Hunter, P. (1999). Aboriginal Community Controlled Health Services (ACCHS): Keynote address, 5th National Rural Health Conference, Adelaide.

Hurley, K. F., McKay, D. W., Scott, T. M. & James, B. M. (2003). 'The Supplementary Instruction Project: Peer Devised and Delivered Tutorials'. *Medical Teacher*, 25: 404–7.

Iacono, T. & Murray, V. (2003). 'Issues of Informed Consent in Conducting Medical Research Involving People with Intellectual Disability'. *Journal of Applied Research in Intellectual Disabilities*, 16: 41–51.

Irons, A. (2008). *Enhancing Learning through Formative Assessment and Feedback*. Routledge, London and New York.

Isles, R. C., Nitz, J. C. & Low Choy, N. L. (2004). 'Normative Data for Clinical Balance Measures in Women Aged 20 to 80'. *Journal of the American Geriatric Society*, 52(8): 1367–72.

Jantzen, D. (2008). 'Reframing Professional Development for First-line Nurses'. *Nursing Inquiry*, 15(1): 21–9.

Jette, D. U., Bertoni, A., Coots, R., Johnson, H., McLaughlin, C. & Weisbach, C. (2007). 'Clinical Instructors' Perceptions of Behaviors that Comprise Entry Level Clinical Performance in Physical Therapy Students: A Qualitative Study'. *Physical Therapy*, 87: 833–43.

Johnson, D. & Johnson, R. (1999). *Learning Together and Alone: Cooperative, Competitive, and Individualistic Learning*. Allyn & Bacon, Boston.

Johnson, D. W. & Johnson R. T. (2009). 'Energizing Learning: The Instructional Power of Conflict'. *Educational Researcher*, 38(1): 37–51.

Johnstone, R. (2004). *Occupational Health and Safety Law and Policy: Texts and Materials*. Law Book, Sydney.

Junco, R. & Cole-Avent, G. A. (2008). 'An Introduction to Technologies Commonly Used by College Students'. *New Directions for Student Services*, 124: 3–17.

Kadushin, A. & Harkness, D. (2002). *Supervision in Social Work*. (4th edn). Columbia University Press, New York.

Kamel Boulos, M. N., Hetherington, L. & Wheeler, S. (2007). 'Second Life: An Overview of the Potential of 3-D Virtual Worlds in Medical and Health Education'. *Health Information and Libraries Journal*, 24: 233–45.

Kamel Boulous, M. N. & Wheeler, S. (2007). 'The Emerging Web 2.0 Social Software: An Enabling Suite of Sociable Technologies in Health and Health Care Education'. *Health Information and Libraries Journal*, 24: 2–23.

Kilminster, S. M., & Jolly, B. C. (2000). 'Effective Supervision in Clinical Practice Settings: A Literature Review'. *Medical Education*, 34: 827–40.

Kinsella, P. (2000). *Person Centred Risk Assessment*. Paradigm, Liverpool.

Knowles, M. S., Elwood, F., Holton R, III. & Swanson, A. (2005). *The Adult Learner: The Definitive Classic in Adult Education and Human Resource Development* (6th edn). Elsevier, Amsterdam & Boston.

Kramer, P. & Hinojosa, J. (1999). *Frames of Reference for Pediatric Occupational Therapy*. Lippincott Williams & Wilkins, Philadelphia.

Laws, P., Abeywardan, S., Walker, J. & Sullivan, E. A. (2007). *Australia's Mothers and Babies 2005*, Australian Institute of Health and Welfare National Perinatal Statistics Unit, Sydney.

Leap, N. (2009). 'Woman-centred or Women-centred Care: Does It Matter?' *British Journal of Midwifery*, 17(1): 12–16.

Lee, S. & Mackenzie, L. (2003). 'Starting Out in Rural New South Wales: The Experiences of New Graduate Occupational Therapists'. *Australian Journal of Rural Health*, 11: 36–43.

Letendre, P. (2008). Perils and joys of blogging: Electronic letter to the editor. *Canadian Medical Association Journal*. <http://www.cmaj.ca/cgi/eletters/179/3/292#19949> accessed 18 February 2009.

Levett-Jones, T. & Bourgeois, S. (2007). *The Clinical Placement: An Essential Guide for Nursing Students*. Churchill Livingstone, Sydney.

Lincoln, M. A., Adamson, B. J., & Cant, R. V. (2001). 'The Importance of Managerial Competencies for New Graduates in Speech Pathology'. *Advances in Speech-Language Pathology*, 3(1): 25–36.

Lloyd, C., McKenna, K. & King, R. (2005). 'Sources of Stress Experienced by Occupational Therapists and Social Workers in Mental Health Settings'. *Occupational Therapy International*, 12(2), 81–94.

LoCicero, A. & Hancock, J. (2000). 'Preparing Students for Success in Fieldwork'. *Teaching of Psychology*, 27: 117–20.

Lowry, P. B., Curtis, A. & Lowry, M. R. (2004). 'Building a Taxonomy and Nomenclature of Collaborative Writing to Improve Interdisciplinary Research and Practice'. *Journal of Business Communication*, 41: 66–99.

Luft, J. (1969). *Of Human Interaction*. National Press Books, Palo Alto, CA.

Luntz, H., Hambly, D., Burns, K., Dietrich, J. & Foster, N. (2008). *Torts: Cases and Commentary* (LexisNexis, Sydney)

McAllister, L. & Lincoln, M. (2004). *Clinical Education in Speech-Language Pathology*. Whurr, London.

McBride, S. L. (1999). 'Research in Review: Family-centred Practices'. *Young Children*,54(3), 62–70.

McCluskey, A. & Cusick, A. (2002). 'Strategies for Introducing Evidence-based Practice and Changing Clinician Behaviour: A Manager's Toolbox'. *Australian Occupational Therapy Journal*, 49: 63–70.

McCulloch, P., Mishra, A, Handa, A., Dale, T. Hirst, G. & Catchpole, K. (2009). 'The Effects of Aviation-style Non-technical Skills Training on Technical Performance and Outcome in the Operating Theatre'. *Quality and Safety in Health Care,* 18, 109–15, doi:10.1136/qshc.2008.032045.

McInstry, C. (2005). 'From Graduate to Practitioner: Rethinking Organisational Support and Professional Development'. In G. Whiteford & V. Wright-St Clair (eds), *Occupation and Practice in Context*. Elsevier, Sydney: 129–42.

McKenna, K., Scholtes, A., Fleming, J. & Gilbert, J. (2001). 'The Journey through an Undergraduate Occupational Therapy Course: Does It Change Students' Attitudes, Perceptions and Career Plans?' *Australian Occupational Therapy Journal*, 48(4): 157–69.

McKenzie, K., Matheson, E., Paxton, D., Murray, G. C. & McKaskie, K. (2001). 'Health and Social Care Worker's Knowledge and Application of the Concept of Duty of Care'. *Journal of Adult Protection*, 3(4): 29–37.

McLean, R., Richards, B. H. & Wardman, J. (2007). 'The Effect of Web 2.0 on the Future of Medical Practice and Education: Darwikian Evolution or Folksonomic Revolution?' *IT and Health*, 187(3): 174–7.

Maidment, J. (2003). 'Problems Experienced by Students on Field Placement: Using Research Findings to Inform Curriculum Design and Content'. *Australian Social Work*, 56(1), 50–60.

Maloney, P. (2009). Barriers and enablers to clinical placement in rural public and private practice. Unpublished honours thesis. Deakin University, Geelong.

Meads, G., Ashcroft, J., Barr, H., Scott, R. & Wild, A. (2008). *The Case for Interprofessional Collaboration*. Wiley-Blackwell, Oxford.

Mendelson, D. (2007). *The New Law of Torts* (Oxford University Press, Melbourne).

Meyer, B., Fletcher, T. & Parker, S. (2004). 'Enhancing Emotional Intelligence in the Health Care Environment'. *Health Care Manager*, 23(3), 225–34.

Mezirow, J. (1991). *Transformative Dimensions in Adult Learning*. Jossey-Bass, San Francisco.

Mezirow, J. (2000). *Learning as Transformation: Critical Perspectives on a Theory in Progress*. Jossey-Bass, San Francisco.

Miller, P. A., Solomon, P., Giacomini, M. & Abelson, J. (2005). 'Experience of Novice Physiotherapists Adapting to their Role in Acute Care Hospitals'. *Physiotherapy Canada*, 57: 145–153.

Mitchell, T. (2008). 'Utilization of the Functional Capacity Evaluation in Vocational Rehabilitation'. *Journal of Vocational Rehabilitation*, 28: 21–8.

Molloy, E. & Clarke, D. (2005). 'The Positioning of Physiotherapy Students and Clinical Supervisors in Feedback Sessions'. *Focus on Health Professional Education: A Multi-Disciplinary Journal*, 7(1): 79–90.

Moore, B. (2004). *Australian Oxford Dictionary* (2nd edn). Oxford University Press, Melbourne.

Moore, J., McMillan, D., Rosenthal, M. & Weishaar, M. (2005). 'Risk Determination for Patients with Direct Access to Physical Therapy in Military Health Care Facilities.' *Journal of Orthopedic Sports Physical Therapy*, 35, 674–8.

Murray, R. B. & Wronski, I. (2006). 'When the Tide Goes Out: Health Workforce in Rural, Remote and Indigenous Communities'. *Medical Journal of Australia*, 185(1): 37–8.

Murray-Harvey, R., Slee, P., Lawson, M., Silins, H., Banfield, G. & Russell, A. (2000). 'Under Stress: The Concerns and Coping Strategies of Teacher Education Students'. *European Journal of Teacher Education*, 23(1), 19–35.

National Centre for Cultural Competence (2005). *Cultural Awareness: Teaching Tools, Strategies and Resources* <http://www.nccccurricula.info/awareness/D16.html> accessed 12 January 2009.

Nelson, D. B. & Low, G. R. (2003). *Emotional Intelligence: Achieving Academic and Career Excellence*. Prentice Hall, Upper Saddle River, NJ.

Nemeth, E. (2008). Learning from failure: Speech pathology students experiences of failure in a clinical placement. Unpublished Master of Health Science (Honours) thesis, Charles Sturt University.

Nimon, S. (2007). 'Generation Y and Higher Education: The Other Y2K'. *Journal of Institutional Research*, 13(1): 24–41.

Nitz, J. C. & Hourigan, S. R. (2004). 'Physiological Changes With Ageing'. In J. C. Nitz & S. R. Hourigan (eds) *Physiotherapy Practice in Residential Aged Care*. Butterworth Heinemann, Edinburgh.

Oblinger D. G. & Hawkins, B. L. (2005). 'The myth about Students: "We Understand Our Students"'. *Educause*, 40(5): 12–13.

Oblinger, D. G. & Oblinger, J. L. (2005). *Educating the Net Generation*. Educause, Washington, DC.

O'Connor, P. (1992). 'Workplace Literacy in Australia: Competing Agenda'. In A. Welch and P. Freebody, *Knowledge, Culture and Power: International Perspectives on Literacy as Policy and Practice*. Routledge, London.

O'Reilly, T. (2005). *What Is Web 2.0? Design Patterns and Business Models for the Next Generation of Software*. <http://oreillynet.com/pub/a/oreilly/tim/news/2005/09/30/what-is-web-20.html> accessed 1 May 2008.

OT Australia (1994). *The Australian Competency Standards for Entry-Level Occupational Therapists* <http://www.ausot.com.au/inner.asp?relid=11&pageid=22> accessed 27 January 2009.

Overton, A., Clark, M. & Thomas, Y. (2009). 'A Review of Non-Traditional Occupational Therapy Practice Placement Education: A Focus on Role-Emerging and Project Placements'. *British Journal of Occupational Therapy*, 72: 294–301.

Pardue, K. T. & Morgan, P. (2008). 'Millennials Considered: A New Generation, New Approaches, and Implications for Nursing Education'. *Nursing Education Perspectives*, 29(2): 74–9.

Paschal, K. A. (2002). 'Techniques for Teaching Students in Clinical Settings'. In K. F. Shepard & G. M. Jensen (eds). *Handbook of Teaching for Physical Therapists* (2nd edn). Butterworth Heinemann, New Jersey: 255–85.

Paterson, M. L., McColl, M. & Paterson, J. A. (2004). 'Preparing Allied Health Students for Fieldwork in Smaller Communities'. *Australian Journal of Rural Health*, 12: 32–3.

Patrick, C., Peach, D., Pocknee, C., Webb, F., Fletcher, M. & Pretto, G. (2008). *The WIL Report. Work Integrated Learning. A National Scoping Study.* Australian Learning and Teaching Council (ALTC) Final Report. Queensland University of Technology, Brisbane <www.altc.edu.au and www.acen.edu.au>.

Peck, E. & Norman, I. (1999). 'Working Together in Adult Community Mental Health Services: Exploring Inter-Professional Role Relations'. *Journal of Mental Health*, 8(3): 231–42.

Pereira, R. B. (2008). 'Learning and Being a First-Time Student Supervisor: Challenges and Triumphs'. *Australian Journal of Rural Health*, 16: 47–8.

Pickvance, D. (1997). 'Becoming a Supervisor'. In G. Shipton (ed.), *Supervision of Psychotherapy and Counselling: Making a Place to Think*. Open University Press, Buckingham: 131–42.

Playford, D., Larson, A. & Wheatland, B. (2006). 'Going Country: Rural Student Placement Factors Associated with Future Rural Employment in Nursing And Allied Health'. *Australian Journal of Rural Health*, 14(1): 14–19.

Potts, H. W. W. (2006). 'Is E-health Progressing Faster than E-health Researchers?' (electronic version). *Journal of Medical Internet Research*, 8. <http://www.jmir.org/2006/3/e24/> accessed 1 May 2008.

Powers, C. L., Allen, R. M., Johnson, V. A. & Cooper-Witt, C. M. (2005). 'Evaluating Immediate and Long-Range Effect of a Geriatric Clerkship Using Reflections and Ratings from Participants as Students and as Residents'. *Journal of the American Geriatric Society*, 53(2): 331–5.

Prensky, M. (2001). 'Digital Natives, Digital Immigrants'. *On the Horizon*, 9(5): 1–6.

Razack, N. (2002). *Transforming the Field: Critical Antiracist and Anti-oppressive Perspectives for the Human Services Practicum*. Fernwood Publishing, Halifax.

Reynolds, F. (2005). *Communication and Clinical Effectiveness in Rehabilitation*. Elsevier, Edinburgh.

Rodger, S. & Ziviani, J. (2006). *Occupational Therapy with Children: Understanding Children's Occupations and Enabling Participation*. Blackwell, Melbourne.

Rugg, S. (1996). 'The Transition of Junior Occupational Therapists to Clinical Practice: Report of a Preliminary Study'. *British Journal of Occupational Therapy*, 59(4), 165–8.

Ryan, J. (2003). 'Continuous Professional Development along the Continuum of Lifelong Learning'. *Nurse Education Today*, 23(7): 498–508.

Sadock & Sadock (2007). *Kaplan and Sadock's Synopsis of Psychiatry/Behavioral Sciences/Clinical Psychiatry* (10th edn). Wolters Kluwer Health/Lippincott Williams & Wilkins, Philadelphia, PA.

Schalock, R. L. (1997). 'The Conceptualization and Measurement of Quality of Life: Current Status and Future Considerations'. *Journal of Developmental Disabilities*, 5: 1–21.

Schaper, L. & Pervan, G. (2007). 'ICT and OTs: A Model of Information and Communication Technology Acceptance and Utilisation by Occupational Therapists (Part 2). *International Journal of Medical Informatics*, 76: 212–21.

Schembri, A. M. (2008). 'Why Social Workers Need to Embrace Web 2.0'. *Australian Social Work*, 61(2): 119–123.

Schim, S., Doorenbos, A. & Borse, N. (2005). 'Cultural Competence among Ontario and Michigan Healthcare Providers'. *Journal of Nursing Scholarship*, 37(4), 354–60.

Schon, D. (1983). *The Reflective Practitioner*. Temple Smith, London.

Schon, D. (1987). *Educating the Reflective Practitioner*. Jossey-Bass, San Francisco.

Schon, D. (1991). *The Reflective Practitioner: How Professionals Think in Action*. Basic Books, New York.

Schon, D. (1995). *Reflective Practitioner: How Professionals Think In Action* (new edn). Arena, Aldershot.

Schon, D. A. (2003). *The Reflective Practitioner*. Ashgate, Aldershot, Hants.

Schoo, A. M. M., McNamara, K. & Stagnitti, K. E. (2008). 'Clinical Placement and Rurality of Career Commencement: A Pilot Study'. *Rural and Remote Health*, 8: 964.

Scottish Public Mental Health Alliance (2002). *With Health in Mind: Improving Mental Health and Wellbeing in Scotland: A Document to Support Discussion and Action.* Scottish Development Centre for Mental Health, Edinburgh.

Seeman, N. (2008). 'Web 2.0 and Chronic Illness: New Horizons, New Opportunities' (electronic version). *Healthcare Quarterly*, 6: 104–110. <http://www.electronichealthcare.net> accessed 1 May 2008.

Shannon, S. J., Walker-Jeffreys, M., Newbury, J. W. Cayetano, T., Brown, K. & Petkov, J. (2006). 'Rural Clinician Opinion of Being a Preceptor'. *Rural and Remote Health*, 6(490).

Shapiro, D. A., Ogletree, B. T. & Brotherton, W. D. (2002). 'Graduate Students with Marginal Abilities in Communication Sciences and Disorders: Prevalence, Profiles and Solutions'. *Journal of Communication Disorders*, 35: 421–51.

Siporin, M. (1982). 'The Process of Field Instruction in Quality Field Instruction in Social Work'. In B. W. Sheafor & L. E. Jenkins (eds). *Quality Field Instruction in Social Work: Program Development and Maintenance.* Longman, New York: 175–97.

Sladyk, K. (2002). *The Successful Occupational Therapy Fieldwork Student.* Slack Incorporated, Thorofare, NJ.

Smith, J. K. (2007). 'Promoting Self-awareness in Nurses to Improve Nursing Practice'. *Nursing Standard*, 21(32): 47–52.

Smith, R. & Anderson, L. (2008). 'Interprofessional Learning: Aspiration or Achievement?' *Social Work Education*, 27(7): 759–76.

Smull, M. (1996). *Helping Staff Support Choice.* Support Development Associates, Kensington.

Stagnitti, K. (2005). 'The Family as a Unit in Postmodern Society'. In G. Whiteford and V. Wright St Clair (eds). *Occupation and Practice in Context.* Elsevier, Sydney, 213–29.

Stagnitti, K., Schoo, A., Reid, C. & Dunbar, J. (2005). 'Retention of Allied Health Professionals in the South-West of Victoria'. *Australian Journal of Rural Health*, 13: 364–5.

Stebnicki, M. A. (1997). 'A Conceptual Framework for Utilizing a Functional Assessment Approach for Determining Mental Capacity: A New Look at Informed Consent in Rehabilitation'. *Journal of Rehabilitation*, 63: 32–6.

Stone, N. (2006a). 'Evaluating Interprofessional Education: The Tautological Need for Interdisciplinary Approaches'. *Journal of Interprofessional Care*, 20(3): 260–75.

Stone, N. (2006b). 'The Rural Interprofessional Education Project'. *Journal of Interprofessional Care*, 20(1): 79–81.

Stone, N. & Curtis, C. (2007). *Interprofessional Education in Victorian Universities.* Report for the Department of Human Services: Victoria. Available from the author.

Sweeney, G., Webley, P. & Treacher, A. (2001). 'Supervision in Occupational Therapy, Part 2: The Supervisee's Dilemma'. *British Journal of Occupational Therapy*, 64(8): 380–6.

Takahashi, S., Killette, D. & Eftekari, T. (2003). *Exploring Issues Related to the Qualifications Recognition of Physical Therapists.* World Confederation of Physical Therapy, London.

Tassone, M. R. & Heck, C. S. (1997). 'Motivational Orientations of Allied Health Care Professionals Participating in Continuing Education'. *Journal of Continuing Education in the Health Professions*, 17(2): 97–105.

Taylor, J., Wilkinson, D. & Cheers, B. (2008). *Working with Communities in Health and Human Services.* Oxford University Press, South Melbourne.

Thomas, Y., Penman, M. & Williamson, P. (2005). 'Australian and New Zealand Fieldwork: Charting the Territory for Future Practice'. *Australian Occupational Therapy Journal*, 52: 78–81.

Townsend, E., Sheffield, S., Stadnyk, R. & Beagan, B. (2006). 'Effects of Workplace Policy on Continuing Professional Development: The Case of Occupational Therapy in Nova Scotia, Canada'. *Canadian Journal of Occupational Therapy*, 73(2): 98–108.

Tryssenaar, J. & Perkins, J. (2001). 'From Student to Therapist: Exploring the First Year of Practice'. *American Journal of Occupational Therapy*, 55: 19–27.

Ubachs-Moust, J., Houtepen, R., Vos, R. & ter Meulen, R. (2008). 'Value Judgements in the Decision-Making Process for the Elderly Patient'. *Journal of Medical Ethics*, 34: 863–8.

Urdang, E. (1999). 'Becoming a Field Instructor: A Key Experience in Professional Development'. *Clinical Supervisor*, 18(1): 85–103.

van Ginkel, H. (1999). 'Networks and Strategic Alliances within and between Universities and the Private Sector'. In W. Hirsch & L. Weber (eds), *Challenges Facing Higher Education at the Millennium*. American Council of Education. Oryx Press, Phoenix: 85–92.

van Manen, M. (1990). *Researching Lived Experience: Human Science for an Action Sensitive Pedagogy*. University of Western Ontario, London, Ontario.

Veitch, C., Underhill, A. & Hays, R. B. (2006). 'The Career Aspirations and Location Intentions of James Cook University's First Cohort of Medical Students: A Longitudinal Study at Course Entry and Graduation'. *Rural & Remote Health*, 6(537): 1–8.

Villamanta Legal Service (1996). *Duty of Care: Who's Responsible? A Guide for Carers Supporting People with Disabilities*. Villamanta Publishing Service, Geelong West.

Wade, G. H. (1998). 'A Concept Analysis of Personal Transformation'. *Journal of Advanced Nursing*, 28(4): 713–19.

Wakerman, J., Matthews, S., Hill, P. & Gibson, O. (2000). Beyond Charcoal Lane. Aboriginal and Torres Strait Islander health managers: issues and strategies to assist recruitment, retention and professional development. Menzies School of Health Research and Indigenous Health Program. University of Queensland, Alice Springs.

Worksafe Victoria (2008). *Annual Report 2008* <worksafe.vic.gov.au> accessed 24 January 2009.

World Health Organization (2002). *Towards a Common Language for Functioning, Disability and Health: ICF The International Classification of Functioning, Disability and Health*. World Health Organization, Geneva.

World Health Organization (WHO) (2009). *Mental Health*. <http://www.who.int/topics/mental_health/en/> accessed 30 January 2009.

Worley, P., Prideaux D., Strasser, R., March, R. & Worley, E. (2004). 'What Do Medical Students Actually Do On Clinical Rotations?' *Medical Teaching*, 26(7): 594–8.

Yaphe, J. & Street, S. (2003). 'How Do Examiners Decide?: A Qualitative Study of the Process of Decision Making in the Oral Examination Component of the MRCGP Examination'. *Medical Education*, 37: 764–71.

Zupiria Gorostidi, X., Huitzi Egilegor, M., Jose Alberdi Erice, M., Jose Uranga Iturriotz, I., Eizmendi Garate, M. et al. (2007). 'Stress Sources in Nursing Practice. Evolution During Nursing Training'. *Nurse Education Today*, 27(7), 777.

USEFUL WEBSITES

All Things Socialwork: http://socialworkpodcast.com

Australian Bureau of Statistics, *Population Projections, Australia, 2006 to 2101*: www.abs.gov.au/
AUSSTATS/abs@.nsf/Lookup/3222.0Main+Features12006 to 2101?OpenDocument

Australian Department of Health and Ageing: www.health.gov.au

Australian Institute of Health and Welfare (AIHW)—Publications: www.aihw.gov.au/
publications

Australian Federal Police: http://www.afp.gov.au/business/national_police_checks.html#crim

Blogger: www.blogger.com/start

Bloglines: www.bloglines.com

CNET Podcast Central: www.cnet.com/podcasts

Comcare: www.comcare.gov.au

Commoncraft: www.commoncraft.com

CRS Australia: www.crsaustralia.gov.au

Department of Justice: www.justice.vic.gov.au/workingwithchildren

Department of Human Services: www.dhs.vic.gov.au

Facebook: http://facebook.com

Get a Note from Your Doctor: www.ganfyd.org

Google Documents: http://docs.google.com

Google Reader: www.google.com/reader

Healthcare Blogger Code of Ethics: http://medbloggercode.com/the-code

Health Evidence Search Wiki: http://healthevidencesearch.pbworks.com

HONCode: www.hon.ch/index.html

How to Create a Podcast: www.how-to-podcast-tutorial.com

MedReader: www.medreader.com

MediaWiki: www.mediawiki.org/wiki/MediaWiki

Midwives and Second Life SLENZ project: http://sarah-stewart.blogspot.com/search/label/
second%20life

MyCareer: www.mycareer.com.au

MySpace: www.myspace.com

National Indigenous Health Equality Summit in March 2008: www.hreoc.gov.au/social_Justice/
health/targets/index.html

National Aboriginal Community Controlled Health Organisation, *Annual Report 2007–2008*:
www.naccho.org.au/Files/Documents/NACCHO_AR08_final_press.pdf

Ning: www.ning.com

Office of the Victorian Privacy Commissioner: www.privacy.vic.gov.au

PB Wiki user manual: http://pbwikimanual.pbwiki.com

Podcast.com: http://podcast.com

RSS in Plain English: www.commoncraft.com/rss_plain_english

Second Life: http://secondlife.com

Self-directed learning modules on cultural awareness and cultural competency for health
professionals: www.nccccurricula.info/modules.html

Top educational locations in Second Life: http://healthcybermap.org/sl.htm

Useful Websites

Victoria Police: www.police.vic.gov.au
WebCite: www.webcitation.org/5aDEkONrK
Wordpress: http://wordpress.org
YouTube: http://Youtube.com
Zoho Writer: http://writer.zoho.com

INDEX

Aboriginal and Torres Strait Islanders   27–8, 125, 128
Aboriginal community-controlled health service   124–6
Aboriginal health services   124–7
Aboriginal health workers (AHWs)   121, 128–9
absent, what to do if you are   59
accommodation supervision style   340
acute care setting, working in   50–61
    absent, what to do if you are   59
    communication   58–9
    emergencies   59–60
    fieldwork placement   56–60, 138–9
    infection control   58
    pace of work   57
    pre-fieldwork placement   52–6
    preparation list   56
    types of placement and settings   51–2
    work intensity   57
acute hospital wards   69
acute setting   39, 50–61, 206
administrative function (supervisory function)   147–9
adult learning principles   148–9
alternative fieldwork placements   186–97
    active participation   190
    background   187–8
    educator visits   192
    evaluation   192–3
    goals and aims   190
    independent learner   188–9
    learning experience   189–93
    managing stress   188
    OWLS program   193–4
    peer mentors   192
    professional identity   189
    self-directed learning   188
    supervision and facilitation   191
    tutorials   191
appearance and fieldwork placement, professional   55, 294
apprenticeship approach (supervision)   150–1
arrest trolley   60
articulated model (supervisory practice)   150
assessment
    fieldwork placement   50, 172–3, 174, 287–8
    peer assessment/comparison   182
    performance data collection   182–3
    ratings of performance   177–8
    self   179–81, 182–3

    see clinical learning, assessment of
Australian Association of Social Work (AASW)   5, 253
Australian healthcare system   13–17
    community-based health services   16–17
    overall structure   13–14
    private systems   15–16
    public hospitals   14–15
Australian Nursing Council   5
Australian Red Cross   14
Australian Rural Health Education Network   120
autism spectrum disorder (ASD)   38, 45–6
avatar   239

babies *see* mothers and babies
behaviours, professional   97, 113–14, 163–5, 219, 292, 293–5
blind quadrant (Johari window)   166, 167
blogs   234–6
body language   24, 67, 68, 131

Canada   103
capacity   268–9
child and family health nurse   35
childhood illnesses   42
children, working with
    acute settings   39
    clinical reasoning process   46–8
    common assessments   42
    community settings   39–40
    development, knowledge of typical   42
    developmental disabilities   42
    and families   44–6
    fieldwork settings   38–40, 41–4
    frames of reference   42
    general skills and considerations   46–8
    intervention strategies   42–3
    private practice   40
    school-based settings   40
    screening tools   42
    working effectively   41
    your role in a fieldwork setting   43–4
chronic condition self-management (CCMS)   73
client-health professional interactions   302–3, 304
client-therapist fieldwork placement   306
clinical learning, assessment of   171–84
    criteria and marking scales   175–7
    fieldwork placement   172–3, 174

clinical learning, assessment of (*continued*)
  performance data collection 182–3
  ratings of performance 177–8
  role of 174–5
  self-assessment 179–81, 182–3
clinical reasoning 46–8, 64, 66, 71, 82, 190, 191, 350
collaborative writing 236–7
communication
  body language 24, 67, 68, 131
  and fieldwork placement 27, 50, 58–9, 66–8, 164–5, 189, 311
  interference 67
  and older people 65, 66–8
community geriatric fieldwork placements 72–3
community projects 186
community-based health services 16–17, 302
community-based settings 39–40, 206
  and legal issues 302, 304
community-building project work 189
community-level healthcare 16
competency-based approach (supervision) 152
confidentiality and consent
  and fieldwork placement 19, 97, 105, 236, 284, 291–2, 295, 304–6
  mothers and babies 28, 31–2
  older people 68
  professional interactions 306
  and students 304–6
  workplace practice 97
consulting therapist 40
continuing professional development 315, 316, 320–1
conventional fieldwork placements 186
core business 255
critical incident 155–6
critical incident analysis 157
critical reflection (supervision) 152–4, 155–7
cultural competence 22–3

decision-making
  influences on competence and 269–72
  model of supported 272–4
  pathway 275
Department of Education, Employment and Workplace Relations (DEEWR) 90
Diagnostic and Statistical Manual of Mental Disorders 82
discipline-specific fieldwork educator visits 187, 192
discipline-specific intervention 39
discipline-specific knowledge/skills 41, 129, 157, 161, 163, 165, 166, 175, 294, 332, 350
discipline-specific standards of performance 175
discipline-specific supervision 187, 190, 191, 192
diversity and cultural competence 22–3
documentation for fieldwork placement 54–5
doughnut principle 265–6

duty of care 147, 263–5, 268, 269, 274, 275, 295, 306, 309

educative function (supervisory function) 146
emergencies in acute settings 59–60
emotional intelligence (EI) 8–9
ethical decision-making 263–79, 309
ethical practice in supervision 342
ethical responsibility 263
evidence-based approach to fieldwork practice 165
experiential learning 4
exploration supervision style 340

facilitation and alternative fieldwork 191
failure, learning from 218–29
  fieldwork placement difficulties 218–24
  fieldwork setting difficulties 226–7
  readiness to learn 225–6
  transformative learning 226
families and children 37–49
  acute settings 39
  community settings 39–40
  fieldwork settings 38–40, 41–4
  working effectively with 41
family-centred practice 38, 41, 44
feelings, managing 9–10
fieldwork, international 258–9
fieldwork contract 65, 300, 335
fieldwork education
  placement contract 65, 300, 335
  supervision within 330
fieldwork educator 4, 65, 292–3, 295–6, 323–7, 334, 339–40, 350, 355–6
fieldwork learning framework 160–5, 190
fieldwork parameters 285–8
fieldwork partnerships
  development 288–95
  importance of 255–9
  stakeholders 252–5, 282, 288–95
  why do they matter? 257–8
  your role in 259
fieldwork placement 4–5
  acute care settings 56–60, 138–9
  absent, what to do if you are 59
  agency (stakeholders) 282, 284–5, 288–95, 296–7
  areas 96–7
  and assessment 50, 172–3, 174
  checklist 246–8, 309–12, 355–6
  common information 289–90
  and communication 27, 50, 58–9, 66–8, 164–5, 189
  concerns, addressing 295–7
  and confidentiality 19, 97, 304–6
  costs 292
  day-to-day dynamics 251–2
  documentation 54–5
  families and children 41–3
  general control and discipline 292
  generational attributes 162–3

fieldwork placement (*continued*)
  getting ready for   5–7, 41–3, 52–6,
    114–15
  goals and objectives   54
  Indigenous health   120–4, 125, 129–34,
    141–2
  interviews   6
  key stakeholders   252–5
  learning opportunities   166–9
  legal issues   299–301
  mental health   79–80, 82, 140
  older people   64–6, 139–40
  organisation   288–95
  orientation to new settings   17–19
  parameters   286–7
  personal attributes   161–2
  planning and organising   6, 7, 52–6
  pre-fieldwork organisation   52–6
  preparation   96–7
  preparation list   56, 137–42
  preparation sessions   53
  private practice   100–6, 140
  professional appearance/behaviours   55,
    97, 112, 113–14, 163–5, 293–5
  reflection   316–17
  reflecting on practice   166
  requirements   281
  rural and remote settings   108, 111–13,
    346–8
  student behaviour   97, 113–14, 163–5,
    292, 293–5
  student difficulties   218–24, 226–7, 292,
    295–6
  student's choice of workplace
    setting   345–6
  transport   52
  the venue   53–4
  workplace practice   96–7, 140
fieldwork planning   190
forcefield analysis   260

generational attributes and fieldwork
  placement   162–3
generic knowledge and skills   41, 111, 160, 161,
  163, 166
generic role   39
generic staff   187, 192
geriatric care   62–4
goal-setting   168–9
goals for placement   54
government (stakeholder)   253–4
government funding, federal   14
governance   5
growth therapeutic approach (supervision)   151
guided practice   274–7

Handy, Charles   265
health professionals   87–8
  client-health interactions (legal issues)
    302–3, 304
  role with families and children   43–4

in rural and remote areas   110–11, 113
  skills required for workplace
    practice   94–6
health promotion   16, 66, 131, 206
health services, community-based   16–17
hospital settings and legal issues   301, 304
health workforce recruitment   345–52
  rural placements   346–8
  and workplaces   349–51
Healthcare Blogger Code of Ethics   232–3
healthcare professional
  confidentiality   19, 97, 304–6
  role in a fieldwork setting   43–4, 51
  work practice   87–8, 94–6
healthcare services   14, 108–11
healthcare system, Australian   13–17
  community-based health services   16–17
  overall structure   13–14
  private systems   15–16
  public hospitals   14–15
  rural and remote areas   110–11
hermeneutic phenomenological
  approach   220
hidden quadrant (Johari window)   166
Home and Community Care (HACC)
  Program   14
HONcode   232–3
horizontal partnerships   256
host centres   187

immunisations for fieldwork placement   54
impression management   237
independent learning   188–9
indigenous health
  context of   121–2
  multiple language groups   120
  outcomes   119, 122–3
  rural and remote settings   126
  strategies   123–4
  workforce   128–9
Indigenous health settings, fieldwork
  placements
  Aboriginal community-controlled health
    service   125, 131–2
  checklist   141–2
  curriculum and learning objectives
    129–34
  field trips   132–3
  guiding principles   120–4
  personal development   130–1
  placement success   133
  student challenges and benefits   134
  student support   133–4
Indigenous populations   110
infection control in acute settings   58
informed consent   265
information packs   190
insurance (professional indemnity)   290–1
interdisciplinary team   20–1
integrated fieldwork practice   251

International Classification of Functioning, Disability and Health 269–72
International Private Practice Association (IPPA) 101
international fieldwork 258–9
interprofessional education (IPE) 201, 202
  Leicester model 334
interprofessional fieldwork 199–214
  assessing 212–13
interprofessional knowledge 213
interprofessional learning (IPL) 199
  definition 201–3
  does it work? 206–8
  effects of successful 207–8
  in-placement review 214–15
  myths and realities 203, 204
  placement debrief 216
  why? 203–6
interprofessional skills 213
interpreters 23–4
intervention strategies, common 42–3
interviews, placement 6

Johari window 166–7
journals 157

learning
  fieldwork 166–9, 190
  personal and professional resources for 161–5
legal issues 299–307, 312
  client-health professional interactions 302–3
  community-based settings 302
  hospital settings 301
  student confidentiality 304–6
  and universities 299–301, 303–4
lifelong learning 169, 316
line management 321

maternity care workforce 32–4
MediaWiki 242
medical emergency equipment 60
Medicare 14, 15, 16, 103
mental health 76–85
  definition 77
  fieldwork placement 79–80, 82, 140
  knowing yourself 79–80
  stigma, labels and myths 78
mental health practice
  and clinical reasoning 82
  settings 81
  and stress 81–2
  team work and role blurring 82–5
mentoring 121, 129, 320–1, 323
midway feedback 172
mothers and babies 26–35, 138
  Australia 27–8
  challenges when working with 35
  child and family health nurse 35
  communication 27, 28, 31

in the community 35
  confidentiality 28, 31–2
  continuity of care 28, 29–30
  key skills of health professionals 28
  maternity care workforce 32–4
  maternity unit 34
  the unwell baby 34
  women-centred care 28, 29

narrative inquiry 220
narrative record 157
National Aboriginal Community Controlled Health Organisation (NACCHO) 125
negligence in fieldwork placement 303–4
neonatal intensive care unit (NICU) 34

objectives for placement 54
Occupation Wellness Life Satisfaction (OWLS) program 193–4
occupational health and safety 55, 58, 88, 95, 96, 97, 290, 293, 295, 299–301
occupational rehabilitation 88–90
older people, working with 62–74
  acute hospital wards 69
  communication 65, 66–8
  community fieldwork placements 72–3
  discharge planning 70–2
  fieldwork placement 64–6, 139–40
  fieldwork settings 63
  form of address 66–7
  institutional settings 69–70
  palliative care wards 70
  rehabilitation hospital wards 69–70
  transitional care wards 69–70
  types of contact 67
  work-integrated learning 64–6
older persons care 14
online social networks 237
online technology 231–42
  avatar 239
  blogs 234–6
  collaborative writing 236–7
  key tools to support/enhance learning 233–4
  MediaWiki 242
  online social networks 237
  PBWorks 240
  podcasts 238
  reliability of 232–3
  syndication feeds (RSS) 238–9
  useful websites 244–5
  virtual worlds 239
  Web 2.0 231–2, 240–1
  wikis 239–42
open quadrant (Johari window) 166
orientation to new settings (fieldwork placement) 17–19

paediatrics 37, 39, 41, 42, 43
palliative care wards 70
parent support group (PSG) meetings 40

partnering models   256–7
    triple helix   256–7
partnerships
    development   288–95
    fieldwork   255–9, 288–95
    horizontal   256
    vertical   256
peer assessment/comparison   182
peer mentors   192
peer skill performance evaluation   192
performance data collection
    (assessment)   182–3
performance evaluation   192–3
performance ratings (assessment)   177–8
personal attributes and fieldwork
    placement   161–2
personal authority   339
person-centred care   20
person-centred risk assessment   266, 267, 277
perspective transformation   222
Pharmaceutical Benefits Scheme (PBS)   16
placement see fieldwork placement
podcasts   238
Police Record Checks (PRC)   6, 55, 284,
    286–7
practice-reflection-theory-reflection
    process   156
pre-fieldwork organisation   52–6
preparation sessions for fieldwork
    placement   53
Primary Care Partnership (PCP)   16
privacy   31, 68, 97, 105, 235, 236–7, 284,
    291–2, 295, 305, 306
private health system   15–16
private practice   40
    challenges and opportunities   102–6
    fieldwork placement   100–6, 140
    work-integrated learning and the
        student   101–2
profession, scope of the   4–5
professional appearance for fieldwork
    placement   55, 97, 112, 113–14, 163–5
professional associations   5, 253
professional authority   339
professional characteristics   166–7
professional development   315, 316, 319, 320–1
professional identity   189, 253
professional interactions and
    confidentiality   306
professional job, preparation for   317–19
professional stereotypes   211–12
professionals, individual   254
public hospitals   14–15

readiness to learn   220, 225–6
Really Simple Syndication (RSS)   238–9
Regional Health Services   14
reflecting on practice   166–7
regulation   5
rehabilitation
    occupational   88–90

    vocational   90–1
rehabilitation hospital wards   69–70
remote supervisor   187
risk of lost opportunities   266
role authority   339
role blurring and mental health   82–5
role emerging fieldwork   187
role system approach (supervision)   151–2
roles, rights and responsibilities   281–97,
    309–11
    assessment and evaluation   287–8
    common information   289–90
    confidentiality and privacy   291
    field-based parameters   286–8
    general control and discipline   292
    insurance   290–1
    non-payment of students   291–2
    placement agency   292–3
    placement concerns   295–7
    placement costs   292
    placement organisation   288–95
    stakeholders   282, 283–5
    students   293–5
    university parameters   286
Royal Flying Doctor Service (RFDS)   14, 116
rural and remote settings   108–18
    accommodation and leisure   115–16
    fieldwork placement   108, 111–13
    health   109–10
    health professionals   110–11, 113
    Indigenous health   126
    populations   109
    professional behaviour and surviving
        113–14
    Royal Flying Doctor Service (RDFS)   116
    workforce recruitment   346–8

school-based settings   40
Scottish Public Mental Health Alliance   77
self-assessment   179–81, 182–3
self-awareness   166
self-directed learning   188
sexual harassment   303
SMART goal   168–9
Smull, Michael   265
stakeholders   252–5, 282, 283–5, 288–97
standards of practice   174
stereotypes   211–12
stress and mental health practice   81–2
stress management   188
student, work-integrated learning and the   101–
    2
student behaviour   97, 113–14, 163–5, 219,
    292, 293–5
student supervision in fieldwork
    administrative function   147–9
    checklist   148
    definition   146
    educative function   146

student supervision in fieldwork (*continued*)
    and fieldwork educator   4, 65, 292–3, 295–6
    placement difficulties   218–24, 226–7, 292
    supportive function   146–7
students
    assessment and evaluation   287–8
    and confidentiality   304–6
    experiencing fieldwork placement difficulties   218–24, 226–7, 292, 295–6
    and fieldwork educator   4, 65, 292–3, 295–6
    and negligence in fieldwork placement   303–4
    non-payment of   291–2
    readiness to learn   220, 225–6
    role of   293–5
    as stakeholders   254–5, 282, 283, 284–5, 289, 295–6
    workplace setting (fieldwork placement)   345–6
supervisee levels of independence   337
supervision
    and alternative fieldwork   191
    apprenticeship approach   150–1
    becoming a supervisor   329–30
    competency-based approach   152
    and continuing professional development   321
    critical reflection   152–4
    emotional awareness   339–40
    ethical practice in   342
    in fieldwork education   330–2
    focus of   330–43
    growth therapeutic approach   151
    managing power and authority   338–9
    relationship   331, 332–3, 342–3
    review and ending   342–3
    role system approach   151–2
    stages model of   337
    student and practitioner (key differences)   336
    see also student supervision in fieldwork
supervisory practice   149–52
supported decision-making model   272–3
supportive function (supervisory function)   146–7
syndication feeds (RSS)   238–9

teamwork
    and interprofessional learning   208–9
    and mental health   82–5
think sheet   157
thoughts, managing   9–10
three Rs (roles, rights and responsibilities)   281, 309–11
transdisciplinary team   39
transformative learning   220, 226
transition   316

transitional care wards   69–70
transport and fieldwork placement   52
triple helix partnering model   256–7
tutorials   191

United States   101, 103, 104
university
    assessment and evaluation   287–8
    and fieldwork placement   288–95, 303–4
    fieldwork parameters   286
    and insurance   290–1
    and legal issues   299–301, 303–4
    and placement organisation   188–95
    as stakeholder   253, 254, 281, 283, 284–5, 286, 289
unknown quadrant (Johari window)   166, 167

venue for fieldwork placement   53–4
vertical partnerships   256
vicarious liability   303
virtual worlds   239
vocational rehabilitation   90–1
Vocational Rehabilitation Services (VRS)   90–1
vulnerable decision makers   264

Web 2.0   231–2, 240–1
websites, useful   25, 99, 136, 244–5, 298, 367–8
wikis   239–42
women-centred care   28, 29
workforce recruitment *see* health workforce recruitment
work-integrated learning   xi, xii, 3, 100, 106, 149–50, 155–6, 165, 252, 257
    with older people   64–6
    parameters   285
    scope and purpose of   4–5
    and the student   101–2
workplace literacy   7–9
workplace practice, work in   87–98
    fieldwork placement areas   96–7, 140
    occupational rehabilitation   88–90
    preparation for fieldwork   96–7
    skills required   94–6
    student behaviour   97
    vocational rehabilitation   90–1
workplace setting (fieldwork placement)   345–6
working in the field
    as a beginning fieldwork educator   323–7
    newly qualified practitioner   319–23
Working With Children Check (WWC)   6, 55, 286
World Confederation of Physical Therapy   5, 101, 103
World Federation of Occupational Therapists   100
World Health Organization (WHO)   77, 269